ELSEVIER

1600 John F. Kennedy Boulevard ● Suite 1800 ● Philadelphia, Pennsylvania, 19103-2899

http://www.theclinics.com

SURGICAL PATHOLOGY CLINICS Volume 16, Number 1
March 2023 ISSN 1875-9181, ISBN-13: 978-0-323-96073-1

Editor: Taylor Hayes
Developmental Editor: Diana Grace Ang

Surgical Pathology Clinics (ISSN 1875-9181) is published quarterly by Elsevier Inc., 360 Park Avenue South, New York, NY 10010. Months of issue are March, June, September, and December. Business and Editorial Office: Elsevier Inc., 1600 John F. Kennedy Blvd., Ste. 1800, Philadelphia, PA 19103-2899. Accounting and Circulation Offices: Elsevier Inc., 3251 Riverport Lane, Maryland Heights, MO 63043. Periodicals postage paid at New York, NY and at additional mailing offices. Subscription prices are $246.00 per year (US individuals), $354.00 per year (US institutions), $100.00 per year (US students/residents), $294.00 per year (Canadian individuals), $402.00 per year (Canadian Institutions), $295.00 per year (foreign individuals), $402.00 per year (foreign institutions), and $120.00 per year (international students/residents), $100.00 per year (Canadian students/residents). Foreign air speed delivery is included in all *Clinics'* subscription prices. All prices are subject to change without notice. **POSTMASTER:** Send address changes to *Surgical Pathology Clinics*, Elsevier, 3251 Riverport Lane, Maryland Heights, MO 63043. **Customer Service: 1-800-654-2452 (US). From outside the United States, call 1-314-447-8871. Fax: 1-314-447-8029. E-mail:** JournalsCustomerServiceusa@elsevier.com **(for print support)** and JournalsOnlineSupport-usa@elsevier.com **(for online support)**.

Reprints. For copies of 100 or more, of articles in this publication, please contact the Commercial Reprints Department, Elsevier Inc., 360 Park Avenue South, New York, NY 10010-1710. Tel. 212-633-3874; Fax: 212-633-3820; E-mail: reprints@elsevier.com.

Surgical Pathology Clinics of North America is covered in *MEDLINE/PubMed (Index Medicus)*.

Contributors

CONSULTING EDITOR

JASON L. HORNICK, MD, PhD
Director of Surgical Pathology and
Immunohistochemistry, Brigham and Women's
Hospital, Professor of Pathology, Harvard
Medical School, Boston, Massachusetts, USA

EDITOR

NICOLE A. CIPRIANI, MD
Associate Professor, Co-Director of Surgical
Pathology and Director of Anatomic Pathology
Informatics, Department of Pathology, The
University of Chicago, Pritzker School of
Medicine, Chicago, Illinois, USA

AUTHORS

EMAD ABABNEH, MD
Department of Pathology, Massachusetts
General Hospital, Boston, Massachusetts,
USA

JUSTINE A. BARLETTA, MD
Department of Pathology, Brigham and
Women's Hospital, Harvard Medical School,
Boston, Massachusetts, USA

JORDAN M. BROEKHUIS, MD
Harvard Medical School, Department of
Surgery, Beth Israel Deaconess Medical
Center, Boston, Massachusetts, USA

LINDSAY W. BRUBAKER, MD
Department of Obstetrics and Gynecology,
Division of Gynecologic Oncology, University
of Colorado School of Medicine, Aurora,
Colorado, USA

YING-HSIA CHU, MD
Department of Pathology, Chang Gung
Memorial Hospital, Chang Gung University,
Taoyuan City, Taiwan

NICOLE A. CIPRIANI, MD
Associate Professor, Co-Director of Surgical
Pathology and Director of Anatomic Pathology
Informatics, Department of Pathology, The
University of Chicago, Pritzker School of
Medicine, Chicago, Illinois, USA

VINCENT CRACOLICI, MD
Associate Staff Head and Neck Pathologist,
Assistant Professor, Cleveland Clinic
Lerner College of Medicine, Cleveland,
USA

JAMES M. DOLEZAL, MD
Department of Medicine, Section of
Hematology/Oncology, University of Chicago
Medical Center, The University of Chicago
Medicine and Biological Sciences, Chicago,
Illinois, USA

LORI A. ERICKSON, MD
Department of Laboratory Medicine and
Pathology, Mayo Clinic, Rochester, Minnesota,
USA

HAILEY L. GOSNELL, MD
Resident in Pathology, Cleveland Clinic,
Cleveland, Ohio, USA

RAYMON H. GROGAN, MD, MS, FACS
Professor of Surgery, Michael E. DeBakey
Department of Surgery, Baylor College of
Medicine, Houston, Texas, USA

SOUNAK GUPTA, MBBS, PhD
Department of Laboratory Medicine and
Pathology, Mayo Clinic, Rochester, Minnesota,
USA

ALIYA N. HUSAIN, MBBS
Department of Pathology, The University of
Chicago Medicine, Chicago, Illinois,
USA

PARI JAFARI, MD
Department of Pathology, The University of
Chicago Medicine, Chicago, Illinois, USA

BENJAMIN C. JAMES, MD, MS
Harvard Medical School, Department of
Surgery, Beth Israel Deaconess Medical
Center, Boston, Massachusetts,
USA

CARL CHRISTOFER JUHLIN, MD, PhD
Department of Oncology-Pathology,
Karolinska Institutet, Department of Pathology
and Cancer Diagnostics, Karolinska University
Hospital, Stockholm, Sweden

DARCY A. KERR, MD
Department of Pathology and Laboratory
Medicine, Dartmouth-Hitchcock Medical
Center, Lebanon, New Hampshire,
USA; Geisel School of Medicine at Dartmouth,
Hanover, New Hampshire, USA

XAVIER M. KEUTGEN, MD
Associate Professor of Surgery, Division of
General Surgery and Surgical Oncology,
Department of Surgery, The University of
Chicago, The University of Chicago Medicine,
Chicago, Illinois, USA

CHIH-YI LIAO, MD
Assistant Professor of Medicine, Section of
Hematology/Oncology, Department of
Medicine, The University of Chicago, The
University of Chicago Medicine, Chicago,
Illinois, USA

VANIA NOSÉ, MD, PhD
Department of Pathology, Massachusetts
General Hospital, Boston, Massachusetts,
USA

ALEXANDER T. PEARSON, MD, PhD
Department of Medicine, Section of
Hematology/Oncology, The University of
Chicago Medical Center, The University of
Chicago Comprehensive Cancer Center,
The University of Chicago Medicine and
Biological Sciences, Chicago, Illinois,
USA

SIDDHI RAMESH, BA
Department of Medicine, Section of
Hematology/Oncology, The University of
Chicago Medical Center, The University of
Chicago Medicine and Biological Sciences,
Chicago, Illinois, USA

PETER M. SADOW, MD, PhD
Director, Head and Neck Pathology,
Massachusetts General Hospital, Associate
Professor of Pathology, Harvard Medical
School, Boston, Massachusetts,
USA

JASON L. SCHWARZ, MD
General Surgery Resident, Division of General
Surgery and Surgical Oncology, Department of
Surgery, The University of Chicago, The
University of Chicago Medicine, Chicago,
Illinois, USA

NAMRATA SETIA, MD
Department of Pathology, The University of
Chicago Medicine, Chicago, Illinois, USA

LYNELLE P. SMITH, MD
Department of Pathology, University of
Colorado School of Medicine, Aurora,
Colorado, USA

YOULEY TJENDRA, MD
Department of Pathology and Laboratory
Medicine, University of Miami Miller
School of Medicine, Miami, Florida,
USA

JAYLOU M. VELEZ TORRES, MD
Department of Pathology and Laboratory
Medicine, University of Miami Miller
School of Medicine, Miami, Florida,
USA

JELANI K. WILLIAMS, MD
General Surgery Resident, Division of General
Surgery and Surgical Oncology, Department of
Surgery, The University of Chicago, The
University of Chicago Medicine, Chicago,
Illinois, USA

REBECCA J. WOLSKY, MD
Department of Pathology, University of
Colorado School of Medicine, Aurora,
Colorado, USA

KRISTINE S. WONG, MD
Department of Pathology, Brigham
and Women's Hospital, Harvard Medical
School, Boston, Massachusetts,
USA

FOUAD R. ZAKKA, MD
Head and Neck Pathology Fellow, Department
of Pathology, The University of Chicago,
Pritzker School of Medicine, Chicago, Illinois,
USA

Contents

Risk stratification is essential in the preoperative evaluation and management of thyroid nodules, most of which are benign. Advances in DNA and RNA sequencing have shed light on the molecular drivers of thyroid cancer. Molecular testing of cytologically indeterminate nodules has helped refine risk stratification, triage patients for surgery, and determine the extent of surgery. Molecular platforms with high negative predictive values can help identify nodules that may be spared surgery and can be managed conservatively. Here we discuss the importance of integrating cytomorphologic, molecular, and histologic features to help avoid errors and improve patient management.

The use of intraoperative consultation for indeterminate thyroid lesions is not advocated but is still requested by some surgeons. Obscured cytomorphology and nonrepresentative sampling limit the specificity of intraoperative assessment. Formalin fixation of thyroid glands before sectioning also minimizes artifacts introduced by fresh sectioning. Inking of thyroid may vary based on institutional preferences and information desired by clinical teams. Sectioning may occur in the conventional transverse method or the modified transverse vertical method to more thoroughly evaluate the lesion's periphery. Gross examination of thyroid lesions should always consider possible high-grade features, such as necrosis or extrathyroidal extension.

Thyroid pathology is notoriously fraught with high interobserver variability, and follicular-patterned tumors are among some of the most challenging to assess accurately and reproducibly. Given that encapsulated or well-circumscribed follicular-patterned tumors often have similar molecular profiles, that is, frequent RAS or RAS-like alterations, the diagnosis usually relies on histopathologic examination alone. Unfortunately, many of the features that are used for diagnosis and prognosis of these tumors have long been controversial and frequently debated topics, both due to their subjectivity and their evolving (or not yet resolved) definitions. In more recent years, the introduction of noninvasive follicular thyroid neoplasm with papillary-like nuclear features has added further complexity to this discussion. In particular, the criteria and significance of nuclear features of papillary thyroid carcinoma, architectural patterns, and invasive growth still pose significant diagnostic challenges and confusion. This review explores some of the challenges in evaluating encapsulated follicular-patterned tumors, focusing on those histologic elements.

Poorly differentiated thyroid carcinoma (PDTC) and differentiated high-grade thyroid carcinoma (DHGTC) are uncommon thyroid malignancies, recently (re)codified into distinct entities with overlapping clinical significance. Recognizing them may be challenging for the general practitioner and subspecialty pathologist alike. This article will describe the required features to diagnose PDTC and DHGTC, differential diagnostic considerations, molecular findings, and clinical implications. It is intended to be a general synopsis of the most critical elements of PDTC and DHGTC as well as a summary of points in approaching these challenging cases.

This review aims to provide an overview of the molecular pathogenesis thyroid carcinomas, emphasizing genetic alterations that are therapeutically actionable. The main pathways in thyroid carcinogenesis are the MAPK and PI3K pathways. Point mutations and gene rearrangements affecting the pathway effectors and receptor tyrosine kinases are well-known drivers of thyroid cancer. Research over the past few decades has successfully introduced highly effective treatments for unresectable thyroid cancer, evolving from multi-kinase inhibitors to structurally selective agents, with constantly improving toxicity profiles and coverage of resistance mechanisms. The pros and cons of major laboratory techniques for therapeutic target identification are discussed.

Thyroid carcinoma originating in struma ovarii comprises a small minority of all cases of struma ovarii. Given the rarity of this diagnosis, literature to guide evaluation and management is limited. The most common carcinoma originating from struma ovarii is papillary thyroid carcinoma. Treatment includes surgery, including a fertility sparing approach if disease is confined to the ovary, with consideration of total thyroidectomy and radioactive iodine ablation for high-risk pathologic features or disease spread beyond the ovary. This review discusses the histopathologic findings, molecular pathology, clinical implications and management, and prognosis of thyroid carcinomas originating in struma ovarii.

Parathyroid disease typically presents with parathyroid hyperfunction as result of neoplasia or a consequence of non-neoplastic systemic disease. Given the parathyroid gland is a hormonally active organ with broad physiologic implications and serologically accessible markers for monitoring, the diagnosis of parathyroid disease is predominantly a clinical pathologic correlation. We provide the current pathological correlates of parathyroid disease and discuss preoperative, intraoperative, and postoperative pathology consultative practice for optimal patient care.

Emad Ababneh and Vania Nosé

CDC73 alterations are associated with three main parathyroid lesions according to the World Health Organization (WHO) classification of tumors of the endocrine system. These include hyperparathyroidism-jaw tumor (HPT-JT) syndrome-associated adenomas, atypical parathyroid tumors (APTs), and parathyroid carcinomas (PCs). The loss of nuclear parafibromin expression, which serves as a surrogate marker for the underlying CDC73 alteration, encompasses these tumors under the term parafibromin-deficient parathyroid tumors. They have distinct morphologic features of more abundant eosinophilic cytoplasm with perinuclear clearing surrounding a large nucleus as well as prominent dilated branching "hemangiopericytoma-like" vasculature and a thick capsule as well as variably sized cystic spaces. These tumors include cases that show unequivocal histologic features fulfilling the criteria for PCs with growing data indicating a higher rate of recurrence or metastasis compared with parafibromin intact PCs. More importantly, the loss of parafibromin expression can be used in clinical practice to recognize APTs that fall short of a conclusive diagnosis of PCs, but clinically behave akin to them. Moreover, recognizing these tumors can lead to an underlying germline mutation and a diagnosis of HPT-JT, which impacts long-term treatment and surveillance for patients and close family.

Carl Christofer Juhlin

Mutational inactivation of the *DICER1* gene causes aberrant micro-RNA maturation, which in turn may have consequences for the posttranscriptional regulation of gene expression, thereby contributing to tumor formation in various organs. Germline *DICER1* mutations cause *DICER1* syndrome, a pleiotropic condition with an increased risk of various neoplastic conditions in the pleura, ovaries, thyroid, pituitary, pineal gland, and mesenchymal tissues. Somatic *DICER1* mutations are also frequently observed in a wide variety of solid tumors, thereby highlighting the importance of this gene in tumor development. In this review, the importance of *DICER1* inactivation in endocrine tumors is discussed.

Sounak Gupta and Lori A. Erickson

There is increasing recognition of the high prevalence of hereditary predisposition syndromes in patients diagnosed with paraganglioma/pheochromocytoma. It is widely acknowledged that germline pathogenic alterations of the succinate dehydrogenase complex genes (SDHA, SDHB, SDHC, SDHD, SDHAF2) contribute to the pathogenesis of most of these tumors. Herein, we have provided an update on the biology and diagnosis of succinate dehydrogenase-deficient paraganglioma/pheochromocytoma, including the molecular biology of the succinate dehydrogenase complex, mechanisms and consequences of inactivation of this complex, the prevalence of pathogenic alterations, and patterns of inheritance.

Pari Jafari, Aliya N. Husain, and Namrata Setia

Neuroendocrine neoplasms (NENs) span virtually all organ systems and exhibit a broad spectrum of behavior, from indolent to highly aggressive. Historically, nomenclature and grading practices have varied widely across, and even within, organ systems. However, certain core features are recapitulated across anatomic sites, including characteristic morphology and the crucial role of proliferative activity in prognostication. A recent emphasis on unifying themes has driven an increasingly standardized approach to NEN classification, as delineated in the World Health Organization's Classification of Tumours series. Here, we review recent developments in NEN classification, with a focus on NENs of the pancreas and lungs.

Radiolabeled somatostatin analogs are increasingly used in the diagnosis and treatment of neuroendocrine tumors. Diagnostic imaging with 68Ga-DOTATATE PET/CT has demonstrated the improved sensitivity in detecting primary and metastatic neuroendocrine lesions compared with conventional imaging and prior generation somatostatin receptor imaging. Peptide receptor radionuclide therapy with 177Lu-DOTATATE is now frequently included in the management of neuroendocrine neoplasms, with prospective randomized control studies demonstrating its beneficial impact on survival and quality of life. Nonetheless, peptide rector radionuclide therapy is still considered palliative rather than curative and may be accompanied by adverse effects.

Transoral endocrine surgery (TES) is a scarless approach to thyroidectomy and parathyroidectomy for well-selected patients. Criteria for the TES approach to thyroidectomy include thyroid diameter less than or equal to 10 cm, benign nodule less than or equal to 6 cm, or confirmed or suspected malignant nodule less than or equal to 2 cm. Although fragmentation of surgical specimens has been reported in TES, additional studies are needed to evaluate the implications of TES on pathologic examination.

Machine learning methods have been growing in prominence across all areas of medicine. In pathology, recent advances in deep learning (DL) have enabled computational analysis of histological samples, aiding in diagnosis and characterization in multiple disease areas. In cancer, and particularly endocrine cancer, DL approaches have been shown to be useful in tasks ranging from tumor grading to gene expression prediction. This review summarizes the current state of DL research in endocrine cancer histopathology with an emphasis on experimental design, significant findings, and key limitations.

SURGICAL PATHOLOGY CLINICS

SERIES OF RELATED INTEREST

Clinics in Laboratory Medicine
http://www.labmed.theclinics.com/
Medical Clinics
https://www.medical.theclinics.com/

THE CLINICS ARE AVAILABLE ONLINE!
Access your subscription at:
www.theclinics.com

Preface

Endocrine Pathology: Practical Suggestions, Emerging Diagnostics, and New Frontiers

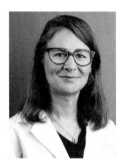

Nicole A. Cipriani, MD
Editor

This issue on Endocrine Pathology in *Surgical Pathology Clinics* tackles common and challenging problems in thyroid and parathyroid pathology, emerging clinically relevant molecular findings in endocrine neoplasms and syndromes, and new horizons in diagnosis and treatment of endocrine tumors.

Starting with (my favorite organ) the thyroid gland, the article, "A Triumvirate: Correlating Thyroid Cytopathology, Molecular Testing, and Histopathology," emphasizes the importance of correlating thyroid cytopathology to preoperative molecular testing to final diagnosis, specifically regarding how to interpret molecular tests for clinical decision making and how they can inform histopathologic diagnosis. The article, "To Freeze or not to Freeze? Recommendations for Intraoperative Examination and Gross Prosection of Thyroid Glands," suggests standard practices for gross handling of thyroid glands, whether sent for intraoperative diagnosis (which should be discouraged) or permanent evaluation, and it provides recommendations for clinically relevant inking, sectioning, and cassette submission. The article, "Challenges in Encapsulated Follicular-Patterned Tumors: How Much is Enough? Evaluation of Nuclear Atypia, Architecture, and Invasion," discusses the age-old (and often frustrating) question of the minimum threshold for a cancer diagnosis (whether it lies in the nuclei, the

architecture, the capsule, the vessels…), identifies common pitfalls, and provides practical recommendations for pathologists. The article, "No Longer Well-Differentiated: Diagnostic Criteria and Clinical Importance of Poorly Differentiated/High-Grade Thyroid Carcinoma," addresses the new WHO category of high-grade follicular-derived thyroid carcinomas, comparing the diagnostic criteria for differentiated high-grade and poorly differentiated thyroid carcinomas and the clinical implications thereof. The article, "This Is Your Thyroid on Drugs: Targetable Mutations and Fusions in Thyroid Carcinoma," transitions to emerging molecular diagnostics in thyroid carcinomas, specifically addressing actionable mutations and how pathologists can play a critical role in the interdisciplinary care team by facilitating targeted therapy for patients. The article, "It Does Exist! Diagnosis and Management of Thyroid Carcinomas Arising in Struma Ovarii," faces a question that endocrine pathologists may find themselves asked by gynecologic pathology colleagues—can we capture the elusive beast of thyroid carcinoma arising in struma ovarii? The articles, "Preoperative, Intraoperative and Postoperative Parathyroid Pathology: Clinical Pathologic Collaboration for Optimal Patient Management" and "Para this, Fibromin that: The Role of CDC73 in Parathyroid Tumors and Familial Tumor Syndromes," move to the small but mighty parathyroid

Surgical Pathology 16 (2023) xiii–xiv
https://doi.org/10.1016/j.path.2022.11.001
1875-9181/23/© 2022 Published by Elsevier Inc.

surgpath.theclinics.com

gland: how to frame an overall diagnostic approach to parathyroid disease during intraoperative evaluation compared with permanent evaluation, and how to conceptualize *CDC73*-mutated parathyroid neoplasms, which may point to a clinical syndrome. The articles, "On the Chopping Block: Overview of DICER1 Mutations in Endocrine and Neuroendocrine Neoplasms" and "Back to Biochemistry: Evaluation for and Prognostic Significance of *SDH* Mutations in Paragangliomas and Pheochromocytomas," are also devoted to the molecular basis of disease in the rare but clinically important *DICER1* and succinate dehydrogenase (*SDH*)-related endocrine/neuroendocrine syndromes. The article, "All Together Now: Standardization of Nomenclature for Neuroendocrine Neoplasms Across Multiple Organs," addresses the protean classification of neuroendocrine tumors (carcinoid? NET? NEN? NEC?) and the push to standardize nomenclature across organ systems, which would facilitate communication and standard of patient care. The last three articles, courtesy of our colleagues in endocrine surgery and internal medicine, aim to facilitate pathologists' understanding of cutting-edge clinical issues: the use of DOTATATE radiotracer for diagnosis and therapy ("Light It Up! The Use of DOTATATE in Diagnosis and Treatment of Neuroendocrine Neoplasms"); transoral surgery for endocrine lesions of the neck ("Scarless Surgery: Clinical Indications for Transoral Endocrine Surgery and Implications for Pathologists"); and how deep learning could be applied to the management of patients with endocrine tumors ("Applications of Deep Learning in Endocrine Neoplasms"). The overall aims of this collection of fourteen articles are to address challenges that pathologists encounter in daily practice as well as to introduce innovations in the interdisciplinary practice of medicine related to endocrine tumors.

I would like to thank Dr Hornick for the invitation to serve as guest editor as well as the article authors for their hard work and interesting contributions to this collection! I hope you find it interesting and educational.

Nicole A. Cipriani, MD
Department of Pathology
The University of Chicago
5841 S Maryland Ave, MC 6101
Chicago, IL 60637, USA

E-mail address:
Nicole.Cipriani@uchospitals.edu

A Triumvirate:
Correlating Thyroid Cytopathology, Molecular Testing, and Histopathology

Jaylou M. Velez Torres, MD[a], Youley Tjendra, MD[a],
Darcy A. Kerr, MD[b,c],*

KEYWORDS

- Thyroid nodule • Thyroid cancer • Molecular alterations • Fine-needle aspiration • Indeterminate
- Probability of malignancy • False-positive diagnoses • False-negative diagnoses

Key points

- Thyroid nodules are very common, and the majority are benign.
- Fine-needle aspiration cytology is a valuable diagnostic tool for the preoperative evaluation of thyroid nodules.
- Thyroid cytology has limitations, including indeterminate thyroid nodules and false-positive and false-negative results.
- Molecular testing has emerged as a reliable ancillary tool to improve preoperative risk stratification of thyroid nodules, and results can help guide patient treatment.
- Correlating cytomorphologic, molecular, and histologic features is helpful to optimize diagnostic accuracy.

ABSTRACT

Risk stratification is essential in the preoperative evaluation and management of thyroid nodules, most of which are benign. Advances in DNA and RNA sequencing have shed light on the molecular drivers of thyroid cancer. Molecular testing of cytologically indeterminate nodules has helped refine risk stratification, triage patients for surgery, and determine the extent of surgery. Molecular platforms with high negative predictive values can help identify nodules that may be spared surgery and can be managed conservatively. Here we discuss the importance of integrating cytomorphologic, molecular, and histologic features to help avoid errors and improve patient management.

OVERVIEW

Fine-needle aspiration cytology (FNAC) plays an essential role in the preoperative evaluation of thyroid nodules. It can reliably distinguish benign versus malignant lesions in many cases and guide patient treatment (e.g., active surveillance, lobectomy, or thyroidectomy). The Bethesda System for Reporting Thyroid Cytopathology (TBSRTC) categorizes samples into six diagnostic categories: non-diagnostic (ND), benign (B), atypia of undetermined significance (AUS), suspicious for a follicular neoplasm (SFN), suspicious for malignancy (SM), and malignant (M), each with an implied risk of malignancy (ROM).[1] Thyroid fine-needle aspiration biopsies (FNAs) have a high positive predictive value (PPV) ranging from 97% to

[a] Department of Pathology and Laboratory Medicine, University of Miami Miller School of Medicine, 1400 NW 12th Avenue, Miami, FL 33136, USA; [b] Department of Pathology and Laboratory Medicine, Dartmouth-Hitchcock Medical Center, One Medical Center Drive, Lebanon, NH 03756, USA; [c] Geisel School of Medicine at Dartmouth, Hanover, NH 03755, USA
* Corresponding author.
E-mail address: Darcy.A.Kerr@hitchcock.org
Twitter: @JaylouVelez (J.M.V.T.); @Y_Tjendra (Y.T.); @darcykerrMD (D.A.K.)

Surgical Pathology 16 (2023) 1–14
https://doi.org/10.1016/j.path.2022.09.003
1875-9181/23/

99%, with sensitivities and specificities ranging from 65% to 99% and 72% to 100%, respectively.[2] However, cytomorphology has its limitations, and potential diagnostic pitfalls exist. A principal limitation is that of cytologically indeterminate thyroid nodules. Furthermore, false-positive (FP) and false-negative (FN) results are possible. FP results may occur due to morphologic overlap between benign and malignant neoplastic and/or non-neoplastic entities. FN results commonly occur in cases with limited cellularity or macrofollicular thyroid lesions.[1,3,4] Molecular testing has emerged as a reliable ancillary tool for preoperative risk assessment of thyroid nodules with indeterminate cytology diagnoses, and results can help guide patient treatment.[5,6] Here we discuss the role and limitations of cytomorphology, molecular testing, and histopathology, highlighting how careful correlation between each branch of this triumvirate can help avoid errors and optimize patient care.

DIAGNOSTIC CHALLENGES IN THYROID CYTOLOGY

INDETERMINATE NODULES

FNAC is among the most commonly used modalities for the evaluation of thyroid nodules. Despite its high specificity for the diagnosis of benign and malignant lesions, it fails to provide a definite diagnosis in approximately 15% to 30% of cases.[7–9] These aspirates are classified in indeterminate diagnostic categories of TBSRTC, including AUS (category III) or SFN (category IV).[8,10] Indeterminate categories pose a diagnostic dilemma and include a heterogeneous group of lesions. TBSRTC defines the AUS category as aspirates that contain follicular cells with architectural and/or cytologic atypia (**Fig. 1**) without sufficient evidence to be classified as SFN, SM, or M (**Fig. 2**).[1] The estimated ROM for the AUS category ranges from 10% to 30%.[1,11–13] Aspirates composed of follicular cells with an altered architectural pattern characterized by significant crowding and/or predominance of microfollicles are classified as SFN.[1] The estimated ROM for the SFN category ranges from 25% to 40%.[1] Management of patients with indeterminate cytology can be challenging. Molecular testing has emerged as a reliable preoperative diagnostic tool that can help refine the risk stratification of indeterminate thyroid nodules and triage patients for surgery.[14]

Select Pitfalls in Thyroid Cytopathology

For a comprehensive discussion of pitfalls in thyroid cytopathology, the authors would refer readers to an excellent recent review by Rossi and colleagues.[2] Herein, we highlight several important pitfalls that particularly illustrate the importance of correlating cytomorphologic, molecular, and histologic features.

PARATHYROID

FNAs of parathyroid lesions are a potential diagnostic pitfall as they are often misclassified as SFN.[15] Such aspirates are composed of crowded and overlapping cells that can resemble follicular cells.[16,17] If there is clinical suspicion that the lesion may be parathyroid, FNA washout fluid can be evaluated for parathyroid hormone.[18] Alternatively, if there are cellular features suggesting that possibility (e.g., tight clusters of small, relatively uniform cells with round to oval nuclei with stippled chromatin and abundant granular or pale cytoplasm), ancillary studies can be performed to help confirm the diagnosis (**Fig. 3**).[19] Immunohistochemistry (IHC) for GATA3 and TTF-1 can help differentiate parathyroid (GATA3+, TTF-1–) versus thyroid (GATA3–, TTF-1+) lesions.[17] Molecular analysis is also useful here for detecting the expression profile of parathyroid cells.[15,20]

MEDULLARY THYROID CARCINOMA

Given its morphologic heterogeneity and cytologic overlap with follicular cell-derived thyroid tumors, FNA diagnosis of medullary thyroid carcinoma (MTC) can be challenging (**Fig. 4**A, B). MTC can mimic a diverse range of other neoplasms and it is commonly mistaken for oncocytic FNs, given that a subset of MTCs can show discohesive cells with eccentric nuclei, abundant granular cytoplasm, and binucleation.[21] However, MTC tends to show salt-and-pepper chromatin and lack the prominent nucleoli seen in oncocytic FNs.[21] Intranuclear pseudoinclusions can be present in ~20% to 50% of cases and can raise the differential diagnosis of papillary thyroid carcinoma (PTC) (**Fig. 4**C, D).[22,23] In contrast to PTC, nuclear grooves are not a feature of MTC.[21] Careful evaluation of cytologic features and use of a panel of IHC such as positivity for calcitonin, synaptophysin, INSM1, and CEA, and negativity for thyroglobulin and monoclonal PAX8 can help confirm the diagnosis (**Fig. 5**).[24–27] Measuring calcitonin in serum or FNA washout specimens can also be a valuable tool for diagnosing MTC.[28] Both familial and sporadic MTC frequently carry *RET* gene point mutations, which can be detected by molecular testing. In addition, finding a *RAS* mutation in combination with a high serum calcitonin level is virtually diagnostic of sporadic MTC.[5,29–31]

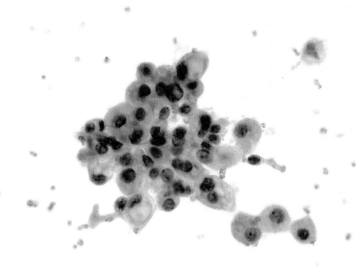

Fig. 1. Fine-needle aspiration of cystic papillary thyroid carcinoma interpreted as atypia of undetermined significance showing a loosely cohesive cluster of hypervacuolated histiocytoid cells with scattered intranuclear pseudo-inclusions (Papanicolaou stain, ThinPrep). ThyroSeq testing revealed a *BRAF* V600E mutation.

HYALINIZING TRABECULAR TUMOR

Hyalinizing trabecular tumor (HTT) is a rare, well-circumscribed thyroid neoplasm characterized by a trabecular growth pattern and inter- and intra-trabecular hyalinization. It shows cohesive groups of cells with spindled nuclei, fine chromatin, nuclear grooves, and intranuclear pseudo-inclusions.[32] The presence of abundant nuclear pseudo-inclusions and grooves make it challenging to differentiate HTT from PTC on FNA specimens (**Fig. 6**).[32] A recent study by Nikiforova and colleagues[33] showed that *GLIS* fusions, including *PAX8::GLIS3* (93%) and *PAX8::GLIS1* (7%), are a genetic hallmark of HTT. Furthermore, none harbored *BRAF* or *RAS* mutations, *RET::PTC*, or any molecular alterations typical for PTC. As *GLIS* fusions are a unique feature of HTT, molecular tools will allow its distinction from PTC.[33] Recognizing cytologic features of HTT becomes key in selecting FNA samples for molecular testing to identify potential HTT cases, avoid an FP

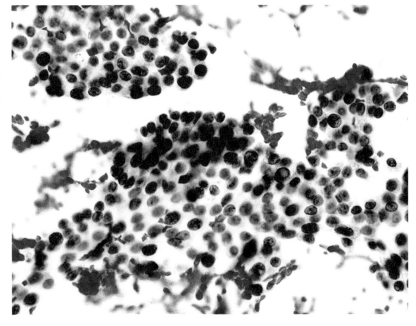

Fig. 2. Fine-needle aspiration of conventional papillary thyroid carcinoma showing large sheets of follicular cells with pale chromatin, nuclear grooves, and intranuclear pseudo-inclusions (Papanicolaou stain, smear).

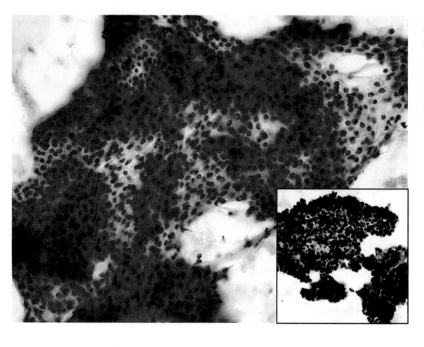

Fig. 3. Hypercellular parathyroid showing a large sheet of relatively uniform cells with round to oval nuclei with stippled chromatin and abundant cytoplasm (Papanicolaou stain, smear). Inset: GATA3 immunohistochemistry.

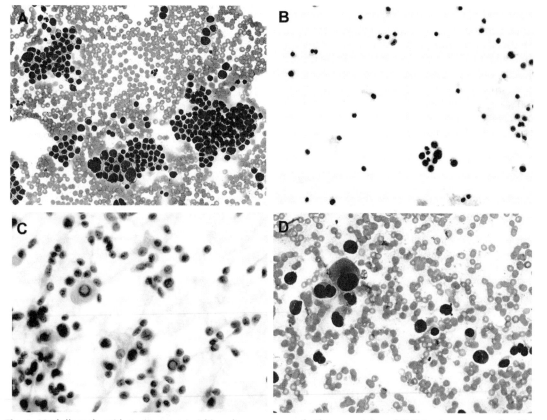

Fig. 4. Medullary thyroid carcinoma mimicking diverse range of other neoplasms. (*A*) Cohesive groups of epithelioid cells with limited cytoplasm mimicking a follicular nodule (Diff-Quik stain, smear). (*B*) Dispersed small cells with scant cytoplasm, raising the differential diagnosis of lymphoma (Papanicolaou stain, ThinPrep). (*C, D*) Intranuclear inclusions reminiscent of papillary thyroid carcinoma (*C*: Papanicolaou stain, smear; *D*: Diff-Quik stain, smear). Note the background dyscohesion, a morphologic clue for medullary thyroid carcinoma.

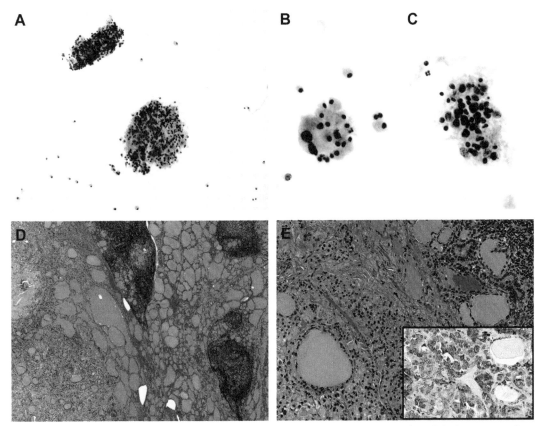

Fig. 5. Medullary thyroid carcinoma in a background of chronic lymphocytic thyroiditis. (*A*) The aspirate shows two distinct groups: small, tightly cohesive cells (upper left) and larger, loosely cohesive cells (lower right) (Papanicolaou stain, ThinPrep). Higher power images of the same specimen showing (*B*) a cluster of oncocytic-appearing cells with scattered single cells in the background and (*C*) germinal center fragments. The overall findings closely mimic chronic lymphocytic thyroiditis. (*D*) Histology shows medullary thyroid carcinoma (left side of image) in a background of chronic lymphocytic thyroiditis (hematoxylin and eosin (H&E) stain). (*E*) The medullary carcinoma is composed of oncocytic cells that morphologically overlap with the background oncocytic follicular cells (H&E stain). Inset: calcitonin immunohistochemistry.

diagnosis, and guide appropriate patient management.[33] Histologically, the diagnosis of HTT can be confirmed by membranous staining with MIB-1 monoclonal antibody or strong nuclear and cytoplasmic staining using antibody to the C-terminus region of GLIS3.[33]

MACROFOLLICULAR NODULES

FNAs of thyroid nodules composed predominantly of macrofollicles without cytologic atypia are typically classified as benign follicular nodules (**Fig. 7**). However, this can lead to the misclassification of a rare macrofollicular subtype of follicular thyroid carcinoma (FTC) that may go undetected unless resected.[3,34] Somatic *DICER1* gene mutations have been reported in this subtype of FTC. The diagnosis is only rendered after

histologic examination, which shows evidence of capsular invasion. Fortunately, these tumors occur rarely and generally have an indolent behavior.[3]

MOLECULAR TESTING

MOLECULAR UNDERPINNINGS OF THYROID CARCINOMA

The Cancer Genome Atlas (TCGA) has provided important insights into the molecular pathogenesis of the most common type of thyroid carcinoma, PTC. The most important finding of the TCGA was the discovery of two molecular subtypes of PTC: *BRAF* V600E-like (BVL) and *RAS*-like (RL) (**Table 1**).[35] The BVL subtype was strongly associated with *BRAF* V600E mutation and diverse fusion genes

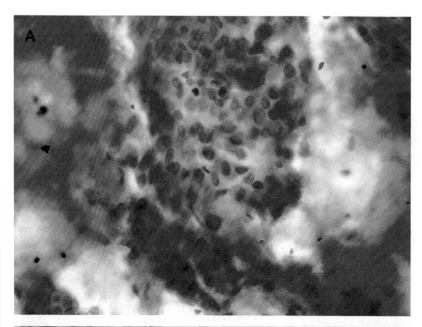

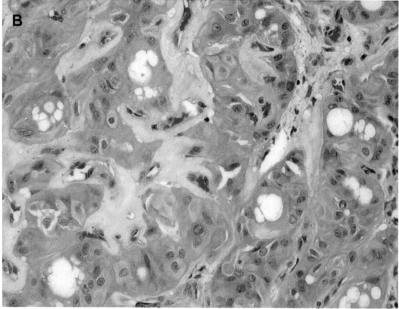

Fig. 6. Hyalinizing trabecular tumor. (*A*) The aspirate shows a cohesive cluster of tumor cells with ovoid to spindled-shaped nuclei, fine chromatin, and intranuclear pseudo-inclusions (Papanicolaou stain, smear). (*B*) Histology shows polygonal-to-spindled tumor cells with ovoid-to-elongated nuclei and nuclear pseudo-inclusions arranged in a trabecular pattern with marked inter- and intra-trabecular hyalinization (hematoxylin and eosin stain).

such as *BRAF, RET,* and *NTRK*1/3. The RL subtype was related to mutations of *RAS* and *EIF1AX* and fusion genes such as *PAX8::PPARG, FGFR2,* and *THADA.* BVL alterations confer a very high probability of cancer, a higher risk of distant metastasis, and early recurrence and are typically seen in PTC. In contrast, RL alterations are associated with a lower probability of cancer and a low risk for recurrence. Generally, they are associated with follicular-patterned cancer or noninvasive follicular thyroid neoplasm with papillary-like nuclear features (NIFTP) and benign adenomas.[36]

TERT promoter mutations have been associated with tumor progression, aggressive behavior, and poor clinical outcomes. The combination of *TERT* promoter mutation and BVL mutations is associated with an increased risk of extrathyroidal extension, lymph node metastases, and a very high probability of thyroid cancer. This combination is also more frequently identified in poorly differentiated thyroid carcinoma (PDTC) and anaplastic thyroid carcinoma (ATC).[37] Overall, TCGA showed a strong correlation between molecular alterations and histopathological diagnosis.[38]

Fig. 7. Benign follicular nodule is composed of a large flat sheet of evenly spaced follicular cells with intact macrofollicles (Diff-Quik stain, smear).

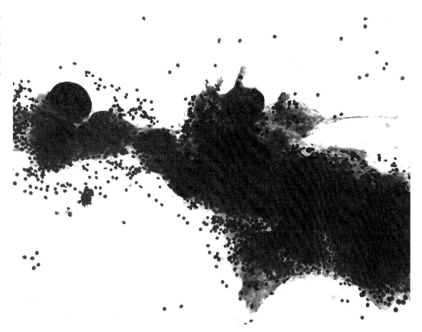

RISK STRATIFICATION OF CYTOLOGICALLY INDETERMINANT NODULES

Several molecular tests are commercially available for testing thyroid FNAC specimens, including ThyroSeq v3 Genomic Classifier (GC), Veracyte Afirma Genomic Sequencing Classifier (GSC), and ThyGeNEXT/ThyraMIR (**Table 2**). The choice of molecular platform depends on institutional preference. However, regardless of the method, the goals of molecular testing are to refine and stratify indeterminate nodules to decrease the frequency of diagnostic surgeries or determine the extent of surgery.[10,39]

ThyroSeq v3 GC uses targeted next-generation sequencing (NGS) to classify test results as *negative* (no alterations), *currently negative* (low-risk and/or low-level alterations), or *positive* (non-low-risk alterations or gene expression alterations). ThyroSeq v3 GC is reported to be a highly sensitive and specific test with an NPV of up to 98%.[5] In tests with high NPV, such as ThyroSeq v3 GC, a negative test result has a ~3% probability of malignancy, comparable to that of a benign FNA.[40] Therefore, patients with a negative result may be spared surgery and can be managed conservatively.[6] In patients with a positive result, Thyroseq v3 GC also provides information regarding specific genetic alterations with distinct cancer probabilities that can help guide individualized patient treatment. Thyroseq v3 GC can also help determine the cellular composition of FNAs and flag aspirates that are suspicious for parathyroid tissue, MTC, and certain metastatic tumors.[9,41]

The Afirma GSC uses RNA sequencing to measure gene expression to further classify indeterminate nodules as either *benign* or *suspicious*. Twelve independent classifiers are used, and seven other components are included.[42,43]

Table 1
Characteristics of molecular subtypes of papillary thyroid carcinoma

	BRAF V600E-like (BVL)	*RAS*-like (RL)
Molecular alterations	*BRAF* V600E mutations Gene fusions—*BRAF, RET,* and *NTRK*1/3	*RAS, BRAF* K601E, *PTEN,* and *EIF1AX* mutations Gene fusions—*PAX8::PPARG, FGFR2,* and *THADA*
Probability of cancer	High	Low
Risk of lymph node metastasis and extrathyroidal extension	High	Low

Table 2
Test and performance characteristics of ThyroSeq v3 GC, Veracyte Afirma GSC, and Interpace Diagnostics ThyGeNEXT/ThyraMIR

ThyroSeq v3 GC	Veracyte Afirma GSC	ThyGeNEXT/ThyraMIR
DNA- and RNA-based next-generation sequencing assay that analyzes 112 genes	RNA-based next-generation sequencing assay that analyzes expression of 10,196 nuclear and mitochondrial genes	Multiplatform test (MPTX) that combines DNA-RNA-based next-generation sequencing panel (ThyGeNEXT) with microRNA risk classifier test (ThyraMIR)

Interrogates five different classes of molecular alterations and two other components:
• Point mutations
• Insertions/deletions
• Gene fusions
• Copy number alterations (CNA)
• Abnormal gene expression (GEA)
  ○ Parathyroid
  ○ Medullary/C-cells
	Includes seven additional components:
	• Parathyroid
	• Medullary thyroid carcinoma
	• *BRAF* V600E mutation
	• *RET::PTC1/PTC3* fusion
	• Follicular cell content index
	• Oncocytic (Hürthle) cell index
	• Oncocytic (Hürthle) cell neoplasm index
		Includes:
		• 10 oncogenic mutations
		• 38 gene fusions
		• Follicular cell content
		• Parathyroid
		• Medullary thyroid carcinoma

Sensitivity (91%—97%) Specificity (75%—85%) PPV (~66%) NPV (~98%)	Sensitivity (91%) Specificity (68%) PPV (~48%) NPV (~96%)	Sensitivity (95%) Specificity (90%) PPV (~75%) NPV (~97%)
Results: • Reports specific mutations with corresponding probability of cancer or NIFTP • *Negative* (3%[a]) • *Currently negative* (5% to 10%[a]) • *Positive* (30% to 99%[a])	Results: • Binary result • *Benign* (low risk ≤ 4% ROM) • *Suspicious* (high risk ≥ 50% ROM) • If suspicious, additional genomic information can be obtained via Afirma Xpression Atlas (XA)	Results: • Reports specific genetic alterations and risk stratification • MPTX result as *negative* (level 1), *moderate* (level 2), and *positive* (level 3) • *Low risk* (3% to 20% POM), *moderate risk* (25% to 75% POM), and *high risk* (>75% POM)
Limitations: • High rate of FP due to *RAS* mutations/*RAS*-like alterations • Validated in patients ≥18 years	Limitations: • Only analyzes transcribed portions of the genome (fails to detect *TERT* promoter mutations)	Limitations: • *TP53* mutation not detected

Abbreviations: FP, false positive; GC, genomic classifier; GSC, genomic sequencing classifier; NIFTP, noninvasive follicular thyroid neoplasm with papillary-like nuclear features; NPV, negative predictive value; POM, probability of malignancy; ROM, risk of malignancy.
[a] Probability of cancer or NIFTP.

Afirma's GSC validation studies showed that it had a 91% sensitivity, 68% specificity, 47% PPV, and 96% NPV.[43] Similar to Thyroseq v3 GC, a high NPV among Bethesda III and IV thyroid nodules can reduce the number of thyroid surgeries.[43] The Afirma Xpression Atlas (XA) is an expanded panel introduced for indeterminate thyroid nodules with suspicious Afirma GSC and those diagnosed as Bethesda V/VI. This panel also uses RNA sequencing to report genomic variants and gene fusions associated with thyroid cancer. Its findings can contribute to individualized patient management regarding systemic targeted therapies and the extent of surgery.[44] This panel only analyzes sequences from transcribed portions of the genome.[9,45]

ThyGeNEXT/ThyraMIR is a multiplatform test (MPTX) that includes an expanded targeted DNA-RNA-based NGS mutational panel (e.g., *ALK*, *RET*, *TERT*, *NTRK*) to identify genetic alterations associated with thyroid cancer and a microRNA risk classifier test. All samples first undergo ThyGeNEXT testing, and samples with strong driver mutations do not undergo microRNA risk classifier. In contrast, those with weak drivers or no detectable mutations are reflexed to ThyraMIR. MPTX test results are recorded as *negative, moderate*, or *positive*. This test risk stratifies patients into low, moderate, or high-risk categories with varying probabilities of malignancy.[46] Its reported sensitivity, specificity, NPV and PPV are 95%, 90%, 97%, and 75%, respectively.[46-48]

MOLECULAR ALTERATIONS WITH POTENTIAL THERAPEUTIC APPLICATIONS

Thyroid carcinomas that harbor actionable kinase fusions account for 10% to 15% of cases. Kinase fusion-related thyroid carcinomas (KFTCs) encompass a spectrum of molecularly diverse tumors with overlapping clinicopathologic features and a tendency for clinical aggressiveness. *RET* rearrangement is the most common, accounting for ~50% of KFTC, followed by less common *NTRK*1/2/3 (~30%), *ALK* (~5%), *MET, ROS1*, and *FGFR*1/2 rearrangements.[49] These oncogenic fusions cause aberrant kinase activation and are crucial drivers in thyroid carcinogenesis.[49,50] Selective kinase inhibitors (e.g., larotrectinib, entrectinib, selpercatinib, and pralsetinib) have shown significant efficacy with favorable side effects in the treatment of KFTCs. Therefore, identifying these tumors becomes an important task.[50] However, given the reported low frequency of kinase rearrangements in thyroid tumors, an algorithmic approach for referring cases to molecular testing becomes essential. Recognizing the distinct morphologic features of these tumors, including multinodular growth, prominent fibrosis, and extensive lymphovascular invasion (**Fig. 8**), can help triage these cases for further testing. Screening these tumors with BRAF IHC, clone VE1, is recommended.[50,51] As *BRAF* V600E mutation is mutually exclusive with kinase fusions, cases with positive staining are unlikely to have kinase fusions and may be excluded from further analysis (**Fig. 9**). However, cases lacking staining should undergo further testing.[49]

ATC represents approximately 1% of all thyroid cancers and is the most aggressive form, being nearly universally lethal and comprising the majority of all thyroid cancer deaths.[52] ATCs may develop through dedifferentiation of a preexisting differentiated thyroid cancer (25–75% of cases) or PDTC.[53-56] The standard treatment of ATC includes a multimodal combination of surgery and external beam radiation with radiosensitizing chemotherapy.[57] In 2018, the FDA approved the first targeted treatment of patients with ATC based on findings from a clinical trial that investigated dabrafenib plus trametinib in *BRAF* V600E-mutated ATC. As this combination showed a response against *BRAF* V600E-mutated ATC, it is now mandatory to test all ATCs for *BRAF* V600E mutation.[53] This testing can be performed using BRAF IHC or molecular testing.

HISTOLOGY

Cytologic-histologic correlation has been used as the gold standard to estimate the ROM associated with indeterminate diagnostic categories; however, this method has its limitations and represents an overestimation of the ROM due to selection bias (as benign thyroid nodules are often spared surgery). Ohori and colleagues[58] recently proposed a new method to approximate ROM by including all indeterminate thyroid cytology cases assessed molecularly, not only those treated surgically. They used ThyroSeq v3 GC results to calculate the molecular-derived ROM (MDROM), showing that this measure correlated well with the TBSRTC-reported ROMs and showing that it could be a reliable preoperative risk assessment tool. Using the same approach, another group validated these findings and further showed that AUS subcategories are associated with specific MDROM, ROM, and genetic alterations.[59]

The benign call rate (BCR) is the proportion of cases with a negative molecular test (MT) result and reflects the percentage of patients that can potentially avoid surgery.[6,39] Conversely, the positive call rate (PCR) is the percentage of patients with positive MT results for which surgery is indicated. In cases with a positive MT, the extent of surgery will depend on the specific genetic alterations, given that different molecular alterations are associated with variable cancer probabilities. In resected tumors with equivocal histology, integration of molecular results, IHC, and cytomorphologic features of prior FNA can be helpful. IHC can be used as a screening tool for specific genetic alterations, including BRAF to detect *BRAF* V600E mutation, pan-RAS Q61R to detect *HRAS/NRAS/KRAS* Q61R mutations, and pan-TRK to detect *NTRK*1/3 fusions.[60-62]

Follicular-patterned thyroid neoplasms are diagnostically challenging. Accurately distinguishing FTC from follicular adenoma requires thorough histologic evaluation. These tumors must show

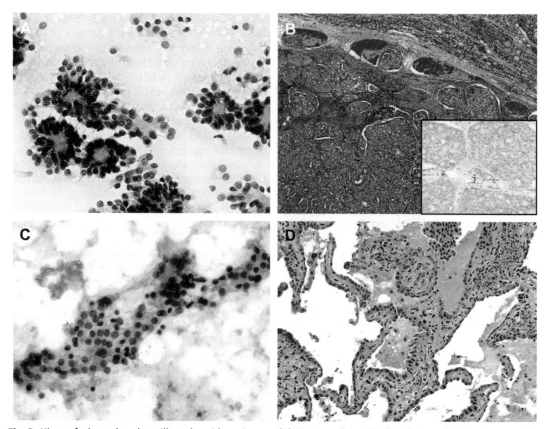

Fig. 8. Kinase fusion-related papillary thyroid carcinoma. (*A*) Fine-needle aspiration shows cohesive clusters of tumor cells with mild nuclear enlargement and powdery chromatin arranged in microfollicles (Papanicolaou stain, smear). Molecular testing showed *EML4::NTRK3*. (*B*) The corresponding papillary thyroid carcinoma shows multinodular growth, cribriform and glomeruloid architecture, fibrosis, and prominent lymphovascular invasion (hematoxylin and eosin stain). Inset: pan-TRK immunohistochemistry shows diffuse, weak cytoplasmic reactivity in tumor cells. (*C*) *NTRK3*-rearranged papillary thyroid carcinoma shows a sheet of tumor cells with mildly enlarged rounded nuclei, pale chromatin, and scattered nuclear grooves (Papanicolaou stain, smear). (*D*). Papillary thyroid carcinoma harboring *ETV6::NTRK3* shows a macrofollicular architecture and granular oncocytoid tumor cells with subtle papillary thyroid carcinoma nuclear features (hematoxylin and eosin stain).

full-thickness capsular or vascular invasion and lack PTC nuclear features to fulfill diagnostic criteria for FTC. They are generally worked up with deeper levels of suspicious areas and application of vascular/lymphatic markers in cases of questionable vascular/lymphatic invasion, but some cases remain indeterminate. The 2022 WHO classification of thyroid neoplasms recommends the term follicular tumor of uncertain malignant potential (FT-UMP) for tumors with questionable capsular or vascular invasion.[53] Although the diagnosis of carcinoma hinges on the identification of unequivocal capsular or vascular invasion, the presence of aggressive mutations such as *TERT* promoter mutation may indicate potentially malignant behavior even in non-invasive neoplasms. FT-UMPs require close clinical follow-up as their biologic potential is uncertain, especially if additional atypical features

(e.g., solid growth and mitoses) are present.[63] Alternatively, a more reassuring genetic profile could help favor a more conservative histologic interpretation.

Classically, the presence of a perilesional fibrous capsule has been used as a morphologic feature indicative of a neoplastic rather than a hyperplastic process. Multinodular goiters show numerous thyroid nodules composed of follicular cells with variable architecture; nodules range from colloid-rich and macrofollicular to hypercellular and microfollicular. Owing to their variable architecture, different terms have been used for these proliferations, including nodular hyperplasia, adenomatoid nodules, etc.[64] These nodules have not generally been classified as neoplasms. However, various studies have shown that many of them are neoplastic, whereas others are hyperplastic.[65,66] Histologically, it may be challenging to distinguish

Fig. 9. (*A*) Conventional papillary thyroid carcinoma (hematoxylin and eosin stain) with (*B*) diffuse strong reactivity for *BRAF* V600E mutation-specific antibody (VE1, immunohistochemistry).

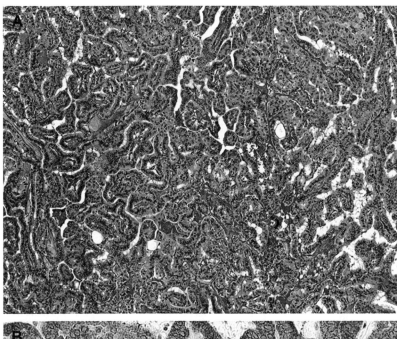

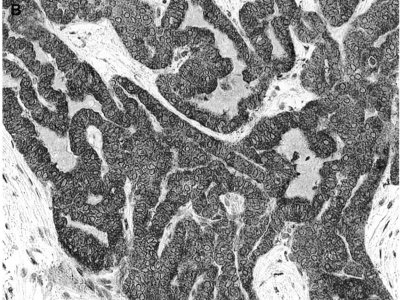

cellular hyperplastic nodules from neoplastic nodules, and the only way to definitively make this distinction is with clonality studies.[66] For this reason, the 2022 WHO of thyroid neoplasms recommends using "thyroid follicular nodular disease" as an alternative terminology because it avoids defining a lesion as hyperplastic or neoplastic.[53,66]

SUMMARY

FNAC and molecular testing help inform the management of patients with thyroid nodules.

Molecular testing can contribute to thyroid cancer risk stratification, impact the selection of targeted therapies, and improve patient management. Integrating histopathology, cytomorphology, molecular results, and immunohistochemical findings is crucial to making the optimal diagnosis and avoiding diagnostic pitfalls.

DISCLOSURE

The authors have nothing to disclose.

REFERENCES

1. Cibas ES, Ali SZ. The 2017 bethesda system for reporting thyroid cytopathology. J Am Soc Cytopathol 2017;6(6):217–22.

2. Rossi ED, Adeniran AJ, Faquin WC. Pitfalls in thyroid cytopathology. Surg Pathol Clin 2019;12(4):865–81.

3. Juhlin CC, Stenman A, Zedenius J. Macrofollicular variant follicular thyroid tumors are DICER1 mutated and exhibit distinct histological features. Histopathology 2021;79(4):661–6.

4. Policarpio-Nicolas ML, Sirohi D. Macrofollicular variant of papillary carcinoma, a potential diagnostic pitfall: a report of two cases including a review of literature. Cytojournal 2013;10:16.

5. Nikiforova MN, Mercurio S, Wald AI, et al. Analytical performance of the ThyroSeq v3 genomic classifier for cancer diagnosis in thyroid nodules. Cancer 2018;124(8):1682–90.

6. Ohori NP, Landau MS, Carty SE, et al. Benign call rate and molecular test result distribution of ThyroSeq v3. Cancer Cytopathol 2019;127(3):161–8.

7. Bose S, Sacks W, Walts AE. Update on molecular testing for cytologically indeterminate thyroid nodules. Adv Anat Pathol 2019;26(2):114–23.

8. Bongiovanni M, Spitale A, Faquin WC, et al. The bethesda system for reporting thyroid cytopathology: a meta-analysis. Acta Cytol 2012;56(4):333–9.

9. Nishino M, Krane JF. Role of ancillary techniques in thyroid cytology specimens. Acta Cytol 2020;64(1–2):40–51.

10. Nishino M, Nikiforova M. Update on molecular testing for cytologically indeterminate thyroid nodules. Arch Pathol Lab Med 2018;142(4):446–57.

11. Kim SJ, Roh J, Baek JH, et al. Risk of malignancy according to sub-classification of the atypia of undetermined significance or follicular lesion of undetermined significance (AUS/FLUS) category in the Bethesda system for reporting thyroid cytopathology. Cytopathology 2017;28(1):65–73.

12. Ho AS, Sarti EE, Jain KS, et al. Malignancy rate in thyroid nodules classified as Bethesda category III (AUS/FLUS). Thyroid 2014;24(5):832–9.

13. VanderLaan PA, Marqusee E, Krane JF. Usefulness of diagnostic qualifiers for thyroid fine-needle aspirations with atypia of undetermined significance. Am J Clin Pathol 2011;136(4):572–7.

14. Vuong HG, Nguyen TPX, Hassell LA, et al. Diagnostic performances of the afirma gene sequencing classifier in comparison with the gene expression classifier: a meta-analysis. Cancer Cytopathol 2021;129(3):182–9.

15. Domingo RP, Ogden LL, Been LC, et al. Identification of parathyroid tissue in thyroid fine-needle aspiration: A combined approach using cytology, immunohistochemical, and molecular methods. Diagn Cytopathol 2017;45(6):526–32.

16. Absher KJ, Truong LD, Khurana KK, et al. Parathyroid cytology: avoiding diagnostic pitfalls. Head Neck 2002;24(2):157–64.

17. Shi Y, Brandler TC, Yee-Chang M, et al. Application of GATA 3 and TTF-1 in differentiating parathyroid and thyroid nodules on cytology specimens. Diagn Cytopathol 2020;48(2):128–37.

18. Trimboli P, D'Aurizio F, Tozzoli R, et al. Measurement of thyroglobulin, calcitonin, and PTH in FNA washout fluids. Clin Chem Lab Med 2017;55(7):914–25.

19. Steen S, Hysek M, Zedenius J, et al. Cyto-morphological features of parathyroid lesions: Fine-needle aspiration cytology series from an endocrine tumor referral center. Diagn Cytopathol 2022;50(2):75–83.

20. Cho M, Oweity T, Brandler TC, et al. Distinguishing parathyroid and thyroid lesions on ultrasound-guided fine-needle aspiration: A correlation of clinical data, ancillary studies, and molecular analysis. Cancer Cytopathol 2017;125(9):674–82.

21. Pusztaszeri MP, Bongiovanni M, Faquin WC. Update on the cytologic and molecular features of medullary thyroid carcinoma. Adv Anat Pathol 2014;21(1):26–35.

22. Kaushal S, Iyer VK, Mathur SR, et al. Fine needle aspiration cytology of medullary carcinoma of the thyroid with a focus on rare variants: a review of 78 cases. Cytopathology 2011;22(2):95–105.

23. Papaparaskeva K, Nagel H, Droese M. Cytologic diagnosis of medullary carcinoma of the thyroid gland. Diagn Cytopathol 2000;22(6):351–8.

24. Suzuki A, Hirokawa M, Takada N, et al. Fine-needle aspiration cytology for medullary thyroid carcinoma: a single institutional experience in Japan. Endocr J 2017;64(11):1099–104.

25. Maleki Z, Abram M, Dell'Aquila M, et al. Insulinoma-associated protein 1 (INSM-1) expression in medullary thyroid carcinoma FNA: a multi-institutional study. J Am Soc Cytopathol 2020;9(3):185–90.

26. Adel Hakim S, Mohamed Abd Raboh N. The diagnostic utility of INSM1 and GATA3 in discriminating problematic medullary thyroid carcinoma, thyroid and parathyroid lesions. Pol J Pathol 2021;72(1):11–22.

27. de Micco C, Chapel F, Dor AM, et al. Thyroglobulin in medullary thyroid carcinoma: immunohistochemical study with polyclonal and monoclonal antibodies. Hum Pathol 1993;24(3):256–62.

28. Trimboli P, Cremonini N, Ceriani L, et al. Calcitonin measurement in aspiration needle washout fluids has higher sensitivity than cytology in detecting medullary thyroid cancer: a retrospective multicentre study. Clin Endocrinol (Oxf) 2014;80(1):135–40.

29. Nikiforova MN, Wald AI, Roy S, et al. Targeted next-generation sequencing panel (ThyroSeq) for detection of mutations in thyroid cancer. J Clin Endocrinol Metab 2013;98(11):E1852–60.

30. Nikiforov YE, Carty SE, Chiosea SI, et al. Impact of the multi-gene thyroseq next-generation sequencing assay on cancer diagnosis in thyroid nodules with atypia of undetermined significance/follicular lesion of undetermined significance cytology. Thyroid 2015;25(11):1217–23.

31. Camacho CP, Lindsey SC, Melo MC, et al. Measurement of calcitonin and calcitonin gene-related peptide mRNA refines the management of patients with medullary thyroid cancer and may replace calcitonin-stimulation tests. Thyroid 2013;23(3):308–16.

32. Podany P, Gilani SM. Hyalinizing trabecular tumor: cytologic, histologic and molecular features and diagnostic considerations. Ann Diagn Pathol 2021; 54:151803.

33. Nikiforova MN, Nikiforov YE, Ohori NP. GLIS rearrangements in thyroid nodules: a key to preoperative diagnosis of hyalinizing trabecular tumor. Cancer Cytopathol 2019;127(9):560–6.

34. Bongiovanni M, Sykiotis GP, La Rosa S, et al. Macrofollicular variant of follicular thyroid carcinoma: a rare underappreciated pitfall in the diagnosis of thyroid carcinoma. Thyroid 2020;30(1):72–80.

35. Cancer Genome Atlas Research N. Integrated genomic characterization of papillary thyroid carcinoma. Cell 2014;159(3):676–90.

36. Chin PD, Zhu CY, Sajed DP, et al. Correlation of thyroseq results with surgical histopathology in cytologically indeterminate thyroid nodules. Endocr Pathol 2020;31(4):377–84.

37. Liu R, Xing M. TERT promoter mutations in thyroid cancer. Endocr Relat Cancer 2016;23(3):R143–55.

38. Song YS, Park YJ. Genomic characterization of differentiated thyroid carcinoma. Endocrinol Metab (Seoul) 2019;34(1):1–10.

39. Ohori NP. A decade into thyroid molecular testing: where do we stand? J Am Soc Cytopathol 2022; 11(2):59–61.

40. Chen T, Gilfix BM, Rivera J, et al. The role of the thyroSeq v3 molecular test in the surgical management of thyroid nodules in the canadian public health care setting. Thyroid 2020;30(9):1280–7.

41. Nikiforov YE, Carty SE, Chiosea SI, et al. Highly accurate diagnosis of cancer in thyroid nodules with follicular neoplasm/suspicious for a follicular neoplasm cytology by ThyroSeq v2 next-generation sequencing assay. Cancer 2014;120(23):3627–34.

42. Zhang L, Smola B, Lew M, et al. Performance of Afirma genomic sequencing classifier vs gene expression classifier in Bethesda category III thyroid nodules: an institutional experience. Diagn Cytopathol 2021;49(8):921–7.

43. Patel KN, Angell TE, Babiarz J, et al. Performance of a genomic sequencing classifier for the preoperative diagnosis of cytologically indeterminate thyroid nodules. JAMA Surg 2018;153(9):817–24.

44. Krane JF, Cibas ES, Endo M, et al. The Afirma Xpression Atlas for thyroid nodules and thyroid cancer metastases: Insights to inform clinical decision-making from a fine-needle aspiration sample. Cancer Cytopathol 2020;128(7):452–9.

45. Kaya C, Dorsaint P, Mercurio S, et al. Limitations of detecting genetic variants from the RNA sequencing data in tissue and fine-needle aspiration samples. Thyroid 2021;31(4):589–95.

46. Sistrunk JW, Shifrin A, Frager M, et al. Clinical performance of multiplatform mutation panel and microRNA risk classifier in indeterminate thyroid nodules. J Am Soc Cytopathol 2020;9(4):232–41.

47. Silaghi CA, Lozovanu V, Georgescu CE, et al. Thyroseq v3, Afirma GSC, and microRNA panels versus previous molecular tests in the preoperative diagnosis of indeterminate thyroid nodules: a systematic review and meta-analysis. Front Endocrinol (Lausanne) 2021;12:649522.

48. Lupo MA, Walts AE, Sistrunk JW, et al. Multiplatform molecular test performance in indeterminate thyroid nodules. Diagn Cytopathol 2020;48(12):1254–64.

49. Chu YH, Sadow PM. Kinase fusion-related thyroid carcinomas: distinct pathologic entities with evolving diagnostic implications. Diagn Histopathol (Oxf) 2021;27(6):252–62.

50. Chu YH, Wirth LJ, Farahani AA, et al. Clinicopathologic features of kinase fusion-related thyroid carcinomas: an integrative analysis with molecular characterization. Mod Pathol 2020;33(12):2458–72.

51. Chu YH, Dias-Santagata D, Farahani AA, et al. Clinicopathologic and molecular characterization of NTRK-rearranged thyroid carcinoma (NRTC). Mod Pathol 2020;33(11):2186–97.

52. Molinaro E, Romei C, Biagini A, et al. Anaplastic thyroid carcinoma: from clinicopathology to genetics and advanced therapies. Nat Rev Endocrinol 2017; 13(11):644–60.

53. Baloch ZW, Asa SL, Barletta JA, et al. Overview of the 2022 WHO classification of thyroid neoplasms. Endocr Pathol 2022;33(1):27–63.

54. Wiseman SM, Loree TR, Rigual NR, et al. Anaplastic transformation of thyroid cancer: review of clinical, pathologic, and molecular evidence provides new insights into disease biology and future therapy. Head Neck 2003;25(8):662–70.

55. McIver B, Hay ID, Giuffrida DF, et al. Anaplastic thyroid carcinoma: a 50-year experience at a single institution. Surgery 2001;130(6):1028–34.

56. Venkatesh YS, Ordonez NG, Schultz PN, et al. Anaplastic carcinoma of the thyroid. A clinicopathologic study of 121 cases. Cancer 1990;66(2):321–30.

57. Smallridge RC, Ain KB, Asa SL, et al. American Thyroid Association guidelines for management of patients with anaplastic thyroid cancer. Thyroid 2012; 22(11):1104–39.

58. Ohori NP, Landau MS, Manroa P, et al. Molecular-derived estimation of risk of malignancy for indeterminate thyroid cytology diagnoses. J Am Soc Cytopathol 2020;9(4):213–20.

59. Gajzer DC, Tjendra Y, Kerr DA, et al. Probability of malignancy as determined by thyroSeq v3 genomic classifier varies according to the subtype of atypia. Cancer Cytopathol 2022. https://doi.org/10.1002/cncy.22617. In press.

60. Parker KG, White MG, Cipriani NA. Comparison of molecular methods and BRAF immunohistochemistry (VE1 Clone) for the detection of BRAF V600E mutation in papillary thyroid carcinoma: a meta-analysis. Head Neck Pathol 2020;14(4): 1067–79.

61. Oishi N, Kondo T, Vuong HG, et al. Immunohistochemical detection of NRAS(Q61R) protein in follicular-patterned thyroid tumors. Hum Pathol 2016;53:51–7.

62. Lee YC, Chen JY, Huang CJ, et al. Detection of NTRK1/3 rearrangements in papillary thyroid carcinoma using immunohistochemistry, fluorescent in situ hybridization, and next-generation sequencing. Endocr Pathol 2020;31(4):348–58.

63. Cracolici V, Ritterhouse LL, Segal JP, et al. Follicular thyroid neoplasms: comparison of clinicopathologic and molecular features of atypical adenomas and follicular thyroid carcinomas. Am J Surg Pathol 2020;44(7):881–92.

64. Derwahl M, Studer H. Hyperplasia versus adenoma in endocrine tissues: are they different? Trends Endocrinol Metab 2002;13(1):23–8.

65. Harrer P, Brocker M, Zint A, et al. The clonality of nodules in recurrent goiters at second surgery. Langenbecks Arch Surg 1998;383(6):453–5.

66. Apel RL, Ezzat S, Bapat BV, et al. Clonality of thyroid nodules in sporadic goiter. Diagn Mol Pathol 1995; 4(2):113–21.

To Freeze or Not to Freeze? Recommendations for Intraoperative Examination and Gross Prosection of Thyroid Glands

Fouad R. Zakka, MD, Nicole A. Cipriani, MD*

KEYWORDS

- Thyroid • Follicular thyroid lesions • Thyroid carcinoma • High-grade features
- Intraoperative consultation • Frozen section • Gross examination

---

Key points

- Intraoperative consultation for thyroid nodules is not recommended in light of diagnostic limitations, freezing artifact, and the superiority of permanent evaluation and thorough sampling.

- The left lobe, right lobe, and isthmus can be differentially inked, with consideration for anterior-posterior differentiation due to increased recurrence risk in posterior tumors.

- Transverse or modified transverse vertical sectioning should be performed after full fixation in order to preserve architectural integrity and nuclear detail.

- Cassette submission should account for the lesion's periphery, possible extension into muscle, and high grade features (fleshy or necrotic cut surface and satellite lesions).

ABSTRACT

The use of intraoperative consultation for indeterminate thyroid lesions is not advocated but is still requested by some surgeons. Obscured cytomorphology and nonrepresentative sampling limit the specificity of intraoperative assessment. Formalin fixation of thyroid glands before sectioning also minimizes artifacts introduced by fresh sectioning. Inking of thyroid may vary based on institutional preferences and information desired by clinical teams. Sectioning may occur in the conventional transverse method or the modified transverse vertical method to more thoroughly evaluate the lesion's periphery. Gross examination of thyroid lesions should always consider possible high-grade features, such as necrosis or extrathyroidal extension.

INTRAOPERATIVE CONSULTATIONS

Intraoperative consultations for thyroid nodules remain prevalent, even though many experts in the field have shown that they may be more detrimental to patient care than they are beneficial.[1,2] The main reason that pathologists are asked to perform frozen sections (FS) on thyroid nodules is to establish a definitive diagnosis for cytologically indeterminate nodules, or those designated atypia of undetermined significance/follicular lesion of undetermined significance (Bethesda

---

Disclosures: None.

Department of Pathology, The University of Chicago, Pritzker School of Medicine, 5841 South Maryland Avenue, MC 6101, Chicago, IL 60637, USA

* Corresponding author.

E-mail address: Nicole.cipriani@uchospitals.edu

Surgical Pathology 16 (2023) 15–26
https://doi.org/10.1016/j.path.2022.09.004

category III, BC3) or suspicious for follicular neoplasm (Bethesda category IV, BC4) on fine-needle aspiration (FNA).[3] An intraoperative diagnosis of "malignant" may prompt completion thyroidectomy and spare the patient a second surgery. However, it has been shown that in BC3 and BC4 lesions, the sensitivity of diagnosing cancer intraoperatively is only 20% and 50%, respectively (even though the specificity is up to 100%). Additionally, FS changed the intraoperative course in only 2.2% and 8% of patients with BC3 and BC4 lesions, respectively.[3] Even if a cancer diagnosis is made intraoperatively (or subsequently on permanent sections), the need for completion thyroidectomy is not necessarily always warranted in low-risk carcinomas in which radioactive iodine therapy is not indicated.[4]

There are several factors that diminish the efficacy of FS for thyroid lesions. When faced with a follicular lesion, common differential diagnoses include follicular adenoma, noninvasive follicular thyroid neoplasm with papillary-like nuclear features (NIFTP), follicular carcinoma, and invasive encapsulated variant of papillary thyroid carcinoma (IEFVPTC). Definitive diagnosis of a follicular neoplasm requires microscopic examination of the nodule's capsule or periphery to assess for capsular and vascular invasion (Fig. 1).[5] Fresh intraoperative sectioning of a follicular neoplasm increases the likelihood that the architectural integrity of the capsule may be compromised. Capsular and vascular distortion, vascular collapse, or dragging of friable tumor cells into vessels mimicking invasion have been documented on FSs.[6,7] The likelihood of finding convincing capsular or vascular invasion on representative FSs, which carries with it suboptimal staining and distorted architecture, is extremely low. Even after fixation, it has been shown that as many as 10 sections are required to identify a focus of capsular invasion.[8] As such, a diagnosis of follicular adenoma or NIFTP cannot be rendered based on a few, potentially suboptimal sections examined intraoperatively. A diagnosis of follicular carcinoma or IEFVPTC can be made if capsular invasion or vascular invasion is identified (see Fig. 1B, D). It can be challenging to confirm capsular invasion on permanent sections, let alone FSs.[5] Features, such as intralesional fibrosis, which mimic a tumor capsule often require multiple tissue levels to discern. Additionally, it is common to encounter situations in which a follicular tumor starts to invade through its capsule but does not breach it entirely. Again, to confidently make this distinction, multiple sections and levels may be required. Furthermore, identification of capsular invasion alone in a follicular

neoplasm without vascular invasion or other high-risk features may not warrant completion thyroidectomy or radioiodine ablation. Lobectomy may be adequate, thereby obviating the utility of FS. Vascular invasion is a finding that would warrant a diagnosis of malignancy and usually completion thyroidectomy but is not always a straightforward diagnosis to make.[9] On permanent sections, the pathologist has the advantage of appropriately fixed tissue, multiple levels, and special or immunohistochemical stains[10] that aid in diagnosis. Features that mimic vascular invasion (such as undermining of endothelial cells by tumor cells or mechanical carryover of friable, detached tumor cells into vascular lumina) are difficult to interrogate on FSs.

The final challenging follicular lesion to address is NIFTP and its malignant counterpart IEFVPTC (see Fig. 1C and D). The diagnostic criteria[11] for NIFTP include but are not limited to encapsulation or clear demarcation (without invasion), nuclear features of papillary thyroid carcinoma (PTC), and predominantly follicular growth pattern with the absence of true papillae, psammoma bodies, tumor necrosis, increased mitoses, and significant solid growth. The ability to adequately assess for these criteria would prove extremely challenging on FSs, again, in the absence of optimal staining and sampling. The nuclear detail that would qualify as PTC-like, such as chromatin clearing, may be confounded by frozen artifact.[12,13] Ultimately, diagnosis of follicular adenoma, follicular carcinoma, NIFTP, and IEFVPTC are best made on permanent histologic sections that allow for adequate fixation and sampling. Many of these lesions are given cytologically indeterminate BC3 or BC4 diagnoses on FNA, and FS is not equipped to play a role in differentiating between them.

The utility of FSs in thyroid pathologic conditions may lie in other areas. Specifically, FSs would be useful in identifying lymph node metastases (thereby confirming malignancy) or parathyroid glands in the field.[14] A pitfall includes exophytic nodules in chronic lymphocytic thyroiditis that may mimic nodal metastases.[15] FSs may have less of a role in managing thyroid nodules. In cases where surgeons think strongly about an intraoperative assessment, a smear or touch imprint can aid in the evaluation of architectural and nuclear features (Fig. 2).[16] In cases of cellular, microfollicular smears, a pathologist can render a diagnosis of a follicular lesion, after which further classification would be deferred to permanent sections.[17,18] Conversely, identification of true intranuclear cytoplasmic pseudoinclusions on smear combined with an infiltrative neoplasm on cryo section may aid in confirmation of PTC.

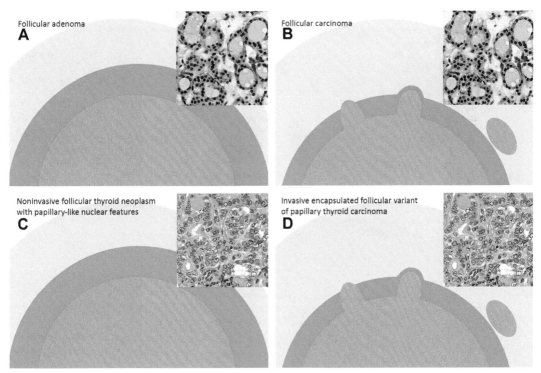

Fig. 1. Follicular neoplasm. Distinction between the various types of follicular neoplasms on frozen section is nearly impossible and is best left to permanent sections. Conceptually, a circumscribed, noninvasive neoplasm with bland nuclei would be regarded as a follicular adenoma (*A*). An invasive neoplasm with bland nuclei would be regarded as a follicular carcinoma (*B*). A circumscribed, noninvasive neoplasm with papillary-like nuclei would be regarded as a noninvasive follicular thyroid NIFTP (*C*). An invasive neoplasm with papillary-like nuclei would be regarded as invasive encapsulated follicular variant of papillary thyroid carcinoma (*D*). Clinical management of adenoma and NIFTP would be observation without additional surgery. Management of carcinoma would depend on additional features (capsular invasion only, angioinvasion, high-grade features) that would not be fully determinable intraoperatively and are best left to permanent sections.

APPROACH TO THYROID GROSSING

Orientation and Inking

Initial gross evaluation of thyroid should include specimen weight, measurement, and orientation. In glands that are not severely distorted, the anterior aspect of the thyroid gland is convex and the posterior aspect is concave. The right and left lobes taper superiorly, and the isthmus is located relatively inferiorly. The posterior surface may contain parathyroid glands, which should be noted and submitted separately. The peri-isthmic region may contain a pyramidal lobe and/or associated central compartment lymph nodes. The thyroid is enveloped by a thin layer of fascia that serves as an anatomic plane during thyroidectomy, sometimes referred to as the "false thyroid capsule."[19] There is no single correct way to ink the outer surface of the gland and approach may vary by institution. As a three-dimensional structure, one may consider the right lobe, left lobe, isthmus, anterior surface, and posterior surface as potential anatomic areas of importance. The lobes and isthmus may be differentially designated by ink colors or by cassette designation. In total thyroidectomies in which the gross pathologist may have to go "back to the bucket" for submission of additional cassettes, a 3-color system to differentially designate right lobe, left lobe, and isthmus is preferred.[20] In lobectomy or hemithyroidectomy specimens, the isthmic margin (which is in continuity with the contralateral isthmus) should be identified and inked differently from the peripheral/outer surface of the lobe. A positive margin at the isthmus may have different clinical implications than a positive margin at the periphery. In cases where both right and left lobes are removed separately within the same procedure, the pathologist should note that the "isthmic margin" in a given lobe is not a true surgical margin because it is continuous with the isthmic portion of the resected contralateral lobe. However, in such

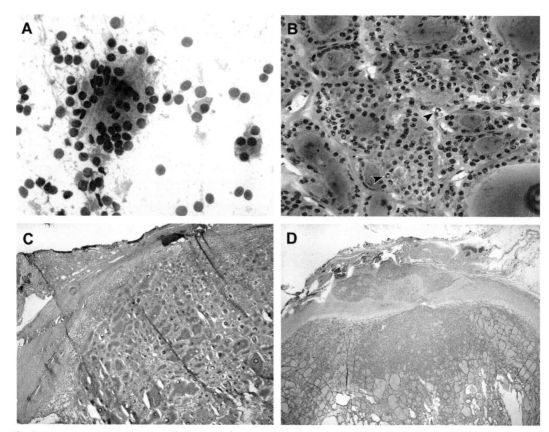

Fig. 2. Intraoperative evaluation. If a request for intraoperative examination of a follicular neoplasm is made, a cytologic preparation (touch prep, smear, or scrimp) can be useful in the evaluation of nuclear features. This smear demonstrates microfollicular clusters with round dark nuclei that are not worrisome for papillary carcinoma (*A*). However, nuclei on cut frozen sections often demonstrate artifactual clear vacuoles due to the freezing process. These artifacts should not be interpreted as pseudoinclusions (*B*). A representative section of the tumor-capsule interface confirms the circumscribed, microfollicular nature of the lesion, and a diagnosis of "follicular neoplasm" can be rendered at the time of frozen (*C*). On complete permanent sampling of the periphery of the lesion, capsular invasion is identified, compatible with a final diagnosis of follicular carcinoma (*D*). This extent of sampling is not feasible intraoperatively. Therefore, confirmation of the follicular nature of the neoplasm by smear (*A*) (with or without cut section [*B/C*]) is adequate, and final diagnosis must be deferred to permanent.

cases, the isthmic margin should still be inked differentially in order to confirm that potential tumor present at isthmic margin is not a true surgical margin.

The more controversial question is whether designation of the anterior versus posterior surface is required. A study comparing the prognostic implications of a microscopically positive anterior versus posterior margin showed that a positive posterior margin was associated with a 23-fold increase in risk of recurrence.[21] Microscopic residual disease (positive margin) in itself was not an independent risk factor for recurrence but location of positive margin was. The proposed reason for this finding is that a final negative anterior margin is easier to obtain, in light of the ability to excise

a portion of the strap muscles along with the anterior aspect of the thyroid, or the potential to resect muscle separately. Obtaining a negative posterior margin is more difficult to achieve due to the presence of structures that are not amenable to being shaved off or partially resected, such as the recurrent laryngeal nerve and the trachea. This potential difference is reflected in the current AJCC staging system, in which T3b is assigned to tumors grossly involving the anterior strap muscles, whereas T4a is assigned to tumors extending posteriorly (to larynx, trachea, esophagus, or recurrent laryngeal nerve) or very far anteriorly (subcutaneous tissue). In clinical settings in which physicians use positive margin location to guide ancillary treatment or predict recurrence risk, it may be useful to differently ink the anterior and posterior surfaces. It bears mentioning that the above study was conducted only on PTC and not other types of primary thyroid malignancies. If differential inking of anterior and posterior surfaces is desired by the clinical team, a 4-color system may be used to differentially label anterior right, anterior left, anterior isthmus, and posterior. Arguably, 6 colors could be used (anterior right, posterior right, anterior left, posterior left, anterior isthmus, posterior isthmus); however, this number of colors can become cumbersome and is not recommended.

Sectioning

Before sectioning thyroid specimens, adequate formalin fixation is advised in order to stabilize anatomic planes and minimize fixation-related nuclear artifacts. Fixation helps prevent "slippage" and preserve the integrity of the outer fascial plane and potential internal tumor capsule. Fresh sectioning may result in architectural distortion or tumor cell fragmentation, mimicking capsular or vascular invasion, as discussed above. Poor fixation may result in artifactual nuclear vacuoles or pseudo-pseudoinclusions, falsely raising suspicion for papillary carcinoma.[22,23] If after overnight fixation, sectioning reveals the tissue to be partially bloody/underfixed, formalin fixation should be continued in order to ensure proper specimen quality before submitting.

In thyroids with clinically relevant nodules, correlation should be made with imaging (usually ultrasound) findings (including location and suspicious features), FNA diagnosis, and molecular findings (if applicable). This information serves as a guide to inform appropriate sectioning and help direct cassette submission. There are 2 main techniques to serially section the specimen, the transverse approach and the modified transverse vertical approach.

The transverse approach is the most commonly used technique and can be performed for most cases with multinodular disease with no dominant nodule, diffuse medical disease (such as Graves or Hashimotos) or a malignant diagnosis on FNA. Using this method, serial transverse sections are made perpendicular to the long axis of the lobe. If the specimen is an intact total thyroidectomy with an appreciable isthmus, the lobes can be sectioned transversely and the isthmus sagittally (**Fig.** 3A). In a total thyroidectomy where the isthmus is short or inconspicuous, the lobes can be sectioned transversely (**Fig.** 3B). In lobectomies/hemithyroidectomies, transverse sectioning allows for visualization of the nodule in relation to the isthmic margin (**Fig.** 3C).

The modified transverse vertical approach can be considered when there is a dominant nodule, especially if indeterminate on FNA (BC3 or BC4). Although there is no specific size guideline, this approach may best be used for nodules measuring 2 cm or larger. This method allows for visualization of the location of the nodule within the lobe and facilitates perpendicular sectioning of the "tips" or poles of nodule.[24] This approach is best used for follicular-patterned neoplasms when thorough examination of the capsule is of paramount importance for diagnosis of benign versus malignant. In this method, the lobe is first bisected longitudinally (in the coronal plane) to expose the lesion (see **Figs.** 3D, **5** and **6**). Once exposed, the "tips" or poles of the dominant nodule can be sectioned perpendicularly in order to maximize ultimate histologic examination of the periphery/capsule. The remaining nonneoplastic thyroid and the "body" of the nodule can be transversely sectioned in the usual transverse way. Using this sectioning method for follicular lesions increased the likelihood of identifying capsular invasion by increasing the amount of examined capsular surface area.[24] However, according to the initial study describing this method, it did not increase the likelihood of identifying vascular invasion. Identification of invasion isolated to the tips of the nodule would certainly result in a diagnosis of malignancy. However, additional studies may be warranted in order to determine if this method results in clinically significant[15] diagnostic changes.

Cassette Submission

Sampling of thyroid specimens can be guided by clinical history, prior biopsies, and gross appearance. In benign processes such as Graves disease or chronic lymphocytic thyroiditis, representative sections may be submitted from the upper, middle, and lower aspects of each lobe as well as from the isthmus. There is no definite consensus regarding the amount of tissue to submit in such cases, and this decision can be left to the discretion of the pathologist and institution. Any areas that vary from the background tissue, such as nodules, lymph nodes, or parathyroid glands can be submitted entirely if possible.

In grossly infiltrative lesions, papillary or medullary thyroid carcinoma is most likely, and prior FNA biopsy may be supportive (**Fig.** 4). PTC often appears white/tan and may show frank papillary architecture or a granular cut surface. Fibrosis may render the tumor firm and calcification is common. Small incidental microcarcinomas may present as pale gray depressed scars. Medullary thyroid

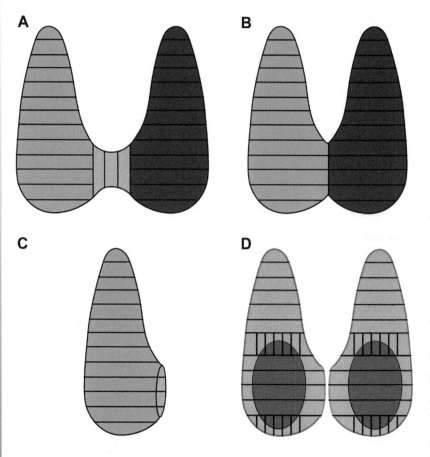

Fig. 3. Sectioning guidelines. Total thyroidectomy specimens can be inked in different colors to differentiate the lobes and isthmus. If a thyroid has an appreciable isthmus, it can be inked differentially (in this case, orange) from the right lobe (blue) and left lobe (black) (*A*). If the isthmus is narrow, one color per lobe can suffice (*B*). Differential inking of the anterior and posterior surfaces is not uniformly recommended but can be done if management is expected to change (namely, if the clinical team uses anterior versus posterior extrathyroidal extension or positive margins as a prognostic or treatment indicator). In this case, a separate color can be used on the posterior surface. Lobectomy or hemithyroidectomy specimens can be inked with one color to denote the external margin (in this case, blue) and another color to denote the isthmic margin (orange) (*C*). The isthmic margin is inked differentially because it is in continuity with the remainder of the thyroid gland rather than the soft tissues of the neck. A positive margin at the isthmus can be remedied by completion thyroidectomy but a positive soft tissue margin may require radioactive iodine therapy. If the thyroid contains a solitary, dominant nodule of appreciable size with an indeterminate cytologic diagnosis, the modified transverse vertical approach can be considered (*D*). In this case, the lobe is bisected longitudinally in order to visualize the extent of the nodule. The "tips" or poles of the nodule can then be sectioned perpendicularly in order to maximize histologic evaluation of the capsule. The remainder of the nodule and adjacent thyroid can be sectioned in the standard transverse method.

carcinoma (MTC) may vary in color and can appear pink, gray, tan-white, or yellow, and the consistency may be soft or firm. Calcifications may be present. Medullary carcinomas usually occur in the upper-middle portions of the lobes (in keeping with the developmental location of C-cell migration) and may sometimes be encapsulated.[25] Sporadic MTC are typically solitary and unilateral, whereas hereditary MTC tend to be multifocal and bilateral. However, all patients with presumed sporadic MTC should be evaluated for *RET* mutation.[26] At least 1 section per centimeter of infiltrative tumors can be submitted but, again, consensus guidelines do not exist. In cases

of known or suspected medullary carcinoma, multiple sections of the contralateral upper-middle lobe should be obtained to assess for C-cell hyperplasia. In cases where a total thyroidectomy is performed prophylactically for MEN syndrome, the entire thyroid should be submitted to examine for C-cell hyperplasia and medullary carcinoma.[27,28]

Solitary dominant nodules are often circumscribed (with or without encapsulation) and may ultimately represent adenomas or carcinomas. A diagnosis of "suspicious for follicular neoplasm" on FNA may alert the prosector to such cases. It is in these lesions that extensive sampling (either

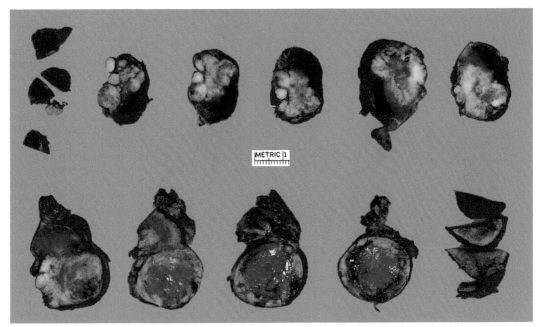

Fig. 4. Transverse sectioning. This thyroid had a diagnosis of papillary carcinoma on FNA. The conventional transverse approach was used in this case, and the changing gross morphology of the carcinoma can be followed from superior pole (top left) to inferior pole (bottom right). Additionally, the superior and inferior poles of the gland can be transversely sectioned in order to more accurately demonstrate the approach of the carcinoma to the polar margins. In this case, the superior pole is uninvolved but the tumor abuts the inferior pole.

upfront or after initial histologic examination) may be warranted. The periphery of the nodule may be bounded by a variably thick capsule. The cut surface of neoplasms with microfollicular growth patterns may seem more solid and pale compared with the background thyroid (Fig. 5), whereas the cut surface of macrofollicular neoplasms rich in colloid is often gelatinous and/or hemorrhagic (Fig. 6). As minimally invasive follicular carcinoma may be grossly indistinguishable from follicular adenoma, the periphery should be adequately sampled in order to search for capsular or vascular invasion. The modified transverse vertical approach outlined previously can be a good starting point. Many authors and institutions advocate for entire sampling of the periphery of such nodules especially if grossly suspicious for invasion.[29,30] Some authors advocate at least 10 sections.[24,31] Arguably, the periphery of a dominant nodule can be sampled extensively upfront, with the opportunity to submit additional sections if worrisome features (such as a thick capsule, solid growth, nuclear atypia) are identified histologically.[20] In cases where NIFTP is suspected based on initial histologic examination, submission of the entire tumor (to evaluate for the presence of well-formed papillae) and periphery (to

evaluate for invasion) should be considered and is recommended by the authors of the NIFTP proposal.[11]

Evaluation of High-Grade Features

High-grade features in thyroid lesions include solid growth, necrosis, satellite nodules (representing intrathyroidal invasion), and extrathyroidal extension. High-grade thyroid carcinomas (including poorly differentiated carcinoma, high-grade differentiated thyroid carcinoma, and anaplastic carcinoma) can show solid, fleshy cut surfaces with yellow-green opaque necrosis and/or hemorrhage (Fig. 7). Differentiated carcinomas may be partially encapsulated but the presence of satellite nodules outside the confines of the main tumor mass is suggestive of intrathyroidal invasion (Fig. 8). Areas demonstrating fleshy growth, potential necrosis, or satellite nodules should be sampled for histologic examination. Additionally, extrathyroidal extension is of importance due to implications for staging. Extrathyroidal extension may be considered an adverse prognostic factor.[9,32,33] Microscopic invasion of adipose tissue or skeletal (strap) muscle with no clinical or macroscopic evidence of invasion does not predict worse biologic behavior and does not necessarily qualify for an

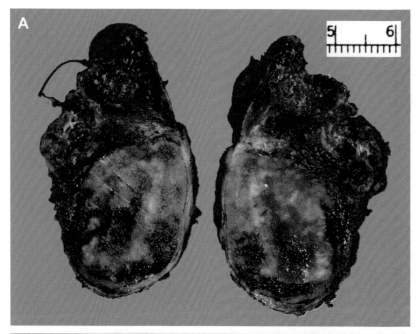

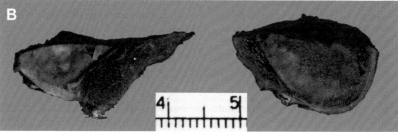

Fig. 5. Modified transverse vertical sectioning, microfollicular lesion. This thyroid nodule received an indeterminate diagnosis on FNA (atypia of undetermined significance/follicular neoplasm of undetermined significance) and the patient underwent hemithyroidectomy. The modified transverse vertical approach was taken. An initial longitudinal section through the lobe exposed the lesion: a relatively solid, focally hemorrhagic, and partly encapsulated nodule occupying the majority of the lower lobe (*A*). The tips or poles of the nodule are clearly demarcated from the nonneoplastic thyroid and can be sectioned perpendicularly to maximize visualization of the capsule to be submitted for histologic sections (*B*). The final diagnosis was a follicular adenoma.

increase in pathologic stage. However, macroscopic ETE into strap muscles (with histologic confirmation) from a tumor of any size qualifies for stage T3b; invasion of larynx, recurrent laryngeal nerve, trachea, or esophagus results in T4a; invasion of prevertebral fascia or encasement of the carotid artery or mediastinal vessels results in T4b.[34] Therefore, the presence of skeletal muscle at the periphery of the gland should be identified by the prosector, and the presence of gross tumor extension into muscle should be documented and sampled (**Fig. 9**). Correlation can be made with the surgeon's intraoperative findings in order to corroborate clinically significant macroscopic ETE. The risk of recurrence with gross ETE is approximately 5 times more than that of minimal ETE.[24] It has also been shown that microscopic ETE has minimal prognostic import and is not a reliably reproducible finding.[9] As such, care must be taken to appropriately document gross ETE for purposes of staging and recurrence risk-prediction.

Considerations for Molecular Testing

Finally, in light of the increasing use of molecular testing on formalin-fixed paraffin-embedded tissue for diagnostic/prognostic purposes and treatment implications, consideration should be given to ensuring preservation of DNA/RNA quality.[35] Some studies suggest that calcifications can be present in almost 40% of thyroid nodules, including approximately 40% of carcinomas and 20% of benign lesions.[36] Conventional hydrochloric acid decalcification solutions, although relatively rapid, sacrifice nucleic acid quality and render specimens ineligible for next generation sequencing.[37,38] However, EDTA-based chelating agents, although slower, have demonstrated better preservation of nucleic acid quality and quantity.[38,39] Therefore, prosectors should ensure submission of representative soft tumor that does not require decalcification or use of EDTA in representative sections of highly-calcified tumors, such that mutational analysis can be performed if subsequently indicated.

Fig. 6. Modified transverse vertical sectioning, macrofollicular lesion. This thyroid nodule received a benign diagnosis on FNA. A modified transverse vertical approach can also be taken in benign cases, if desired, in order to evaluate the full extent of the nodule(s). An initial longitudinal section shows a gelatinous, variably cystic to hemorrhagic lesion occupying the majority of the lower and mid-poles of the lobe. There is no appreciable capsule. In this case, perpendicular sections of the periphery of the unencapsulated nodule can be taken, if desired. The final diagnosis was an adenomatous nodule.

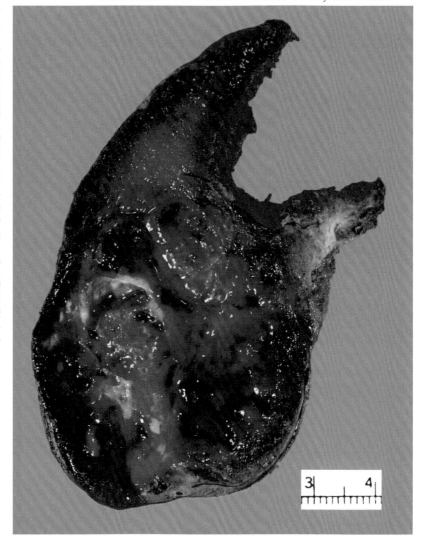

Fig. 7. Cut section of high-grade features. Gross prosectors should be alerted to worrisome or potentially high-grade features of thyroid neoplasms. The cut section of this neoplasm shows fleshy solid-appearing areas, gelatinous possibly necrotic areas, hemorrhagic areas, and small satellite nodules at the bottom right (*arrow*) near the orange-inked isthmus margin. The final diagnosis was poorly differentiated carcinoma.

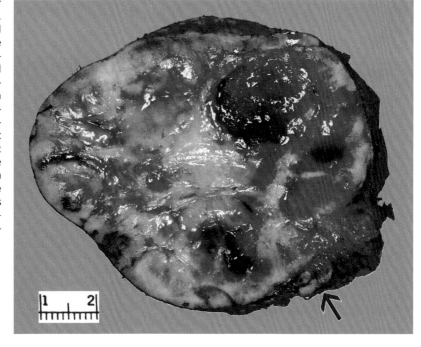

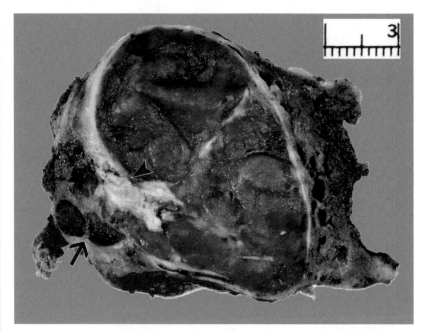

Fig. 8. Cut section of satellite nodules. Although this lesion is partially encapsulated by a thick fibrous band, there are also areas of coarse calcification (*arrowhead*) and satellite nodules (*arrow*) outside the confines of the main lesion. This growth pattern is compatible with invasion. The cut surface of the mass is solid and brown-tan, reflecting the final diagnosis of an oncocytic carcinoma with follicular and poorly differentiated features.

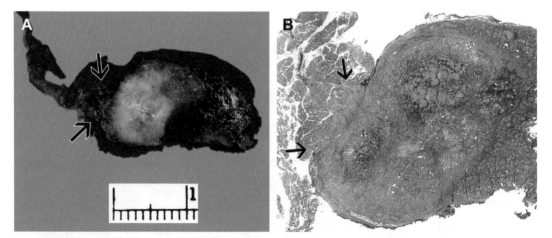

Fig. 9. Extrathyroidal extension. (*A*) As gross extrathyroidal extension may qualify a carcinoma for increase in AJCC T stage, the presence of skeletal muscle at the periphery of the gland (*arrows*) should be documented and evaluated for potential involvement by carcinoma. Prosectors should document possible extrathyroidal extension in their gross description as well as in sections submitted for histology. (*B*) In this case, extrathyroidal extension into skeletal muscle is confirmed microscopically (*arrows*). Extrathyroidal extension identified at gross and/or histologic examination should be corroborated by the intraoperative (and if applicable, radiographic) findings in order to appropriately stage the patient.

CLINICS CARE POINTS

- Intraoperative consultation for indeterminate thyroid nodules does not often provide additional information beyond that obtained by fine needle aspiration biopsy in guiding surgical management. Definitive diagnosis, grading, and staging of malignancy is best performed on permanent evaluation of adequately sampled thyroid neoplasms. If frozen section is still requested, a smear or imprint should be done to better evaluate nuclear morphology in light of freezing artifacts.

- Some studies suggest that posteriorly located thyroid tumors have a higher risk of recurrence compared to anterior. Knowledge of the location of a positive margin (anterior versus posterior) may be desired by some clinical teams. Anywhere between 2 and 4 colors of ink could be utilized depending on the specimen type and desired information.

- Adequate formalin fixation is optimal for preserving architectural features and nuclear detail. Conventional transverse sectioning is appropriate for benign processes and nodules that are known to be malignant or infiltrative. The modified transverse vertical approach allows for more robust examination of the tumor capsule in suspected follicular neoplasms.

- Tissue submission should be dictated by clinical information and gross appearance of the lesion(s). Benign disease processes and overtly invasive neoplasms may be sampled representatively; The periphery of encapsulated lesions should be sampled generously, if not entirely. Features such as solid fleshy cut surface, necrosis, satellite nodules, and extrathyroidal extension should be documented and sampled for grading and staging purposes.

SUMMARY

Intraoperative consultation has not been shown to provide diagnostic information beyond what is gleaned by FNA. Moreover, sectioning of fresh thyroid tissue may hinder the proper assessment of invasion and the tumor capsule. A smear or imprint of the lesion in question may be performed if intraoperative information is needed. Differential inking to allow the assessment of the posterior thyroid margin may be useful because posteriorly located thyroid tumors may have a higher recurrence rate. The modified transverse vertical sectioning approach can be considered for more thorough examination of the tumor capsule.

Evaluation for and documentation of high-grade features, such as necrosis and extrathyroidal extension, should be performed. Decalcification in EDTA may be required for heavily calcified tumors to preserve nucleic acids for potential molecular testing.

ACKNOWLEDGMENTS

The authors would like to acknowledge the residents and pathologists' assistants for diligently taking gross photographs of thyroid lesions.

REFERENCES

1. Sanabria A, Zafereo M, Thompson LDR, et al. Frozen section in thyroid gland follicular neoplasms: it's high time to abandon it. Surg Oncol 2021;36:76–81.
2. Rosário PW, Reis JS, Padrão EL, et al. The utility of frozen section evaluation for follicular thyroid lesions. Ann Surg Oncol 2004;11(9):879.
3. Cotton TM, Xin J, Sandyhya J, et al. Frozen section analysis in the post-Bethesda era. J Surg Res 2016;205(2):393–7.
4. Haugen BR, Alexander EK, Bible KC, et al. 2015 american thyroid association management guidelines for adult patients with thyroid nodules and differentiated thyroid cancer: the american thyroid association guidelines task force on thyroid nodules and differentiated thyroid cancer. Thyroid 2016; 26(1):1–133.
5. Cipriani NA, Nagar S, Kaplan SP, et al. Follicular thyroid carcinoma: how have histologic diagnoses changed in the last half-century and what are the prognostic implications? Thyroid 2015;25(11):1209–16.
6. McHenry CR, Phitayakorn R. Follicular adenoma and carcinoma of the thyroid gland. Oncologist 2011; 16(5):585–93.
7. Mete O, Asa SL. Pathological definition and clinical significance of vascular invasion in thyroid carcinomas of follicular epithelial derivation. Mod Pathol 2011;24(12):1545–52.
8. Leteurtre E, Leroy X, Pattou F, et al. Why do frozen sections have limited value in encapsulated or minimally invasive follicular carcinoma of the thyroid? Am J Clin Pathol 2001;115(3):370–4.
9. Xu B, Ghossein RA. Crucial parameters in thyroid carcinoma reporting – challenges, controversies and clinical implications. Histopathology 2018; 72(1):32–9.
10. Cracolici V, Parilla M, Henriksen KJ, et al. An Evaluation of CD61 immunohistochemistry in identification of vascular invasion in follicular thyroid neoplasms. Head Neck Pathol 2020;14(2):399–405.
11. Nikiforov YE, Baloch ZW, Hodak SP, et al. Change in diagnostic criteria for noninvasive follicular thyroid

neoplasm with papillarylike nuclear features. JAMA Oncol 2018;4(8):1125–6.

12. Grisales J, Sanabria A. Utility of routine frozen section of thyroid nodules classified as follicular neoplasm. Am J Clin Pathol 2020;153(2):210–20.

13. Kim M, Jeon MJ, Oh HS, et al. BRAF and RAS mutational status in noninvasive follicular thyroid neoplasm with papillary-like nuclear features and invasive subtype of encapsulated follicular variant of papillary thyroid carcinoma in korea. Thyroid 2018;28(4):504–10.

14. Antic T, Taxy JB. Thyroid frozen section: supplementary or unnecessary? Am J Surg Pathol 2013;37(2):282–6.

15. Johnson DN, Nash C, Cipriani NA. Chapter 12. Thyroid and Parathyroid. Philadelphia, PA: Wolters Kluwer; p. 295–330.

16. Adhya AK, Mohanty R. Utility of touch imprint cytology in the preoperative diagnosis of malignancy in low resource setting. Diagn Cytopathology 2017;45(6):507–12.

17. Basolo F, Ugolini C, Proietti A, et al. Role of frozen section associated with intraoperative cytology in comparison to FNA and FS alone in the management of thyroid nodules. Eur J Surg Oncol 2007;33(6):769–75.

18. Davoudi MM, Yeh KA, Wei JP. Utility of fine-needle aspiration cytology and frozen-section examination in the operative management of thyroid nodules. Am Surg 1997;63(12):1084–90.

19. Tan YH, Du GN, Xiao YG, et al. The false thyroid capsule: new findings. J Laryngol Otol 2013;127(9):897–901. https://doi.org/10.1017/S0022215113001667.

20. Available at: https://voices.uchicago.edu/grosspathology/head-neck/thyroid/. Accessed June 26, 2022.

21. Lang BHH, Shek TWH, Wan KY. Does microscopically involved margin increase disease recurrence after curative surgery in papillary thyroid carcinoma? J Surg Oncol 2016;113(6):635–9.

22. Ip YT, Dias Filho MA, Chan JKC. Nuclear inclusions and pseudoinclusions: friends or foes of the surgical pathologist? Int J Surg Pathol. 2010;18(6):465-481. doi:10.1177/1066896910385342

23. Petrilli G, Fisogni S, Rosai J, et al. Nuclear bubbles (nuclear pseudo-pseudoinclusions): a pitfall in the interpretation of microscopic sections from the thyroid and other human organs. Am J Surg Pathol 2017;41(1):140–1.

24. Oh HS, Kim SJ, Song E, et al. Modified transverse-vertical gross examination: a better method for the detection of definite capsular invasion in encapsulated follicular-patterned thyroid neoplasms. Endocr Pathol 2019;30(2):106–12.

25. Wenig B. Atlas of head and neck pathology. Philadelphia, PA: Elsevier/Saunders; 2015.

26. Wells SA, Asa SL, Dralle H, et al. Revised American Thyroid Association guidelines for the management of medullary thyroid carcinoma. Thyroid 2015;25(6):567–610.

27. Stamatakos M, Paraskeva P, Stefanaki C, et al. Medullary thyroid carcinoma: the third most common thyroid cancer reviewed. Oncol Lett 2011;2(1):49–53.

28. Ordóñez J, Pérez-Egido L, García-Casillas MA, et al. Management and results of thyroidectomies in pediatric patients with MEN 2 syndrome. J Pediatr Surg 2021;56(11):2058–61.

29. Available at: http://pathology.ucla.edu/workfiles/Education/Residency%20Program/Gross%20Manual/Thyroid.pdf. Accessed June 26, 2022.

30. Available at: https://www.essentialpathology.info/Gross_manual/Index.html?GuidelineAndProcedure24. Accessed June 26, 2022.

31. Anderson CE, McLaren KM. Best practice in thyroid pathology. J Clin Pathol 2003;56(6):401–5.

32. Ortiz S, Rodríguez JM, Soria T, et al. Extrathyroid spread in papillary carcinoma of the thyroid: clinico-pathological and prognostic study. Otolaryngol Head Neck Surg 2001;124(3):261–5.

33. Cipriani NA. Prognostic parameters in differentiated thyroid carcinomas. Surg Pathol Clin 2019;12(4):883–900.

34. Tuttle RM, Morris LF, Haugen BR, et al. Chapter 73. Thyroid-Differentiated and Anaplastic Carcinoma. In: Amin MB, editor. AJCC Cancer Staging Manual. 8th ed. Switzerland: Springer Nature; 2017. p. 873–90.

35. Shonka DC, Ho A, Chintakuntlawar AV, et al. American head and neck society endocrine surgery section and international thyroid oncology group consensus statement on mutational testing in thyroid cancer: defining advanced thyroid cancer and its targeted treatment. Head Neck 2022;44(6):1277–300.

36. Kim BK, Choi YS, Kwon HJ, et al. Relationship between patterns of calcification in thyroid nodules and histopathologic findings. Endocr J 2013;60(2):155–60.

37. Alers JC, Krijtenburg PJ, Vissers KJ, et al. Effect of bone decalcification procedures on DNA in situ hybridization and comparative genomic hybridization. EDTA is highly preferable to a routinely used acid decalcifier. J Histochem Cytochem 1999;47(5):703–10.

38. Choi SE, Hong SW, Yoon SO. Proposal of an appropriate decalcification method of bone marrow biopsy specimens in the era of expanding genetic molecular study. J Pathol Transl Med 2015;49(3):236–42.

39. Schrijver WAME, van der Groep P, Hoefnagel LD, et al. Influence of decalcification procedures on immunohistochemistry and molecular pathology in breast cancer. Mod Pathol 2016;29(12):1460–70.

Challenges in Encapsulated Follicular-Patterned Tumors: How Much Is Enough? Evaluation of Nuclear Atypia, Architecture, and Invasion

Kristine S. Wong, MD[1], Justine A. Barletta, MD[1],*

KEYWORDS

* Follicular-patterned * NIFTP * UMP

Key points

* Nuclear features of papillary thyroid carcinoma should be assessed in all follicular-patterned tumors.
* Follicular-patterned tumors should be assessed for any areas of papillary architecture.
* Assessment of invasion (capsular and vascular invasion) is the most critical component of the evaluation of follicular-pattered tumors.

ABSTRACT

Thyroid pathology is notoriously fraught with high interobserver variability, and follicular-patterned tumors are among some of the most challenging to assess accurately and reproducibly. Given that encapsulated or well-circumscribed follicular-patterned tumors often have similar molecular profiles, that is, frequent RAS or RAS-like alterations, the diagnosis usually relies on histopathologic examination alone. Unfortunately, many of the features that are used for diagnosis and prognosis of these tumors have long been controversial and frequently debated topics, both due to their subjectivity and their evolving (or not yet resolved) definitions. In more recent years, the introduction of noninvasive follicular thyroid neoplasm with papillary-like nuclear features has added further complexity to this discussion. In particular, the criteria and significance of nuclear features of papillary thyroid carcinoma, architectural patterns, and invasive growth still pose significant diagnostic challenges and confusion. This review explores some of the challenges in evaluating encapsulated follicular-patterned tumors, focusing on those histologic elements.

INTRODUCTION

Thresholds and perceived significance of nuclear features of papillary thyroid carcinoma (PTC) are continuing to evolve with our improved understanding of the clinical and biological behavior of follicular-patterned thyroid tumors. Over the past few decades, there was a notable increase in pathologist sensitivity to nuclear features of PTC in follicular-patterned tumors.[1] Initially, the threshold for recognition of nuclear features of PTC was quite high, such that most follicular-patterned tumors diagnosed were follicular adenomas and follicular carcinomas. This threshold lowered over time as greater emphasis was placed on nuclear atypia rather than architectural features. When first gaining traction as a diagnostic entity, follicular variant of PTC (FVPTC) was a relatively uncommon tumor.[2] However, over the next few

Department of Pathology, Brigham and Women's Hospital, Harvard Medical School, Boston, MA, USA
[1]Present address: 75 Francis Street, Boston, MA 02115.
* Corresponding author.
E-mail address: jbarletta@bwh.harvard.edu

surgpath.theclinics.com

decades, the rate of FVPTC sometimes surpassed that of classic PTC. In one study, Jung and colleagues found that ~10% of all PTC diagnosed in 1980 were FVPTC, but by 2009, this rate had risen to ~25%, compared with only 19% classic PTC.[3]

The relaxed threshold for nuclear features of PTC and the lack of defined criteria for FVPTC led to significant interobserver variability in the diagnosis of follicular-patterned tumors. For example, this manifested as frequent overlap with benign lesions when considering the preceding cytologic diagnosis. In a series of 5,469 fine-needle aspirations (FNAs) which had correlation with surgical pathology, Sangalli and colleagues found that over one-third of false-negative fine-needle aspiration biopsies due to diagnostic interpretation were FVPTC on resection.[4] Similarly, in a follow-up of 1,819 cytologically benign nodules, Medici and colleagues identified seven malignancies, all of which were encapsulated or well-circumscribed FVPTC (one tumor had capsular invasion).[5] This variability in diagnosis was also a well-recognized problem in surgical pathology.[6–8] In the evaluation of 21 follicular-patterned lesions, Hirokawa and colleagues found complete agreement in only ~10% of cases (two follicular adenomas). In this study, there was a lack of agreement both in assessment of neoplasia as well as malignancy.[8] This study also highlighted the geographic differences in the diagnosis of FVPTC, which historically has occurred at a much lower frequency in Asia compared with United States and Europe.

The high rates of diagnosis of FVPTC and subjectivity in interpretation of nuclear features became increasingly problematic, as many of these patients were being treated with total thyroidectomy. However, a landmark study by Liu and colleagues helped to establish the differences in clinicopathologic behavior between infiltrative tumors, which behaved more like classic PTC, and encapsulated tumors that were more similar to follicular adenoma or carcinoma.[9] Subsequent studies further supported this concept of distinct subgroups within FVPTC, including molecular studies which demonstrated that infiltrative FVPTC were more often *BRAF*-like, whereas encapsulated or well-circumscribed tumors were more likely to be *RAS*-like.[10,11] Owing to the indolent behavior of the latter, it was ultimately decided that encapsulated or well-circumscribed FVPTC should no longer be considered carcinomas. As such, the term "noninvasive follicular thyroid neoplasm with papillary-like nuclear features" (NIFTP) was adopted with the goal of minimizing the overdiagnosis and overtreatment of these indolent tumors.[12]

This history serves as a backdrop to our current interpretation of follicular-patterned thyroid tumors. In this review, the persistent challenges in evaluating these tumors are explored, with a focus on nuclear atypia, architecture, and invasion.

NUCLEAR ATYPIA: HAS NONINVASIVE FOLLICULAR THYROID NEOPLASM WITH PAPILLARY-LIKE NUCLEAR FEATURES NORMALIZED THE INTERPRETATION OF NUCLEAR FEATURES? OR CAN WE AGREE TO DISAGREE?

The initial NIFTP proposal by Nikiforov and colleagues included a nuclear scoring system for assessment of papillary-like nuclear features (Box 1). Nuclear features were scored on a scale from 0 to 3, with 1 point given for each of the following: (1) nuclear enlargement, (2) nuclear membrane irregularities, and (3) chromatin clearing/pallor. Benign nodules had scores of 0 to 1, whereas NIFTP had scores of 2 to 3.[12] We advise using this scoring system when evaluating nuclear features in all follicular-patterned thyroid tumors. Of note, in the original NIFTP study, the proportion of tumor requiring nuclear features was not included as a criterion, as it was not found to significantly increase the accuracy of the scoring system.[12,13] Moreover, it has been noted that uneven distribution of nuclear atypia and the "sprinkling" phenomenon[14] seen in some FVPTC/ NIFTP (Fig. 1) could potentially lead to over-exclusion of tumors.[13]

With this scoring scheme, there was 85% accuracy in identifying NIFTP when using a molecular endpoint as the reference standard.[12] A subsequent multi-institutional study evaluating the reproducibility of the nuclear scoring system among pathologists in the United States, United Kingdom, and Japan found, not unexpectedly, a lower diagnostic accuracy rate (~75%) compared with the original study's expert panel of endocrine pathologists, who had been primed to assess these nuclear features. Nevertheless, the interobserver variability study by Thompson and colleagues noted good to substantial agreement among the 77 pathologists involved in the study, suggesting that the scoring system could reasonably be applied by pathologists in general practice when diagnosing NIFTP.[15]

Despite the development of the nuclear scoring system, interobserver variability in interpretation of nuclear atypia persists. For example, there are well-established differences in interpretation of nuclear features and rates of NIFTP diagnosis in Asian countries compared with those in North

> **Box 1**
> **Nuclear scoring system**
>
> 1. Size and shape (enlargement, crowding, elongation)
>
> 2. Membrane irregularities (grooves, pseudo-inclusions, irregular contours)
>
> 3. Chromatin (pallor, clearing)

America,[8,12,16–19] with a recent meta-analysis demonstrating an incidence of NIFTP of 2.1% in Asian countries compared with 9.3% in North America.[18] In this study, Rana and colleagues surmised that interobserver variability in the assessment of nuclear features was the main reason for this gap, though other differences likely also contributed. For example, another factor that may be responsible for the lower rate of NIFTP diagnosis in Asia is a lower rate of surgeries for cytologically indeterminate nodules, which are the main source of NIFTP in Western countries. However, institutional differences also result in variation in interpretation of nuclear features. In a 17-site multi-institutional study across the Iberian Peninsula, Paja and colleagues noted rates of NIFTP diagnosis (compared with all PTC) ranging from 0% to ~12%.[20] In the United States, a multi-institutional study which evaluated risk of malignancy among *RAS*-mutant tumors found that the ratio of NIFTP to follicular adenoma/nodular hyperplasia ranged from almost 4:1 to 1:17[21]. Even within one city (such as Boston or New York), academic institutions can vary greatly in the percentage of tumors diagnosed as NIFTP.[18,21] Although NIFTP was initially estimated to comprise ~10% to 20% of PTC based on retrospective reclassification studies,[12] in practice the rates seem to be lower. A study using US SEER registry data from 2000 to 2017 by Kitahara and

colleagues found that NIFTP composed only 1.2% of PTCs in 2017.[22] A subsequent analysis of over 3300 pathology records from 18 hospitals in 6 countries across 2 time points (2015 and 2019) found that NIFTP accounted for just 4.8% of papillary thyroid neoplasms in 2019.[23] Interestingly, the meta-analysis by Rana and colleagues (previously mentioned above) found a 2.5-fold decline in the rate of NIFTP diagnosis from 2016 to 2018 in North America and Europe.[18] The reasons for the lower diagnostic rate of NIFTP compared with what was initially projected are not entirely clear. Although the incidence would be expected to rise based on increased familiarity with the diagnostic criteria, the reverse trend could be due partly to the evolving architectural criteria (discussed further below), or because pathologists have increased their threshold for nuclear features with the introduction of NIFTP. The study by Kitahara and colleagues demonstrated an increase in the diagnosis of encapsulated classic PTC, supporting a role for evolving architectural criteria.[22]

It should be noted that interpretation of nuclear features will not only impact the diagnosis of noninvasive tumors but also impact evaluation of follicular-patterned tumors with invasion (**Table 1**). For example, for an encapsulated follicular-patterned tumor with capsular penetration only and borderline nuclear features, a pathologist that assesses nuclear features of PTC as absent

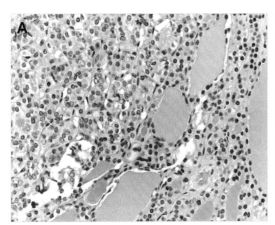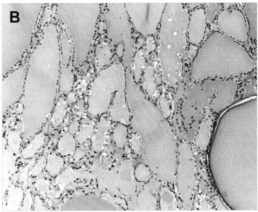

Fig. 1. Nuclear features of NIFTP may be variable, as in this case, where there is minimal nuclear atypia in the right side of the image and more pronounced atypia on the left (*A*). Atypia may also be punctuated throughout the nodule, which has been referred to some as the "sprinkling" sign (*B*).

Table 1
Diagnoses rendered based on nuclear features and extent of invasion

	No Invasion	Questionable Invasion	Capsular Invasion Only	Vascular Invasion (with or without Capsular Invasion)	Wide Invasion[a]
Nuclear features of papillary thyroid carcinoma interpreted as absent	Follicular Adenoma	FT-UMP	Minimally Invasive FTC	Encapsulated Angioinvasive FTC	Widely Invasive FTC
Nuclear features of papillary thyroid carcinoma interpreted as present	NIFTP	WDT-UMP	Minimally Invasive EFVPTC	Encapsulated Angioinvasive FVPTC	Widely Invasive FVPTC

Abbreviations: EFVPTC, encapsulated follicular variant of papillary thyroid carcinoma; FT-UMP, follicular tumor of uncertain malignant potential; FTC, follicular thyroid carcinoma; FVPTC, follicular variant of papillary thyroid carcinoma; NIFTP, noninvasive follicular thyroid neoplasm with papillary-like nuclear features; WDT-UMP, well-differentiated tumor of uncertain malignant potential.
   [a] Wide invasion is based on tumor that grossly invades the thyroid.

will render a diagnosis of minimally invasive follicular thyroid carcinoma (FTC), whereas the same tumor might be diagnosed as a minimally invasive encapsulated FVPTC if a pathologist perceives nuclear features of PTC to be present.

Despite attempts at standardizing the assessment of nuclear features, subjectivity and differences in thresholds between individual pathologists, institutions, and geographic regions will most likely continue to persist. What are the clinical implications of this variability? At this time, there are minimal clinical consequences for a diagnosis of NIFTP compared with follicular adenoma, as less aggressive surveillance has been recommended for NIFTP compared with low-risk PTC.[24,25] Currently, yearly thyroglobulin measurement is recommended by the American Head and Neck Society for patients with NIFTP.[24] This is more follow-up than typically recommended for follicular adenoma or other benign thyroid nodules (and, hence, is deemed as excessive by some).[25] However, given the relatively few prospective studies of NIFTP and the need for more studies on outcome and reproducibility of the diagnosis, NIFTP is still considered in the 2022 World Health Organization (WHO) Classification of Endocrine and Neuroendocrine Tumors as a low-risk neoplasm,[26] and therefore, at least for now, patients should still be monitored following resection. Similarly, the distinction between invasive encapsulated FVPTC and FTC has minimal clinical consequences, as the extent of invasion is the primary driver for prognostication and treatment (as discussed below). In

addition, the biology of invasive encapsulated FVPTC and FTC are similar, with a similar pattern of disease spread (spread is to distant sites such as lung and/or bone instead of lymph nodes) and a similar molecular profile (with RAS and RAS-like genetic alterations).[9,10,27–33]

ARCHITECTURE: WHEN PAPILLAE CAN BECOME A PITFALL

Can noninvasive follicular thyroid neoplasm with papillary-like nuclear features have papillae?

Nuclear atypia is not the only parameter that needs to be considered when evaluating whether a tumor is a NIFTP. NIFTP should have a predominantly follicular architecture (<1% papillae) and be entirely encapsulated or well circumscribed without invasion or infiltrative growth. Other exclusion criteria are listed in Box 2. As indicated, the initial criteria for NIFTP stipulated that these tumors should have less than 1% papillae. True papillae are characterized by a fibrovascular core lined by tumor cells rather than pseudopapillary (abortive, hyperplastic, or Sanderson's polster-like) structures[12,13] (Fig. 2). However, the NIFTP consensus group subsequently took a more conservative approach, excluding tumors with any well-formed papillae.[34] This change was prompted by cases of metastatic disease in rare tumors which reportedly met diagnostic criteria for NIFTP.[35–37] Despite these reports, however, in

> **Box 2**
> **Diagnostic criteria for noninvasive follicular thyroid neoplasm with papillary-like nuclear features**
>
> Nuclear features of PTC (score of 2–3), see **Box 1**
>
> Predominantly follicular architecture (<1% papillae)
>
> Encapsulated or well-circumscribed
>
> Absence of psammoma bodies
>
> No high-grade features (elevated mitotic rate, necrosis)
>
> <30% solid/trabecular/insular growth
>
> Absence of characteristics of other subtypes of PTC (such as, tall cell)

the upcoming 2022 WHO Classification of Endocrine and Neuroendocrine Tumors, NIFTP will retain the original criterion of less than 1% papillae,[26] as many studies using the original cutoff of less than 1% papillae did not find any metastases or adverse outcomes.[12,19,38–41]

Although rare papillae are still allowed in NIFTP, their inclusion emphasizes the importance of careful sampling of the tumor, evaluation of nuclear features, and potential use of molecular testing to exclude classic PTC with a predominantly follicular architecture (**Fig. 3**). As nuclear features of PTC tend to be more pronounced in classic PTC, it was suggested by the NIFTP consensus group that the entire tumor (ie, not just the periphery) should be evaluated in tumors with a nuclear score of 3 in order to exclude papillary structures.[34] In addition, given that classic PTC frequently harbors the *BRAF* V600E mutation,[42] as opposed to the

RAS-like molecular profile of NIFTP,[10–12,43,44] secondary testing for *BRAF* V600E was also suggested by the consensus group as a potential adjunct. However, excluding the presence of *BRAF* V600E is not required to render a NIFTP diagnosis.[34]

A few studies using molecular correlates have highlighted the morphologic overlap between NIFTP and encapsulated classic PTC with predominantly follicular architecture.[35,38,45] Cho and colleagues, who had reported metastases in 3% of NIFTP cases when using a 1% papillae cutoff, found *BRAF* V600E mutation in 10% of cases.[35] In contrast, Xu and colleagues did not find any cases of metastatic disease in unifocal noninvasive encapsulated PTC even when using a 10% cutoff for papillae. Although they did find that 4% of noninvasive cases with less than 1% papillae had *BRAF* V600E mutations, the two cases with

Fig. 2. This case of NIFTP demonstrated scattered hyperplastic-appearing follicles with abortive papillae.

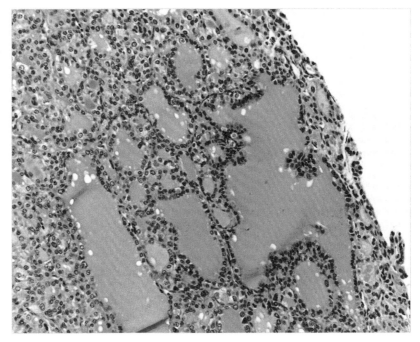

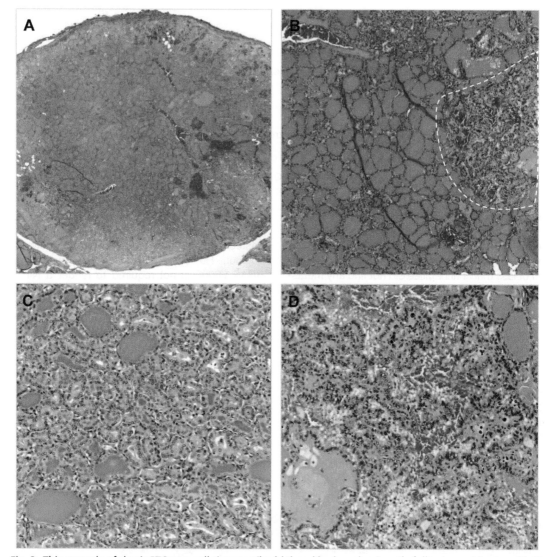

Fig. 3. This example of classic PTC was well circumscribed (*A*) and had predominantly follicular architecture (*B, C*), although a focal area demonstrated well-formed papillary structures (*B*-circled area, *D*).

the mutation were either subcentimeter or had a minor component with a tall cell morphology.[38] In a study evaluating the utility of mutation-specific BRAF immunohistochemistry in 208 cases of follicular-patterned tumors (including NIFTP, encapsulated FVPTC with invasion, and classic PTC with predominantly follicular architecture), BRAF positivity was not detected in any NIFTP, although it was detected in ~15% of FVPTC and ~55% of classic PTC with predominantly follicular architecture.[45] Although these studies suggest that NIFTP can be accurately diagnosed with careful morphologic evaluation, they also highlight that there can be a significant overlap between NIFTP and some classic PTC. An assessment of *BRAF* V600E (by immunohistochemistry or other means)

can be helpful when a differential of NIFTP or encapsulated follicular-predominant classic PTC is being considered (our group routinely uses BRAF V600E immunohistochemistry in this setting).[34,44,45]

Papillae in follicular tumors without nuclear atypia

Although this review has thus far focused primarily on NIFTP and tumors with nuclear atypia, papillae can also become a diagnostic pitfall in encapsulated tumors with prominent follicular architecture when there is minimal to no nuclear atypia. Papillary architecture in benign nodules has been known to be problematic in fine-needle aspiration

(FNA) biopsies,[46–49] as it can be misconstrued as evidence for PTC. However, in contrast to PTC, nuclear atypia should not be a prominent feature. Instead, nuclei are smaller and more hyperchromatic compared with PTC. Papillary groups are also typically admixed with micro- and macrofollicles.[49] Benign nodules with papillary architecture are often more readily recognized in histologic assessment; however, diagnostic uncertainty can occur particularly when the papillary architecture is prominent, or if there is reactive nuclear atypia due to biopsy site changes or inflammation. Although prominent papillary architecture is most often seen as a nonspecific finding (ie, when associated with follicular nodular disease/nodular hyperplasia/goiter), it can also occur in certain settings which may have important clinical implications. Two such scenarios, autonomous hyperfunctioning ("toxic") nodules and adenomatous nodules in DICER1 syndrome, will be briefly described here.

Autonomous hyperfunctioning thyroid neoplasms, described in the 2022 WHO Classification of Endocrine and Neuroendocrine Tumors under follicular adenoma with papillary architecture,[26] are associated with increased thyroid hormone production and radionuclide uptake (the so-called "hot" nodules). These tumors are encapsulated and variably cystic, often with irregularly shaped follicles and/or prominent pseudopapillary (ie, Sanderson's polster-like) as well as true papillary architectures (Fig. 4). Like in papillary hyperplasia, the papillae in these tumors are often oriented toward the center of follicles with a "centripetal" appearance and may be associated with vacuoles at the follicular cell-colloid interface. The follicular cells themselves are typically columnar in shape with a basally located, round, small nucleus. Although there may be slight nuclear crowding, nuclear features of papillary carcinoma should be absent.[47,49,50] Despite these tumors often having a hyperplastic appearance, they have been shown to be neoplastic and frequently harbor TSHR mutations, with a smaller subset associated with GNAS and EZH1 mutations.[51–57] Although most of these neoplasms are adenomas, rare malignancies have been reported.[50,53,58] Interestingly, the three FTCs reported by Mon and colleagues all had TSHR mutations at higher allelic frequencies and demonstrated only focal capsular or vascular invasion (ie, considered low risk by the American Thyroid Association [ATA]).[53] Another case report of an FTC with an activating TSHR mutation demonstrated a concurrent PAX8-PPARγ rearrangement.[58] Although malignancy in this setting is rare, a clinical history or histologic appearance of hyperthyroidism should therefore not deter pathologists from the assessment of features of malignancy (ie, invasion).

DICER1 syndrome, caused by pathogenic germline mutations in DICER1, is an autosomal dominant syndrome associated with the development of tumors in the lung, genitourinary system, central nervous system, and thyroid.[59,60] The most common manifestation in the thyroid is multinodular goiter[61] with multiple hyperplastic- and adenomatous-appearing nodules. The hyperplastic/adenomatous nodules in DICER1 syndrome have been shown to often (though potentially not always) have a second (somatic) hotspot DICER1 mutation.[61–63] Thus, although they have an appearance of hyperplastic nodules, they are clonal neoplasms. For unclear reasons,

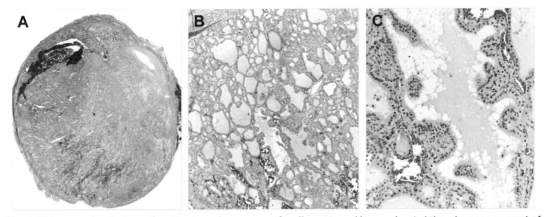

Fig. 4. This example of a hyperfunctioning adenoma was focally cystic and hemorrhagic (*A*) and was composed of variably shaped, irregular follicles (*B*) with reabsorption vacuoles at the interface with the colloid (*C*). The follicular cells are cuboidal to columnar in shape and have a small, round, basally located nucleus. There were frequent small papillary structures oriented toward the center of the follicle, sometimes referred to as a "centripetal" appearance (*C*).

papillary architecture is frequently seen in the nodules in DICER1 syndrome patients,[63] as well as in tumors in nonsyndromic patients with somatic *DICER1* mutations.[64] In these nodules, the papillary architecture can be focal or extensive, but the nuclear features of PTC should be absent (**Fig. 5**). When papillary architecture is prominent, the nodule may be mistaken for PTC, particularly if the cells are crowded with a hyperfunctional appearance (similar to that seen in autonomous hyperfunctioning nodules, see above) or have atypia secondary to prior biopsy. Although thyroid nodules associated with DICER1 syndrome are not frequently encountered in general practice, the prevalence of *DICER1* putative loss of function germline variants was recently estimated to range from 1 in 3700 to 1 in 4600 people, which is comparable to the prevalence of germline *DICER1* variants detected in The Cancer Genome Atlas.[65,66] To put this into context, DICER1 syndrome may have an incidence similar to that of neurofibromatosis type 1 and substantially higher than that of familial adenomatous polyposis, neurofibromatosis type 2, and Von Hippel–Lindau.[65,67] In addition, when including potential germline and somatic variants, Chong and colleagues found *DICER1* hotspot variants in 1.4% of indeterminate thyroid nodules. In a subset of this *DICER1*-altered cohort that was further assessed, 76% of nodules were found to have a second (likely) pathogenic variant (however, future work is needed to determine what percentage of these mutations are germline).[68] Further investigation of the prevalence and histologic features of thyroid nodules in patients with DICER1 syndrome could potentially allow us to help screen for this syndrome when evaluating

thyroidectomy specimens, similar to how PTEN hamartoma tumor syndrome-like findings in thyroidectomy specimens can be used to suggest an underlying predisposition syndrome.

INVASION: CRITICAL BUT COMPLICATED

The final and perhaps most clinically significant histologic feature that will be discussed in this review is invasion. The assessment of invasion is essentially the same in encapsulated tumors regardless of cytomorphology or architecture. For entities in which invasion is used to distinguish malignancy (ie, follicular-patterned tumors including NIFTP/invasive encapsulated FVPTC and follicular adenoma/carcinoma), the entire periphery of the tumor should be submitted for histologic evaluation. In the 2022 WHO Classification of Endocrine and Neuroendocrine Tumors, the patterns of invasion of invasive encapsulated FVPTC are the same as those in FTC, that is, (1) minimally invasive (capsular invasion only), (2) encapsulated angioinvasive (venous invasion with or without capsular invasion), and (3) widely invasive (gross invasion of tumor through the gland).[26] As widely invasive tumors are typically readily recognized as malignant on gross and microscopic examination, only capsular and vascular invasion will be discussed in more detail here.

CAPSULAR INVASION

Capsules in follicular-patterned carcinomas tend to be thicker and more irregular compared with adenomas, although significant variability can be seen.[69–72] Although most pathologists require

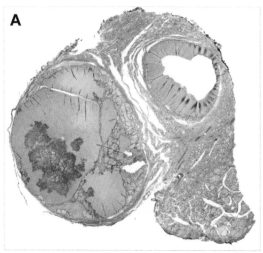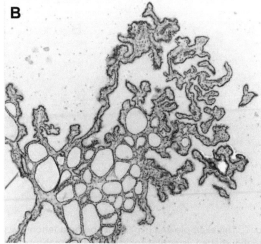

Fig. 5. This patient with DICER1 syndrome had numerous hyperplastic-appearing nodules in the thyroid with variably prominent papillary architecture (*A*). The papillary proliferation was occasionally florid, but the cells had small, hyperchromatic nuclei without overt features of papillary carcinoma (*B*).

complete penetration of tumor through the capsule to be considered invasion, which is consistent with the current WHO and College of American Pathologists (CAP) guidelines,[26,73] some have historically not required complete penetration to constitute invasion.[71,74] If there are foci of tumor protruding into but not through the capsule, or if there are areas of marked capsular irregularity, performing multiple additional levels through the tissue block is suggested to help resolve those foci of incomplete or ambiguous capsular invasion.

The prototypical example of capsular invasion consists of tumor directly transgressing a fibrous capsule, often with a "mushroom"-like appearance (Fig. 6), although this may not always be seen even after extensively leveling the tissue block. As such, tumor present on both sides of the capsule (but still separated in the histologic section by a capsule) is also considered evidence of invasion[26,73] (Fig. 7). Recently, a study using micro-resolution computed tomography (microCT) scanning of whole tissue blocks found that satellite nodules detected on H&E slides were associated with foci of capsular penetration on whole block imaging, supporting that satellite nodules are in fact indicative of capsular invasion.[75] As a caveat, however, satellite nodules should have the same cytomorphology as the tumor to be considered true invasion. This can sometimes be difficult to assess in the setting of multiple adenomatous nodules (Fig. 8); however, the background thyroid and context of the case can help clarify this potential mimic.

Although the evaluation of capsular penetration and/or satellite nodules seems relatively straightforward, in practice this is often not the case. In a study by Franc *and colleagues*, the investigators found that the interobserver agreement (kappa) for capsular invasion in FTC was only 0.27[76]. A more recent study evaluating interobserver variation of capsular invasion in follicular thyroid neoplasms found only fair agreement for a diagnosis of malignancy (kappa of 0.545).[77] Interestingly, the investigators separately analyzed those tumors which had questionable invasion (ie, tumors invading into but not through the capsule, tumors with a thick and irregular capsule "pushed" by tumor cells, or nests of tumor oriented in parallel with the capsule but detached from the main tumor) and found just poor agreement.[77]

The issues with interobserver agreement and questionable invasion stem not only from variable criteria, but also from multiple scenarios that can mimic capsular invasion. Biopsy site changes, for example, can distort the capsule and cause significant hyalinization within the tumor. An iatrogenic breech in the capsule with tumor appearing to be situated outside of the capsule can be especially difficult to interpret. In such cases, the context (ie, features of biopsy site including hemosiderin-laden macrophages, inflammation, and large or irregularly shaped areas of fibrosis) and linear arrangement of the tumor along the capsule may help to suggest biopsy site-related capsular changes rather than true invasion. Not all fibrosis, however, is secondary to biopsy site. For example, invasive tumor may lead to peritumoral fibrosis

Fig. 6. Foci of capsular penetration often have a "mushroom"-like appearance.

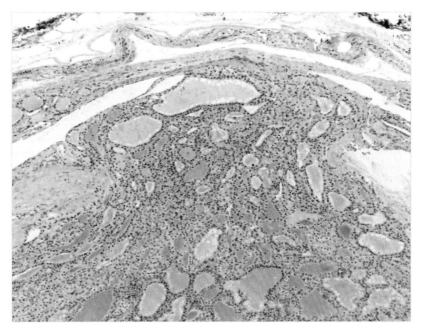

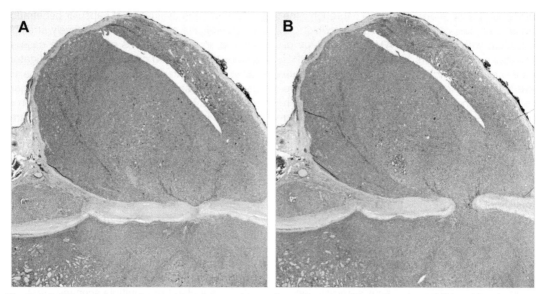

Fig. 7. Satellite nodules can be considered as representative of invasion (*A*). Performing additional levels can occasionally demonstrate the focus of continuity between the satellite and main tumor nodule (*B*), although this is not required to be considered invasion.

and give the appearance of a neocapsule, which should not be confused for the actual capsule (**Fig. 9**).

VASCULAR INVASION

In encapsulated tumors, vascular invasion involves spread of tumor through intracapsular or extracapsular vessels. Consistent with the fact that follicular-patterned tumors spread to distant sites, the vessels within and directly exterior to the capsule represent venous (rather than lymphatic) spaces despite being thin-walled.[78] Other criteria for vascular invasion are highly variable. Some pathologists, as well as the CAP guidelines for thyroid carcinomas, endorse that

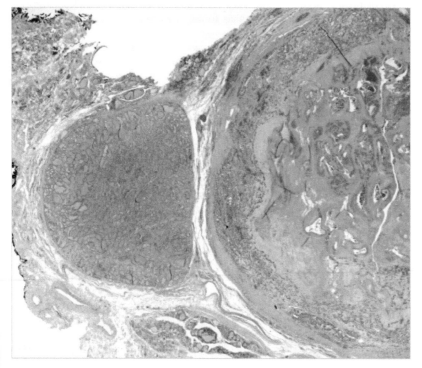

Fig. 8. Multiple adenomatous nodules can be a mimic for capsular invasion and satellite nodules. In this case, there were multiple smaller adenomatous nodules near the main tumor, some of which were abutting each other but were still clearly demarcated.

Fig. 9. This tumor demonstrated a focus of capsular invasion, with the true capsule highlighted by the solid line. However, there was also fibrosis at the pushing edge of the tumor, creating the appearance of a neo-capsule (*dotted line*).

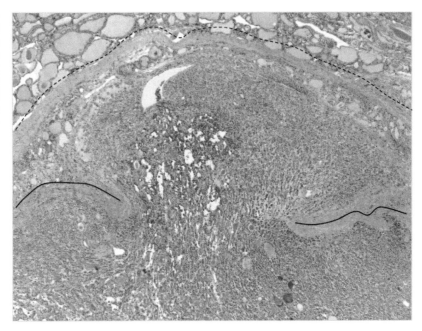

only a tumor thrombus associated with fibrin constitutes unequivocal vascular invasion.[73,79] When using this approach, it was found that 35% of angioinvasive tumors had distant metastases.[79] Although this may help predict which patients are at higher risk for recurrence, it also undoubtedly leads to underdiagnosis in a large subset of patients who have a nonzero risk for metastasis. Most pathologists therefore take the less conservative approach that is supported by the 2022 WHO and International Collaboration on Cancer Reporting, defining vascular invasion as tumor within vessels (in the tumor capsule or beyond) that is attached to the vessel wall, admixed with fibrin, or covered by endothelium[26,78] (**Fig. 10**). To further support this approach, Xu *and colleagues* found that serial sections of a single focus of vascular invasion showed fibrin thrombi only on some histologic levels but not all.[75]

As with capsular invasion, there are multiple potential sources for diagnostic error in assessing vascular invasion. For example, rarely there may be a prominent papillary endothelial hyperplasia ("Masson's tumor") within vascular spaces that may simulate tumor thrombus. Because these endothelial projections are often associated with hyalinized cores or a florid endothelial proliferation rather than tumor, a CD31 or cytokeratin immunohistochemical stain can be performed to resolve challenging cases (**Fig. 11**). When follicular cells are within a vascular space, "push" artifact must also be excluded. This may occur when detached fragments of tumor are pushed into vascular spaces from manipulation during sectioning or

processing, often with tumor appearing to float within the space (**Fig. 12**). Endothelial wrapping around the tumor or associated fibrin can help to distinguish artifact from invasion. Immunohistochemistry for the platelet-associated protein CD61 may also aid in assessment of vascular invasion, as CD61-expressing platelets associated with intravascular tumor can support a diagnosis of vascular invasion.[80] Another potentially challenging scenario is distinguishing whether vessels are simply closely associated with the tumor or in fact invaded by the tumor. Follicular-patterned tumors are often highly vascularized and have numerous vessels at the periphery of the tumor or adjacent to the capsule that the tumor may abut. Merely pushing up against or slightly protruding into a vascular space should not be considered invasion, and some have suggested that at least half of the circumference of the tumor plug should be within the lumen to be considered intravascular.[81] Despite these histologic clues, it can nevertheless be difficult to accurately assess the relationship of vessel and tumor, particularly when the tumor is compressed or entrapped within the capsule.

Given the many potential mimics and subtleties of vascular invasion, it is therefore not surprising that interobserver agreement has been reported as low (kappa of 0.20) and less than that of capsular invasion in FTC.[76] Unfortunately, the issues surrounding diagnosis of vascular invasion not only affect whether a tumor is considered benign or malignant but also impacts prognostication of malignant tumors. In differentiated thyroid

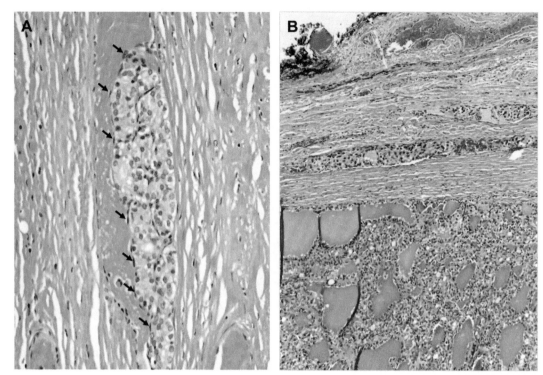

Fig. 10. Examples of vascular invasion. Endothelial cells (highlighted with *arrows*) can be seen "wrapping" around intravascular tumor (*A*). Foci of vascular invasion in adjacent vessels should be counted as separate when determining extent of vascular invasion (*B*).

carcinomas, for example, extensive vascular invasion (four or more foci) has been associated with worse outcomes.[82–85] Although four foci are traditionally the cutoff used for determining focal versus extensive invasion, a recent study by Yamazaki *and colleagues* found that even having only two or more foci of vascular invasion was associated with worse prognosis.[86] Foci of vascular invasion should therefore be enumerated so that tumors can be stratified by extent of invasion (if foci are adjacent, they should be counted separately, see **Fig. 12**). The ATA, for example, considers FTC with extensive vascular invasion as high risk, whereas FTC with focal vascular invasion (<four foci) are considered low risk for recurrence.[87] The extent of vascular invasion therefore may determine whether subsequent treatment (ie, completion thyroidectomy and radioactive iodine) is warranted.

WHEN WE CANNOT DECIDE: TUMORS OF UNCERTAIN MALIGNANT POTENTIAL

For tumors that have equivocal capsular or vascular invasion, a diagnosis of follicular tumor of uncertain malignant potential (FT-UMP) or well-differentiated tumor of UMP (WDT-UMP) may be used, the latter of which has more

pronounced nuclear features of PTC (ie, a nuclear score of 2–3).[26] FT-UMP is an indeterminate category between follicular adenoma and follicular carcinoma, whereas WDT-UMP would fall between NIFTP and invasive encapsulated FVPTC. These terms are preferred over "atypical adenoma" and should be used sparingly in cases where invasion is still ambiguous despite thorough examination. As diagnoses of UMP are uncommon and/or may not be used uniformly across institutions, the overall rate of diagnosis is not well-documented in the literature.

The initial proposal for WDT-UMP included tumors without definite invasion but with equivocal nuclear features of PTC,[88] and other early studies used similar criteria in their evaluation of tumors of UMP (ie, including those cases without invasion but with questionable nuclear features of PTC instead).[89–92] In studies in which only those tumors with questionable invasion could be deduced, the rate of UMP cases among malignant tumors using the current WHO definition ranged from 0.6% (6 of 1009 carcinoma/UMP cases)[90] to 8.6% (17 of 197 carcinoma/UMP cases).[89] In a more recent study using the current WHO definition, Ito *and colleagues* found that 502 of 13,089 patients with thyroid tumors had borderline tumors, including 339 FT-UMP cases (∼8% of all borderline/malignant

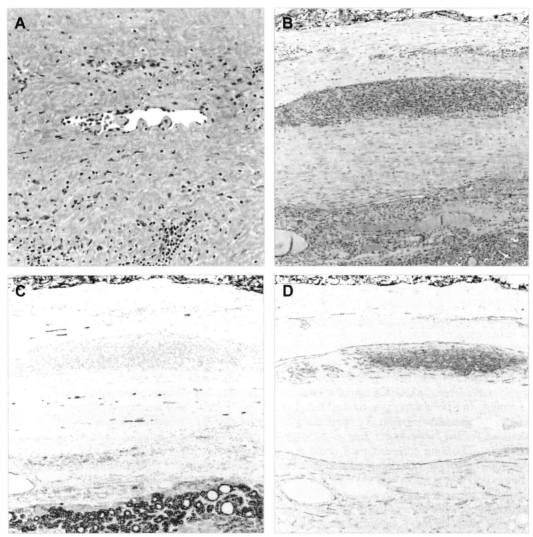

Fig. 11. Prominent endothelial hyperplasia can occasionally mimic vascular invasion, although endothelial cells should be associated with hyalinized cores (*A*) rather than tumor cells. Other cases may have florid intravascular endothelial proliferations that are densely cellular, which a low power can closely mimic tumor (*B*). Cytokeratin (*C*) and CD31 (*D*) stains show that the cells within the vessel are endothelial rather than epithelial.

tumors). Interestingly, the diagnosis of FT-UMP was based on equivocal capsular invasion in the vast majority (~98%) of cases, whereas equivocal vascular invasion only or both vascular and capsular invasions were only found in a handful of cases. At follow-up, the five patients who developed distant metastases had tumors with foci of questionable capsular invasion only.[93]

WHEN WE CAN DECIDE...BUT STILL MISS INVASION

It is not surprising that a small percentage of cases with uncertain capsular invasion recurs or metastasizes, even when those cases did not show

vascular invasion, as in the study by Ito *and colleagues* mentioned above.[93] It has already been recognized that rare FTCs with capsular invasion only may demonstrate distant metastases,[69,74,84,94] although most of these published cases presented with distant metastases at the time of diagnosis.[69,84,94] More disquieting, however, is when metastases have been noted to occur in tumors without any histologic evidence of invasion. Aside from the cases of NIFTP mentioned earlier that had metastasized,[35–37] tumors diagnosed as "follicular adenomas" rarely have been noted to recur as distant disease. Although this may be due to missing focal vascular invasion at the time of initial review,[95] invasion has also been

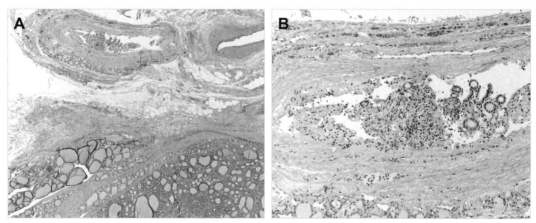

Fig. 12. This case demonstrated push artifact in a large vessel away from the tumor (*A*). On higher power, the fragments of tumor in the vessel appear discohesive and disorganized, without associated endothelial wrapping or thrombus formation (*B*).

noted in subsequent serial sections performed retrospectively.[96] Interestingly, in these select published cases of missed or unsampled invasion, the tumor capsules were found to be thick, with some showing intratumoral fibrosis.[95,96]

As with any area of pathology, there is inevitable sampling error in thyroid tumors. Of the topics discussed in this review, invasion is perhaps the most susceptible to this, leading to a missed focus of vascular or capsular invasion. To help mitigate this issue, some have found that a modified approach to grossing encapsulated thyroid nodules can be useful. Oh and colleagues, for example, found that sectioning the end "caps" of the nodule perpendicularly, in addition to parallel sections through the body of the tumor, improved the yield of invasive foci.[97] Nevertheless, the limitations of evaluating 4 μm sections taken from ~4 mm-thick pieces of tissue still indicates that we are only evaluating ~1/1000 of the tissue. Although some have begun to explore potentially more accurate alternatives, such as microCT scanning of whole tissue blocks, this is currently both impractical for everyday use and has been found to have limitations in the evaluation of vascular invasion.[75] For the immediate future, we will need to continue to rely on routine histologic assessment, although digital pathology and advanced imaging techniques are evolving quickly and could potentially be used to help accurately identify not just invasion but also provide more consistent and uniform thresholds for nuclear atypia and architecture.

SUMMARY

Encapsulated follicular-patterned tumors can be some of the most diagnostically challenging and contentious in thyroid pathology, in large part, because the criteria for nuclear atypia, architecture, and invasion are all subject to individual interpretation. As many follicular-patterned tumors have similar molecular findings, with a high rate of *RAS*-like alterations in follicular adenoma/FT-UMP/follicular carcinoma as well as in their counterparts with more pronounced nuclear atypia (NIFTP/WDT-UMP/invasive encapsulated FVPTC), the distinction between these entities currently still relies on histologic evaluation. Although consensus may never be achievable in all cases, recognition of the pitfalls and problematic issues regarding assessment of these features will hopefully help improve the accuracy of diagnosis.

DISCLOSURE

The authors have nothing to disclose.

REFERENCES

1. Tallini G, Tuttle RM, Ghossein RA. The history of the follicular variant of papillary thyroid carcinoma. J Clin Endocrinol Metab 2017;102(1):15–22.
2. Chen KTK, Rosai J. Follicular variant of thyroid papillary carcinoma: A clinicopathologic study of six cases. Am J Surg Pathol 1977;1(2):123–30.
3. Jung CK, Little MP, Lubin JH, et al. The increase in thyroid cancer incidence during the last four decades is accompanied by a high frequency of BRAF mutations and a sharp increase in RAS mutations. J Clin Endocrinol Metab 2014;99(2): 276–85.
4. Sangalli G, Serio G, Zampatti C, et al. Fine needle aspiration cytology of the thyroid: a comparison of 5469 cytological and final histological diagnoses. Cytopathology 2006;17(5):245–50.

5. Medici M, Liu X, Kwong N, et al. Long- versus short-interval follow-up of cytologically benign thyroid nodules: A prospective cohort study. BMC Med 2016; 14(1):1–9.

6. Lloyd R v, Erickson LA, Casey MB, et al. Observer variation in the diagnosis of follicular variant of papillary thyroid carcinoma. Am J Surg Pathol 2004; 28(10):1336–40.

7. Elsheikh TM, Asa SL, Chan JKC, et al. Interobserver and intraobserver variation among experts in the diagnosis of thyroid follicular lesions with borderline nuclear features of papillary carcinoma. Am J Clin Pathol 2008;130(5):736–44.

8. Hirokawa M, Carney JA, Goellner JR, et al. Observer Variation of Encapsulated Follicular Lesions of the Thyroid Gland. Am J Surg Pathol 2002;26(11):1508–14.

9. Liu J, Singh B, Tallini G, et al. Follicular variant of papillary thyroid carcinoma: A clinicopathologic study of a problematic entity. Cancer 2006;107(6):1255–64.

10. Rivera M, Ricarte-Filho J, Knauf J, et al. Molecular genotyping of papillary thyroid carcinoma follicular variant according to its histological subtypes (encapsulated vs infiltrative) reveals distinct BRAF and RAS mutation patterns. Mod Pathol 2010; 23(9):1191–200.

11. Howitt BE, Jia Y, Sholl LM, et al. Molecular Alterations in Partially-Encapsulated or Well-Circumscribed Follicular Variant of Papillary Thyroid Carcinoma. Thyroid 2013;23(10):1256–62.

12. Nikiforov YE, Seethala RR, Tallini G, et al. Nomenclature revision for encapsulated follicular variant of papillary thyroid carcinoma a paradigm shift to reduce overtreatment of indolent tumors. JAMA Oncol 2016;2(8):1023–9.

13. Seethala RR, Baloch ZW, Barletta JA, et al. Noninvasive follicular thyroid neoplasm with papillary-like nuclear features: A review for pathologists. Mod Pathol 2018;31(1):39–55.

14. Vanzati A, Mercalli F, Rosai J. The "sprinkling" sign in the follicular variant of papillary thyroid carcinoma: A clue to the recognition of this entity. Arch Pathol Lab Med 2013;137(12):1707–9.

15. Thompson LDR, Poller DN, Kakudo K, et al. An International Interobserver Variability Reporting of the Nuclear Scoring Criteria to Diagnose Noninvasive Follicular Thyroid Neoplasm with Papillary-Like Nuclear Features: a Validation Study. Endocr Pathol 2018;29(3):242–9.

16. Lee SE, Hwang TS, Choi Y la, et al. Molecular profiling of papillary thyroid carcinoma in korea with a high prevalence of BRAFV600E mutation. Thyroid 2017;27(6):802–10.

17. Bychkov A, Jung CK, Liu Z, et al. Noninvasive Follicular Thyroid Neoplasm with Papillary-Like Nuclear Features in Asian Practice: Perspectives for Surgical Pathology and Cytopathology. Endocr Pathol 2018; 29(3):276–88.

18. Rana C, Vuong HG, Nguyen TQ, et al. The Incidence of Noninvasive Follicular Thyroid Neoplasm with Papillary-Like Nuclear Features: A Meta-Analysis Assessing Worldwide Impact of the Reclassification. Thyroid 2021;31(10):1502–13.

19. Thompson LD. Ninety-four cases of encapsulated follicular variant of papillary thyroid carcinoma: A name change to Noninvasive Follicular Thyroid Neoplasm with Papillary-like Nuclear Features would help prevent overtreatment. Mod Pathol 2016;29(7): 698–707.

20. Paja M, Zafón C, Iglesias C, et al. Rate of noninvasive follicular thyroid neoplasms with papillary-like nuclear features depends on pathologist's criteria: a multicentre retrospective Southern European study with prolonged follow-up. Endocrine 2021;73(1):131–40.

21. Marcadis AR, Valderrabano P, Ho AS, et al. Interinstitutional variation in predictive value of the Thyro-Seq v2 genomic classifier for cytologically indeterminate thyroid nodules. Surgery (United States) 2018;0:1–8.

22. Kitahara CM, Sosa JA, Shiels MS. Influence of nomenclature changes on trends in papillary thyroid cancer incidence in the united states, 2000 to 2017. J Clin Endocrinol Metab 2020;105(12). https://doi.org/10.1210/clinem/dgaa690.

23. Caulley L, Eskander A, Yang W, et al. Trends in Diagnosis of Noninvasive Follicular Thyroid Neoplasm with Papillarylike Nuclear Features and Total Thyroidectomies for Patients with Papillary Thyroid Neoplasms. JAMA Otolaryngol - Head Neck Surg 2022; 148(2):99–106.

24. Ferris RL, Nikiforov Y, Terris D, et al. AHNS Series: Do you know your guidelines? AHNS Endocrine Section Consensus Statement: State-of-the-art thyroid surgical recommendations in the era of noninvasive follicular thyroid neoplasm with papillary-like nuclear features. Head Neck 2018;40(9):1881–8.

25. Rosario PW, Mourão GF. Follow-up of noninvasive follicular thyroid neoplasm with papillary-like nuclear features (NIFTP). Head Neck 2019;41(3):833–4.

26. WHO Classification of Tumours Editorial Board. Endocrine and neuroendocrine Tumours. 5th edition. International Agency for Research on Cancer; 2022.

27. Pereira M, Williams VL, Hallanger Johnson J, et al. Thyroid cancer incidence trends in the United States: Association with changes in professional guideline recommendations. Thyroid 2020;30(8): 1132–40.

28. Sugino K, Kameyama K, Ito K, et al. Does Hürthle cell carcinoma of the thyroid have a poorer prognosis than ordinary follicular thyroid carcinoma? Ann Surg Oncol 2013;20(9):2944–50.

29. Jeong SH, Hong HS, Kwak JJ, et al. Analysis of RAS mutation and PAX8/PPARγ rearrangements in follicular-derived thyroid neoplasms in a Korean

population: Frequency and ultrasound findings. J Endocrinol Invest 2015;38(8):849–57.

30. Vivero M, Kraft S, Barletta JA. Risk stratification of follicular variant of papillary thyroid carcinoma. Thyroid 2013;23(3):273–9.

31. Rivera M, Tuttle RM, Patel S, et al. Encapsulated papillary thyroid carcinoma: a clinico-pathologic study of 106 cases with emphasis on its morphologic subtypes (histologic growth pattern). Thyroid 2009;19(2):119–27.

32. Kim TH, Lee M, Kwon AY, et al. Molecular genotyping of the non-invasive encapsulated follicular variant of papillary thyroid carcinoma. Histopathology 2018;72(4):648–61.

33. Odate T, Oishi N, Vuong HG, et al. Genetic differences in follicular thyroid carcinoma between Asian and Western countries: a systematic review. Gland Surg 2020;9(5):1813–26.

34. Nikiforov YE, Baloch ZW, Hodak SP, et al. Change in diagnostic criteria for noninvasive follicular thyroid neoplasm with papillarylike nuclear features. JAMA Oncol 2018;4(8):1125–6.

35. Cho U, Mete O, Kim MH, et al. Molecular correlates and rate of lymph node metastasis of non-invasive follicular thyroid neoplasm with papillary-like nuclear features and invasive follicular variant papillary thyroid carcinoma: The impact of rigid criteria to distinguish non-invasive follicular thyroid neoplasm with papillary-like nuclear features. Mod Pathol 2017;30(6):810–25.

36. Kim MJ, Won JK, Jung KC, et al. Clinical Characteristics of Subtypes of Follicular Variant Papillary Thyroid Carcinoma. Thyroid 2018;28(3):311–8.

37. Parente DN, Kluijfhout WP, Bongers PJ, et al. Clinical Safety of Renaming Encapsulated Follicular Variant of Papillary Thyroid Carcinoma: Is NIFTP Truly Benign? World J Surg 2018;42(2):321–6.

38. Xu B, Serrette R, Tuttle RM, et al. How many papillae in conventional papillary carcinoma? A clinical evidence-based pathology study of 235 unifocal encapsulated papillary thyroid carcinomas, with emphasis on the diagnosis of noninvasive follicular thyroid neoplasm with papillary-like nuclear features. Thyroid 2019;29(12):1792–803.

39. Xu B, Reznik E, Tuttle RM, et al. Outcome and molecular characteristics of non-invasive encapsulated follicular variant of papillary thyroid carcinoma with oncocytic features. Endocrine 2019;64(1):97–108.

40. Xu B, Farhat N, Barletta JA, et al. Should subcentimeter non-invasive encapsulated, follicular variant of papillary thyroid carcinoma be included in the noninvasive follicular thyroid neoplasm with papillary-like nuclear features category? Endocrine 2018;59(1):143–50.

41. Xu B, Tallini G, Scognamiglio T, et al. Outcome of Large Noninvasive Follicular Thyroid Neoplasm with Papillary-Like Nuclear Features. Thyroid 2017;27(4):512–7.

42. Agrawal N, Akbani R, Aksoy BA, et al. Integrated Genomic Characterization of Papillary Thyroid Carcinoma. Cell 2014;159(3):676–90.

43. Zhao L, Dias-Santagata D, Sadow PM, et al. Cytological, molecular, and clinical features of noninvasive follicular thyroid neoplasm with papillary-like nuclear features versus invasive forms of follicular variant of papillary thyroid carcinoma. Cancer Cytopathology 2017;125(5):323–31.

44. Paulson VA, Shivdasani P, Angell TE, et al. Noninvasive Follicular Thyroid Neoplasm with Papillary-Like Nuclear Features Accounts for More Than Half of "Carcinomas" Harboring RAS Mutations. Thyroid 2017;27(4):506–11.

45. Johnson DN, Sadow PM. Exploration of BRAFV600E as a diagnostic adjuvant in the non-invasive follicular thyroid neoplasm with papillary-like nuclear features (NIFTP). Hum Pathol 2018;82:32–8.

46. Mai KT, Landry DC, Thomas J, et al. Follicular Adenoma with Papillary Architecture: A Lesion Mimicking Papillary Thyroid Carcinoma. Histopathology 2001;39(1):25–32.

47. Jing X, Michael CW. Potential pitfalls for false suspicion of papillary thyroid carcinoma: A Cytohistologic Review of 22 Cases. Diagn Cytopathol 2012;40(SUPPL. 1). https://doi.org/10.1002/dc.21726.

48. Gorla S, di Bella C, Leone B, et al. Cytological and histological findings of thyroid florid papillary hyperplasia. Cytopathology 2012;23(6):417–9.

49. Pusztaszeri MP, Krane JF, Cibas ES, et al. FNAB of benign thyroid nodules with papillary hyperplasia: A cytological and histological evaluation. Cancer Cytopathology 2014;122(9):666–77.

50. LiVolsi VA, Baloch ZW. The Pathology of Hyperthyroidism. Front Endocrinol 2018;9(737). https://doi.org/10.3389/fendo.2018.00737.

51. Esapa C, Foster S, Johnson S, et al. Protein and Thyrotropin Receptor Mutations inThyroid Neoplasia. J Clin Endocrinol Metab 1997;82(2):493–6. https://academic.oup.com/jcem/article/82/2/493/2823338.

52. Trülzsch B, Krohn K, Wonerow P, et al. Detection of thyroid-stimulating hormone receptor and Gsα mutations: In 75 toxic thyroid nodules by denaturing gradient gel electrophoresis. J Mol Med 2001;78(12):684–91.

53. Mon SY, Riedlinger G, Abbott CE, et al. Cancer risk and clinicopathological characteristics of thyroid nodules harboring thyroid-stimulating hormone receptor gene mutations. Diagn Cytopathol 2018;46(5):369–77.

54. Calebiro D, Grassi ES, Eszlinger M, et al. Recurrent EZH1 mutations are a second hit in autonomous thyroid adenomas. J Clin Invest 2016;126(9):3383–8.

55. Guan H, Matonis D, Toraldo G, et al. Clinical significance of thyroid-stimulating hormone receptor gene mutations and/or sodium-iodine symporter gene

overexpression in indeterminate thyroid fine needle biopsies. Front Endocrinol 2018;9(SEP). https://doi.org/10.3389/fendo.2018.00566.

56. Stephenson A, Eszlinger M, Stewardson P, et al. Sensitive Sequencing Analysis Suggests Thyrotropin Receptor and Guanine Nucleotide-Binding Protein G Subunit Alpha as Sole Driver Mutations in Hot Thyroid Nodules. Thyroid 2020;30(10):1482–9.

57. Landau MS, Nikiforov YE, Ohori NP, et al. Impact of molecular testing on detecting mimics of oncocytic neoplasms in thyroid fine-needle aspirates diagnosed as follicular neoplasm of Hürthle cell (oncocytic) type. Cancer Cytopathology 2021;129(10): 788–97.

58. Lado-Abeal J, Celestino R, Bravo SB, et al. Identification of a paired box gene 8-peroxisome proliferator-activated receptor gamma (PAX8-PPARγ) rearrangement mosaicism in a patient with an autonomous functioning follicular thyroid carcinoma bearing an activating mutation in the TSH receptor. Endocrine-Related Cancer 2010;17(3):599–610.

59. Stewart DR, Best AF, Williams GM, et al. Neoplasm Risk Among Individuals With a Pathogenic Germline Variant in DICER1. J Clin Oncol 2019;37:668–76.

60. González IA, Stewart DR, Schultz KAP, et al. DICER1 tumor predisposition syndrome: an evolving story initiated with the pleuropulmonary blastoma. Mod Pathol 2022;35(1):4–22.

61. Khan NE, Bauer AJ, Schultz KAP, et al. Quantification of thyroid cancer and multinodular goiter risk in the DICER1 syndrome: A family-based cohort study. J Clin Endocrinol Metab 2017;102(5):1614–22.

62. de Kock L, Bah I, Revil T, et al. Deep sequencing reveals spatially distributed distinct hot spot mutations in DICER1-related multinodular goiter. J Clin Endocrinol Metab 2016;101(10):3637–45.

63. Gullo I, Batista R, Rodrigues-Pereira P, et al. Multinodular Goiter Progression Toward Malignancy in a Case of DICER1 Syndrome. Am J Clin Pathol 2018; 149(5):379–86.

64. Juhlin CC, Stenman A, Zedenius J. Macrofollicular variant follicular thyroid tumors are DICER1 mutated and exhibit distinct histological features. Histopathology 2021;79(4):661–6.

65. Mirshahi UL, Kim J, Best AF, et al. A Genome-First Approach to Characterize DICER1 Pathogenic Variant Prevalence, Penetrance, and Phenotype. JAMA Netw Open 2021;4(2). https://doi.org/10.1001/jamanetworkopen.2021.0112.

66. Kim J, Schultz KAP, Hill DA, et al. The prevalence of germline DICER1 pathogenic variation in cancer populations. Mol Genet Genomic Med 2019;7(3). https://doi.org/10.1002/mgg3.555.

67. Evans DG, Howard E, Giblin C, et al. Birth incidence and prevalence of tumor-prone syndromes: Estimates from a UK family genetic register service. Am J Med Genet A 2010;152(2):327–32.

68. Chong AS, Nikiforov YE, Condello V, et al. Prevalence and spectrum of DICER1 mutations in adult-onset thyroid nodules with indeterminate cytology. J Clin Endocrinol Metab 2021;106(4):968–77.

69. Evans HL. Follicular Neoplasms of the Thyroid A Study of 44 Cases Followed for a Minimum of 10 Years, With Emphasis on Differential Diagnosis. Cancer 1984;54(3):535–40.

70. Yamashina M. Follicular neoplasms of the thyroid. Total circumferential evaluation of the fibrous capsule. Am J Surg Pathol 1992;16(4):392–400.

71. Baloch ZW, LiVolsi VA. Our approach to follicular-patterned lesions of the thyroid. J Clin Pathol 2007; 60(3):244–50.

72. Sobrinho-Simões M, Eloy C, Magalhães J, et al. Follicular thyroid carcinoma. Mod Pathol 2011;24:S10–8.

73. Mete O, Seethala R, Asa S, et al. Protocol for the examination of specimens from patients with carcinomas of the thyroid gland, version 4.2.0.0. College of American Pathologists Cancer Protocols; 2019. Published online.

74. Thompson LDR, Wieneke JA, Paal E, et al. A Clinicopathologic Study of Minimally Invasive Follicular Carcinoma of the Thyroid Gland with a Review of the English Literature BACKGROUND. The criteria for minimally invasive (low grade) follicular carcinoma. Cancer 2001;91(3):505–24.

75. Xu B, Teplov A, Ibrahim K, et al. Detection and assessment of capsular invasion, vascular invasion and lymph node metastasis volume in thyroid carcinoma using microCT scanning of paraffin tissue blocks (3D whole block imaging): a proof of concept. Mod Pathol 2020;33(12):2449–57.

76. Franc B, de La Salmonière P, Lange F, et al. Interobserver and Intraobserver Reproducibility in the Histopathology of Follicular Thyroid Carcinoma. Hum Pathol 2003;34(11):1092–100.

77. Zhu Y, Li Y, Jung CK, et al. Histopathologic Assessment of Capsular Invasion in Follicular Thyroid Neoplasms—an Observer Variation Study. Endocr Pathol 2020;31(2):132–40.

78. Ghossein R, Barletta JA, Bullock M, et al. Data set for reporting carcinoma of the thyroid: recommendations from the International Collaboration on Cancer Reporting. Hum Pathol 2021;110:62–72.

79. Mete O, Asa SL. Pathological definition and clinical significance of vascular invasion in thyroid carcinomas of follicular epithelial derivation. Mod Pathol 2011;24(12):1545–52.

80. Cracolici V, Parilla M, Henriksen KJ, et al. An Evaluation of CD61 Immunohistochemistry in Identification of Vascular Invasion in Follicular Thyroid Neoplasms. Head Neck Pathol 2020;14(2): 399–405.

81. Nishino M, Jacob J. Invasion in thyroid cancer: Controversies and best practices. Semin Diagn Pathol 2020;37(5):219–27.

82. Ghossein RA, Hiltzik DH, Carlson DL, et al. Prognostic factors of recurrence in encapsulated Hurthle cell carcinoma of the thyroid gland: A clinicopathologic study of 50 cases. Cancer 2006;106(8): 1669–76.

83. Ito Y, Hirokawa M, Masuoka H, et al. Prognostic factors of minimally invasive follicular thyroid carcinoma: Extensive vascular invasion significantly affects patient prognosis. Endocr J 2013;60(5): 637–42.

84. Xu B, Wang L, Tuttle RM, et al. Prognostic impact of extent of vascular invasion in low-grade encapsulated follicular cell-derived thyroid carcinomas: A clinicopathologic study of 276 cases. Hum Pathol 2015;46(12):1789–98.

85. Matsuura D, Yuan A, Wang LY, et al. Follicular and Hurthle Cell Carcinoma: Comparison of Clinicopathological Features and Clinical Outcomes. Thyroid 2022;32(3):245–54.

86. Yamazaki H, Katoh R, Sugino K, et al. Encapsulated Angioinvasive Follicular Thyroid Carcinoma: Prognostic Impact of the Extent of Vascular Invasion. Ann Surg Oncol 2022. https://doi.org/10.1245/s10434-022-11401-x. Published online February 15.

87. Haugen BR, Alexander EK, Bible KC, et al. 2015 American Thyroid Association Management Guidelines for Adult Patients with Thyroid Nodules and Differentiated Thyroid Cancer. Thyroid 2016;26(1). https://doi.org/10.1089/thy.2015.0020.

88. Williams ED, Abrosimov A, Bogdanova T, et al. Guest editorial: two proposals regarding the terminology of thyroid tumors. Int J Surg Pathol 2000; 8(3):181–3.

89. Hofman V, Lassalle S, Bonnetaud C, et al. Thyroid tumours of uncertain malignant potential: Frequency and diagnostic reproducibility. Virchows Archiv 2009;455(1):21–33.

90. Piana S, Frasoldati A, Felice E di, et al. Encapsulated Well-Differentiated Follicular-Patterned Thyroid Carcinomas Do Not Play a Significant Role in the Fatality Rates From Thyroid Carcinoma. Am J Surg Pathol 2010;34(6):868–72. www.ajsp.com.

91. Liu Z, Zhou G, Nakamura M, et al. Encapsulated follicular thyroid tumor with equivocal nuclear changes, so-called well-differentiated tumor of uncertain malignant potential: A morphological, immunohistochemical, and molecular appraisal. Cancer Sci 2011;102(1):288–94.

92. Baser H, Topaloglu O, Tam AA, et al. Comparing Clinicopathologic and Radiographic Findings Between TT-UMP, Classical, and Non-Encapsulated Follicular Variants of Papillary Thyroid Carcinomas. Endocr Pathol 2016;27(3):233–42.

93. Ito Y, Hirokawa M, Hayashi T, et al. Clinical outcomes of follicular tumor of uncertain malignant potential of the thyroid: real-world data. Endocr J 2022. https://doi.org/10.1507/endocrj.ej21-0723. Published online.

94. O'Neill CJ, Vaughan L, Learoyd DL, et al. Management of follicular thyroid carcinoma should be individualised based on degree of capsular and vascular invasion. Eur J Surg Oncol 2011;37(2):181–5.

95. Baloch ZW, Livolsi VA. Encapsulated Follicular Variant of Papillary Thyroid Carcinoma with Bone Metastases. Mod Pathol 2000;13(8):861–5.

96. Lee YJ, Kim DW, Shin GW, et al. Unexpected Lung and Brain Metastases 9 Years After Thyroid Lobectomy for Follicular Adenoma: A Case Report. Front Endocrinol 2019;10. https://doi.org/10.3389/fendo.2019.00783.

97. Oh HS, Kim SJ, Song E, et al. Modified Transverse-Vertical Gross Examination: a Better Method for the Detection of Definite Capsular Invasion in Encapsulated Follicular-Patterned Thyroid Neoplasms. Endocr Pathol 2019;30(2):106–12.

No Longer Well-Differentiated

Diagnostic Criteria and Clinical Importance of Poorly Differentiated/High-Grade Thyroid Carcinoma

Vincent Cracolici, MD

KEYWORDS

• Poorly differentiated thyroid • Thyroid cancer • High-grade • Turin • WHO

Key points

- Recent modifications in the 2022 WHO Classification of Endocrine Tumors clarify 2 related diagnoses: poorly differentiated thyroid carcinoma and differentiated high-grade thyroid carcinoma. These entities correlate with previously described, partially overlapping systems for diagnosing aggressive thyroid lesions.

- Poorly differentiated thyroid carcinoma and differentiated high-grade thyroid carcinoma are clinically important forms of thyroid cancer that portend an intermediate prognosis between more typical differentiated thyroid carcinomas and anaplastic thyroid carcinoma.

- Clinical management of aggressive thyroid carcinomas may require special surveillance and therapeutic modalities.

ABSTRACT

Poorly differentiated thyroid carcinoma (PDTC) and differentiated high-grade thyroid carcinoma (DHGTC) are uncommon thyroid malignancies, recently (re)codified into distinct entities with overlapping clinical significance. Recognizing them may be challenging for the general practitioner and subspecialty pathologist alike. This article will describe the required features to diagnose PDTC and DHGTC, differential diagnostic considerations, molecular findings, and clinical implications. It is intended to be a general synopsis of the most critical elements of PDTC and DHGTC as well as a summary of points in approaching these challenging cases.

INTRODUCTION

Thyroid cancer exists on a spectrum of low-risk forms to high-risk forms reflected by certain reproducible pathologic findings. A subset of these cancers demonstrates specific morphologic features that predict aggressive clinical behavior. Recently, the WHO Classification of Endocrine Tumors fifth edition has revisited the microscopic criteria necessary to recognize aggressive tumor subgroups that are classified between conventional low-risk well-differentiated thyroid malignancies and anaplastic thyroid carcinoma.[1]

The WHO now defines 2 distinct tumor subgroups that share a clinical phenotype but only partially overlap histologically. Under the umbrella of high-grade follicular cell-derived thyroid carcinomas are 2 distinct diagnoses: poorly differentiated thyroid carcinoma (PDTC) and differentiated high-grade thyroid carcinoma (DHGTC). These reflect the partially overlapping, independently validated diagnostic systems previously recognized for aggressive lesions. The WHO Endocrine Pathology fifth edition clarifies some historical ambiguity that was related to these systems.[1–3] Because the 2 diagnoses converge clinically, the different designations exist to capture these aggressive tumors

Cleveland Clinic Lerner College of Medicine, 9500 Euclid Avenue, L25, Cleveland, OH 44195, USA
E-mail address: cracolv@ccf.org

Surgical Pathology 16 (2023) 45–56
https://doi.org/10.1016/j.path.2022.09.006

while clarifying their precise and distinct microscopic nature with different terms.

For the purposes of this discussion, in keeping with the recent WHO recommendations, the term "poorly differentiated thyroid carcinoma" refers to malignant lesions of thyroid follicular cell derivation that meet specific diagnostic criteria as originally proposed by the Turin criteria and previously adopted by the WHO.[1] The term "differentiated high-grade thyroid carcinoma" refers to malignant lesions of thyroid follicular cell derivation that demonstrate high-grade features but do not fulfill the Turin criteria. These lesions, however, do meet independently validated criteria proposed by the Memorial Sloan Kettering Cancer Center group.[4] The differences between these systems will be elucidated subsequently. A comprehensive review of anaplastic thyroid carcinoma is beyond the scope of this article, although discussions of this entity will be provided particularly in contrast to the diagnostic and clinical features of PDTC and DHGTC.

CLINICAL AND EPIDEMIOLOGIC FACTORS

PDTC and DHGTC are intermediate forms of thyroid cancer that are classified between differentiated thyroid carcinomas and anaplastic thyroid carcinoma. PDTC and DHGTC likely represent less than 5% of all thyroid malignancies diagnosed in the United States, although incidence may be slightly higher in areas of Europe and Latin America.[5,6] PDTC generally affects patients in the fifth to sixth decade of life with a slight female predominance.[5,7,8]

PDTC and DHGTC may originate in long-standing goiter-like conditions or as new/enlarging discrete nodules. On ultrasonic examination, tumors may be solid and hypoechoic with poorly defined borders. Many of these tumors are cold on scintigraphy and FDG-PET avid but lack RAI uptake.[9] Approximately 20% to 50% of patients have metastatic disease, including those with metastasis at the time of initial presentation. Some patients present with a distant metastasis from an otherwise occult primary thyroid malignancy.[1,10] Concordant with their intermediate prognostic nature, these tumors may be associated with locally advanced disease, including extrathyroidal extension.[9] PDTC and DHGTC can originate in the thyroid proper, thyroglossal duct, mediastinal thyroid tissue, or, rarely, in struma ovarii (see Smith and colleagues' article, "It does exist! Diagnosis and Management of Thyroid Carcinomas arising in Struma Ovarii," in this issue).[11]

Much of the available molecular and histologic data support a possible shared lineage of many PDTCs and DHGTCs with differentiated thyroid carcinomas (ie, these represent "de-differentiation" of more conventional papillary or follicular thyroid carcinomas). PDTC and DHGTC may also originate de novo, perhaps in association with iodine deficiency.[1] Radiation exposure is not an established risk factor for these diseases.[11]

GROSS FEATURES

These tumors may demonstrate complete or partial encapsulation. Often gross infiltration is evident, including extrathyroidal extension. Correlation with clinical/surgical extrathyroidal extension is recommended for accurate staging purposes. There is substantial variation in reported tumor sizes but the majority is at least 5 cm in greatest dimension.[9] Tumors are often firm, solid, and white-tan. Grossly evident necrosis should be documented with corresponding histologic sections submitted.

Many PDTCs and DHGTCs reflect a pattern of disease progression in which a differentiated tumor takes on an aggressive phenotype with associated manifest histologic changes. In order to definitively rule out PDTC, an adequate volume of tumor must be evaluated. Generally, for encapsulated lesions, most/all of the tumor capsule will have already been submitted in order to diagnose capsular/vascular invasion diagnostic of malignancy. In otherwise overtly invasive neoplasms, one section per centimeter of tumor may be appropriate. If worrisome features insufficient for the diagnosis of PDTC are initially identified, submission of additional tumor sections may be warranted.

MICROSCOPIC FEATURES

Microscopic recognition of PDTC and DHGTC requires familiarity with the validated diagnostic systems, recently revisited and updated by the WHO.[11]

DIAGNOSING POORLY DIFFERENTIATED THYROID CARCINOMA

PDTC is recognized using criteria previously defined by the WHO and established in the Turin consensus proposal (the "Turin criteria"; Fig. 1).[1,11,12] Importantly, the criteria have not changed between the previous and most recent WHO editions.

The Turin criteria define PDTC as a thyroid tumor of follicular thyrocyte-derivation that either entirely or in part

1. demonstrates diagnostic features of malignancy (invasion),
2. demonstrates solid, insular, or trabecular architecture, and

Fig. 1. Poorly differentiated thyroid carcinoma. This thyroid carcinoma has a "blue" appearance from low-power examination, partially attributable to solid growth and scant colloid production (*A*). This pattern may raise suspicion for PDTC even before high-power examination. Solid growth with variable nuclear atypia is noted (*B*). Away from and intermingled with areas of solid-growth, there is tumor-type necrosis

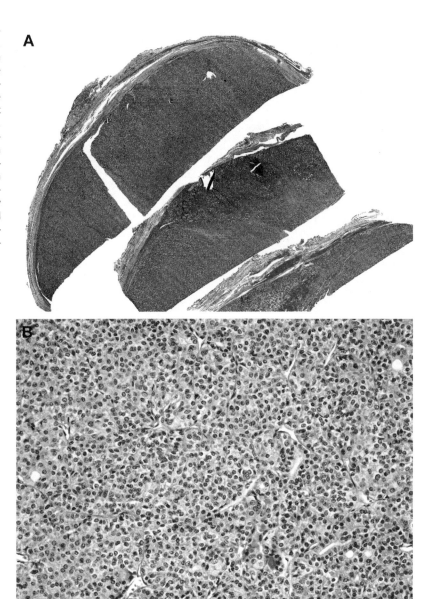

3. is devoid of the conventional nuclear atypia indicative of papillary thyroid carcinoma and also has *3* or greater *mitoses per 10 high-powered fields (2 mm² in the 2022 WHO update) and/or tumor-type necrosis and/or convoluted tumor nuclei.*

THE TURIN CRITERIA IN PRACTICE: PATHOLOGIC CONSIDERATIONS FOR POORLY DIFFERENTIATED THYROID CARCINOMA

Solid growth is distinguished from microfollicular growth by the near absence of colloid production and the lack of well-defined cytoplasmic borders between cells. Rare cases with clear cell, mucinous, signet-ring, or rhabdoid areas have been described.[11]

Occasionally these tumors will be nearly entirely poorly differentiated, that is, they may only demonstrate minute residual components of readily recognizable differentiated thyroid carcinomas. Poorly differentiated areas can also be identified as a minor component of a differentiated thyroid carcinoma. In these instances, it is helpful to note that the basophilic nature of these lesions (owing to their small, monotonous, hyperchromatic nuclei, and solid architecture relatively devoid of colloid) may give a low-power

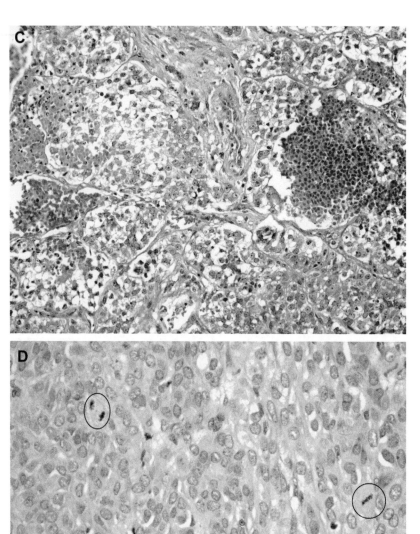

Fig. 1. (continued). (C) and increased mitotic activity (≥3 mitotic figures/ 2 mm²) that are further diagnostic for PDTC (1D) (*mitotic figure circled*).

impression of a "second population." Solid growth can also serve as a clue to more closely interrogate a lesion for focal necrosis or increased mitotic activity that may otherwise not be apparent.

Tumor cell nuclei may be designated "convoluted" if they demonstrate some degree of nuclear atypia distinct from what is expected in conventional papillary thyroid carcinoma (Fig. 2). Specifically, convoluted nuclei are defined as "small, round hyperchromatic nuclei with convolution of the nuclear membranes," which includes "raisin-like" contours and a lack of intranuclear cytoplasmic pseudoinclusions.[7]

Recognition of convoluted nuclei is arguably the most subjective and challenging of the Turin criteria. Generally, a poorly differentiated invasive lesion with solid growth that lacks papillary thyroid carcinoma nuclei will have at least necrosis or increased mitotic activity in addition to convoluted nuclei. The literature reports that it is relatively uncommon to establish a diagnosis of PDTC on convoluted tumor nuclei alone.[2] Furthermore, some expert

Fig. 2. Spectrum of nuclei in thyroid neoplasms. Nuclei in benign and malignant thyroid processes demonstrate a spectrum of changes. Follicular thyroid adenomas/carcinomas generally have small nuclei with a round contour and homogenous dark chromatin (*A*). Nuclei of conventional/classic papillary thyroid carcinoma are enlarged with chromatin clearing, overlapping, contour irregularity, and occasional intracytoplasmic nuclear pseudoinclusions (*B*). Oncocytic thyroid nuclei are generally round with prominent, centrally located nucleoli and associated abundant eosinophilic cytoplasm

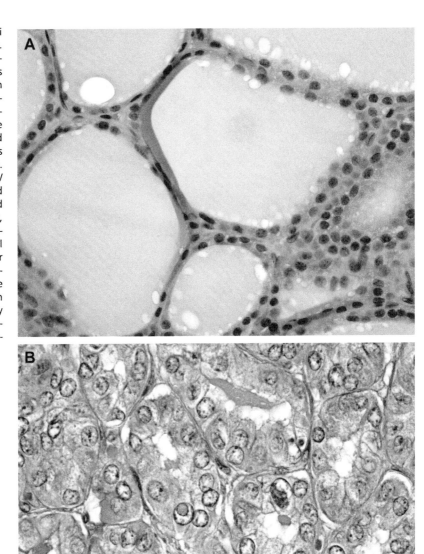

pathologists devalue the role that convoluted nuclei play in the Turin criteria and primarily render the diagnosis based on invasion, solid growth, necrosis, and increased mitotic activity.[8] Some studies call into question the prognostic value of convoluted nuclei, including the relative challenge in confidently recognizing such a change.[2]

However, recognition of nuclei as "convoluted" rather than as "papillary-like" acknowledges a degree of nuclear change that occurs in PDTC and allows it to be separated from solid papillary thyroid carcinoma. Although important in its own right, solid papillary thyroid carcinoma (in the absence of increased mitoses/necrosis) should be distinguished from PDTC because its prognosis may be more favorable.[8,13,14] Specifically, in tumors with solid growth, nuclear features typical of conventional papillary thyroid carcinoma are

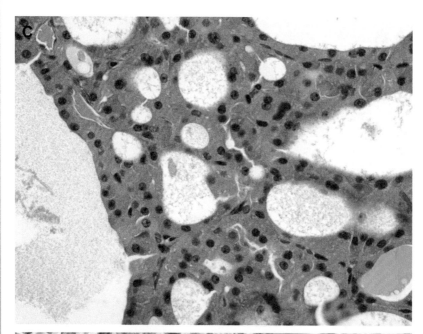

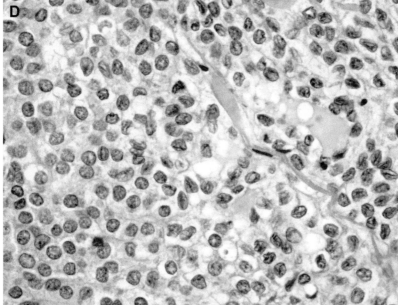

Fig. 2. (continued). (C). Some amount of enlargement or membrane irregularity may be seen. Convoluted or "raisin-like" nuclei of PDTC share some features with conventional papillary thyroid carcinoma (including nuclear contour irregularity) but may be more monomorphic and shrunken-appearing (D). Other features of conventional papillary thyroid carcinoma (chromatin clearing, pseudoinclusions) are absent in convoluted nuclei.

consistent with solid papillary thyroid carcinoma, whereas nuclear irregularities not characteristic of papillary carcinoma do not exclude the diagnosis of PDTC (see **Fig. 2**).

DIAGNOSING DIFFERENTIATED HIGH-GRADE THYROID CARCINOMA

The WHO newly defines DHGTC as a thyroid malignancy of follicular thyrocyte-derivation that retains distinctive architectural and/or cytologic features of differentiated carcinoma of follicular cells (papillary, follicular, or oncocytic) and

1. has 5 mitoses or greater per 10 high-powered fields (2 mm^2 in the 2022 WHO) and/or
2. demonstrates tumor-type necrosis.

Although both DHGTC and PDTC incorporate mitoses and necrosis, the recognition of solid growth and the somewhat nebulous distinction of "convoluted" nuclei are not considerations in DHGTC[1,3,4,15] (Fig. 3). Both DHGTC and PDTC should not have more than moderate nuclear pleomorphism, a useful feature for distinguishing them from anaplastic thyroid carcinoma.[11]

The Turin criteria may more closely capture aggressive forms of follicular patterned lesions including follicular variant of papillary thyroid carcinoma and follicular thyroid carcinoma. Aggressive conventional papillary thyroid carcinomas may be

Fig. 3. Differentiated high-grade thyroid carcinoma. This thyroid carcinoma demonstrates conventional papillary architecture from low-power examination (*A*). There are no areas of solid-growth. Regions of tumor-type necrosis are identified within the carcinoma (*B*) as well as mitotic figures (*circled*) (*C*). In the absence of necrosis, increased mitoses ($\geq$5 mitotic figures/2 mm^2) would be diagnostic for DHGTC.

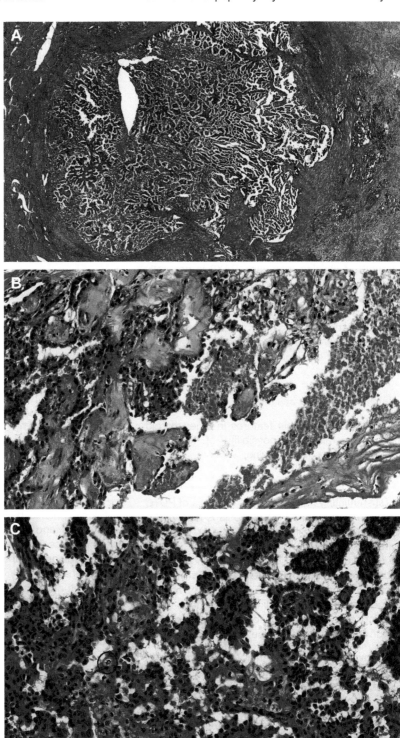

better captured as DHGTC as these lesions may not develop solid growth or may retain nuclei of papillary thyroid carcinoma (solid papillary thyroid carcinoma) that would be exclusionary from the Turin criteria.[3] Known aggressive papillary thyroid carcinoma subtypes such as tall cell, columnar, or hobnail may also be associated with progression to DHGTC.[11] Progression to poorly differentiated/high-grade morphology may be found in lymph node metastases or at distant sites.[11]

IMMUNOHISTOCHEMISTRY

Often, immunohistochemistry factors into the diagnosis of PDTC and HGTC as a means of excluding other entities in the differential. Because these lesions represent a point on the continuum of follicular-thyrocyte–derived malignancies, there is some overlap in immunophenotype.

In PDTC, thyroglobulin staining can vary from entirely negative to focally positive including staining isolated cells in a dot-like pattern. Diffuse TTF-1 nuclear expression is expected, although strength of staining may vary. PAX8 is generally positive. Cytokeratin expression is retained. Focal p53 staining may be identified, although this finding is nonspecific. Neuroendocrine markers and calcitonin are negative.[9] Ki-67 is generally elevated (10%–30%).[1] Exclusion of metastases or parathyroid carcinomas may be worthwhile in some cases.[1]

DIFFERENTIAL DIAGNOSIS

Some histomorphologic features in other thyroid neoplasms raise the possibility of PDTC or DHGTC, such as the following:

1. Infarct (post-FNA) type necrosis

Differentiating true tumor-type necrosis of PDTC or DHGTC from post-FNA necrosis is highly relevant. Tumor necrosis is coagulative or comedo-type and contains identifiable nuclear debris. Individual cell necrosis scattered throughout the tumor is a feature of PDTC/DHGTC. In infarct-type or post-FNA-type necrosis, the presence of hemorrhage/hemosiderin including hemosiderin-laden macrophages and areas of fibrosis or neovascularization favor a secondary type of necrosis.[3]

2. Conventional papillary thyroid carcinoma with solid growth (solid subtype of papillary thyroid carcinoma)

By Turin criteria for PDTC, recognition of "convoluted nuclei" and the absence of readily identifiable nuclei of papillary thyroid carcinoma distinguishes PDTC from papillary thyroid carcinomas with solid growth (solid subtype of papillary thyroid carcinoma). The nuclei of PDTC should not closely resemble those of papillary thyroid carcinoma (enlargement, chromatin clearing, contour irregularity, intranuclear cytoplasmic pseudoinclusions). Solid subtype of papillary thyroid carcinoma may achieve designation as DHGTC if nuclear features of papillary thyroid carcinoma are retained and necrosis and/or increased mitoses are present.

3. Medullary thyroid carcinoma

PDTC and DHGTC only reflect lesions of follicular-thyrocyte derivation. Exclusion of medullary thyroid carcinoma is therefore essential, which may include studies with calcitonin, synaptophysin, and/or other neuroendocrine markers. Amyloid production is associated with medullary thyroid carcinoma. PDTC and DHGTC will often label with thyroglobulin (although possibly in a dot-like fashion) and are generally positive for TTF-1 and PAX8.[3]

4. Anaplastic thyroid carcinoma

Anaplastic thyroid carcinoma is more pleomorphic with striking cytonuclear irregularity when compared with PDTC or DHGTC. Anaplastic thyroid carcinomas are only rarely positive for thyroglobulin and may demonstrate TTF-1 positivity focally (in contrast to the diffuse positivity expected in PDTC).[3] Suspicion for anaplastic thyroid carcinoma may be raised when there is deviation from the monomorphic "small round blue cell" appearance of PDTC or when the diffuse changes of papillary thyroid carcinoma in DHGTC develop into a more pleomorphic and bizarre phenotype. This can include the possibility of sarcomatous/mesenchymal elements.[8]

Although PDTC and DHGTC are intermediate histologic phases between differentiated thyroid carcinomas and anaplastic thyroid carcinomas, their presence is certainly not a histologic prerequisite to diagnose anaplastic thyroid carcinoma. That is, anaplastic thyroid carcinoma can be diagnosed without needing to identify a strict poorly differentiated or differentiated high-grade precursor.

5. Oncocytic follicular thyroid neoplasms

Multiple studies have validated application of the Turin criteria to oncocytic lesions.[6,16,17] Accurate recognition of poorly differentiated features in oncocytic follicular thyroid carcinomas may be difficult because these lesions are composed of large cells occasionally arranged in a microfollicular pattern that may simulate solid growth. The abundant eosinophilic cytoplasm seen in these lesions may also somewhat obscure solid growth as the low-power impression is "less blue" than in nononcocytic poorly differentiated carcinomas. Further reports of a second population of "small cells" perhaps more closely resembling conventional PDTCs have been described.[16]

It may be worth noting that the nuclear features of papillary thyroid carcinoma may overlap with oncocytic lesions (enlargement, nuclear membrane irregularities; see Fig. 2). Therefore, interpreting nuclei as oncocytic (with prominent nucleoli, with associated granular eosinophilic cytoplasm) may be difficult but allows for inclusion of relevant lesions into both the PDTC and DHGTC categories depending on additional architectural features (solid vs follicular growth) and high-grade features (necrosis or mitoses).[18] Interpreting nuclei as papillary-like only allows for inclusion of relevant lesions into the DHGTC category.

STAGING

Pathologic stage classification for PDTCs and DHGTCs is the same as for other follicular thyrocyte-derived carcinomas.

MOLECULAR

In recent history, there has been a great expansion of molecular data to inform our understanding of thyroid neoplasms. The molecular signatures of PDTC and DHGTC further elucidate the diagnoses and have potential prognostic implications.

Briefly, there are 2 broad pathways by which follicular thyrocyte-derived carcinomas typically originate: the RAS-like pathway and the BRAF V600E-like pathway. These pathways are comprehensively described elsewhere.[19–21] To summarize, high-grade carcinomas (generally PDTCs) originating from precursor follicular-patterned lesions (follicular thyroid carcinoma, follicular variant of papillary thyroid carcinoma) often harbor RAS-like driver mutations. Conversely, BRAF V600E-like driver mutations are more commonly identified in DHGTC originating from precursor conventional papillary thyroid carcinomas. This dichotomy is consistent with the new paradigm for categorizing high-grade thyroid carcinomas in the WHO fifth edition. In prior organizational methods, the Turin criteria, as strictly enforced, may have underrepresented aggressively behaving lesions with BRAF V600E-like driver mutated thyroid carcinoma precursors (now largely captured as DHGTC). These driver mutations occur early in tumorigenesis and remain identifiable in poorly differentiated and high-grade tumors.[19–21] Although the molecular signature of a differentiated tumor component may be recognized in a PDTC, the associated histology may not itself be present.

DHGTCs and PDTCs proceed toward a shared clinical phenotype and further converge with "late" phase nondriver mutations (TP53 and TERT promoter mutations most notably). TERT promoter mutations are also a significant prognostic indicator, being associated with aggressively behaving lesions and present in up to 50% of poorly differentiated neoplasms.[20,22] "Late" molecular changes that accumulate with disease progression and "dedifferentiation" also include mutations in the PI3K/PTEN/AKT pathway. Changes in SWI/SNF remodeling genes and mismatch repair proteins are associated with anaplastic morphology.[20]

PROGNOSIS

High-grade follicular cell-derived thyroid carcinomas are an intermediate subtype of thyroid cancer that, although rare, account for many thyroid cancer-related deaths.[6,23] At presentation, these patients tend to be older with advanced local regional disease (including extrathyroidal extension) and metastasis.[23] Worse prognosis is associated with greater tumor size, age greater than 45 years, extrathyroidal extension, and metastasis.[24,25] Oncocytic PDTCs tend to affect older patients with a male predominance and, as some studies suggest, have a more aggressive clinical course, especially as related to disease recurrence.[16,18,26]

PDTC and DHGTC represent common causes of radioiodine refractory thyroid carcinoma because they are generally less avid for RAI.[1,25,27] Clinicians may thus need to adjust the method of follow-up to include other modalities (such as FDG-PET, as recommended by the American Thyroid Association) that may modify the initial staging practices.[28] Monitoring serum thyroglobulin can also be less effective for disease follow-up in PDTC. In concordance with its histologic and immunophenotypic profile, PDTCs may not secrete appreciable quantities of thyroglobulin.[28]

Minor histologic components of PDTC arising in a background of differentiated thyroid carcinoma can affect prognosis. When the poorly differentiated tumor volume reaches approximately 10% of the total, the overall prognostic implications become similar to lesions of predominantly poorly differentiated morphology.[17,20,29,30] Therefore, recognizing any amount of poorly differentiated morphology within a thyroid malignancy should be reported and may be important to quantify, if possible.

Some microscopic features beyond the diagnosis of PDTC are clinically significant. Some data suggest that not simply the presence of capsular/vascular invasion but the extent of such invasion is prognostically relevant for PDTC.[6,31] Specifically, disease-free survival significantly declines in patients with extensive vascular invasion (4 or more foci of vascular invasion) and wide local invasion (57% and 10% at 5 years, respectively).[6] In contrast, patients with PDTCs with focal capsular and/or vascular invasion demonstrate a more indolent clinical course (5 year disease-free survival of 83%–100%).[6] Disease-specific survival is also diminished in patients with extensive invasion versus those with focal invasion.[6] Overall, 5-year survival ranges from 62% to 85% with a 5-year disease-specific survival of 66% and a 10-year survival of approximately 50%.[23,25]

Total thyroidectomy with central and possible lateral neck dissection is a mainstay of therapy. Adjuvant treatment modalities are frequently used; however, definitive standardized management guidelines are not universally used.[23,32] External beam radiation therapy may be considered in patients with advanced disease. Following a several year course, distant metastatic disease represents the major cause of death.[23]

The recognition of specific molecular alterations in thyroid neoplasms will likely become increasingly important as, even now, approximately 50% of PDTCs harbor mutations in drug targetable pathways.[20] These mutations include BRAF V600 E drivers that could be targeted by currently available BRAF inhibitors. Other therapeutics include monoclonal antibodies that target immune checkpoint molecules as well as tyrosine kinases targeting growth factors and growth factor receptors. Tyrosine kinase inhibitors for advanced thyroid carcinomas have also been used in the past for disease progression, particularly in radioiodine-resistant lesions.[20]

POORLY DIFFERENTIATED THYROID CARCINOMA IN PEDIATRIC AND YOUNG PATIENTS

Most PDTCs are diagnosed in adults, generally middle-aged or older. However, rarely, PDTC may originate in younger patients including children and adolescents. Given the variation of diagnostic standardization used over time and the relative rarity of the diagnosis in young individuals, it is difficult to comprehensively evaluate this demographic group.[33]

In a recent study of 6 PDTC cases in patients aged 14 to 19 years, there was a female predominance and aggressive clinical behavior, including death in multiple patients.[33] A concurrent literature review also suggests potentially worse outcomes in young patients with PDTC. In this cohort, the majority of tested cases (83%) harbored mutations in the DICER1 gene, including an example of a possible germline DICER1 mutation. None of the patients in this group seemed to have a syndromic DICER1 clinical phenotype or family history.[33] The authors explain that the DICER1 mutations seen in thyroid neoplasms outside of DICER1 syndrome are usually associated with differentiated, low-risk carcinomas, in contrast to the aggressive cases noted in their review of young patients.[33,34]

These findings suggest that PDTC in young patients is a unique clinico-pathologic and molecular entity that may proceed aggressively, in contrast to what might be predicted by its mutational profile.[33,35] If the features meeting the Turin criteria are identified in an adolescent or young adult patient, a diagnosis of PDTC may be prudent despite the lack of standardized reporting guidelines and relative rarity of the diagnosis. PDTC in young children (aged 13 years and younger) remains extremely rare.

SUMMARY

Intermediate risk thyroid malignancies of follicular-thyrocyte derivation are important to recognize. The 2022 WHO classification system includes diagnostic categories to capture different morphologies that predict increased risk for patients: PDTC and DHGTC, that, broadly speaking, correlate with aggressive diseases originating in follicular-patterned (RAS-like driver mutated) and papillary (BRAF V600E-like driver mutated) carcinomas, respectively. Identifying these tumors and relevant histologic components including the proportion of aggressive disease and the quantity of capsular/vascular invasive foci is important for ensuring appropriate management. Advances in molecular data will likely provide further insight into these entities and may offer avenues for novel therapeutics.

CLINICS CARE POINTS

- Familiarity with the recently revisited criteria for diagnosing PDTC and DHGTC is essential for pathologists who sign-out thyroid specimens.

- If possible, the percentage of PDTC originating in conjunction with a differentiated thyroid carcinoma should be reported; a minor component of even 10% can have meaningful clinical impact.

- The number of foci of vascular and/or extent of capsular invasion should be reported because this is a critical element for prognosticating patients with PDTC.

- There is no single molecular aberration that is uniquely diagnostic for PDTC or DHGTC; however, mutations in *TERT* promoter are correlated with aggressively behaving lesions. In young patients, *DICER1* mutations are common in PDTC.

- Avoid using the phrase "poorly differentiated" as purely descriptive in thyroid pathology because this may be confusing to both clinicians and pathologists. The phrase "poorly differentiated" should be reserved for tumors that meet Turin criteria.

DISCLOSURE

The author has nothing to disclose.

ACKNOWLEDGMENTS

The author would like to thank Dr. C. Griffith, MD, PhD of the Cleveland Clinic for his thoughtful contributions in reviewing an earlier draft of this manuscript.

REFERENCES

1. Baloch ZW, Asa SL, Barletta JA, et al. Overview of the 2022 WHO classification of thyroid neoplasms. Endocr Pathol 2022;33(1):27–63.
2. Gnemmi V, Renaud F, Do Cao C, et al. Poorly differentiated thyroid carcinomas: application of the Turin proposal provides prognostic results similar to those from the assessment of high-grade features. Histopathology 2014;64(2):263–73.
3. Xu B, Ghossein R. Poorly differentiated thyroid carcinoma. Semin Diagn Pathol 2020;37(5):243–7.
4. Hiltzik D, Carlson DL, Tuttle RM, et al. Poorly differentiated thyroid carcinomas defined on the basis of mitosis and necrosis: a clinicopathologic study of 58 patients. Cancer 2006;106(6):1286–95.
5. Asioli S, Erickson LA, Righi A, et al. Poorly differentiated carcinoma of the thyroid: validation of the Turin proposal and analysis of IMP3 expression. Mod Pathol 2010;23(9):1269–78.
6. Wong KS, Lorch JH, Alexander EK, et al. Prognostic significance of extent of invasion in poorly differentiated thyroid carcinoma. Thyroid 2019;29(9): 1255–61.
7. Volante M, Collini P, Nikiforov YE, et al. Poorly differentiated thyroid carcinoma: the Turin proposal for the use of uniform diagnostic criteria and an algorithmic diagnostic approach. Am J Surg Pathol 2007;31(8):1256–64.
8. Wong KS, Barletta JA. Thyroid Tumors You Don't Want to Miss. Surg Pathol Clin 2019;12(4):901–19.
9. Wenig B. Neoplasms of the thyroid gland. In: Atlas of head and neck pathology. Philadelphia: Elsevier; 2016. p. 1381–8.
10. Cracolici V, Kadri S, Ritterhouse LL, et al. Clinicopathologic and molecular features of metastatic follicular thyroid carcinoma in patients presenting with a thyroid nodule versus a distant metastasis. Am J Surg Pathol 2019;43(4):514–22.
11. Tallini G, Asa SL, Barletta JA, Kondo T, Lam AK, Piani S. Follicular-derived carcinomas, high-grade. In: Tallini G, editor. WHO Classification of Endocrine Tumors, 5th edition. 2023. Epub ahead of print: tumourclassification.iarc.who.int.
12. Wong KS, Dong F, Telatar M, et al. Papillary thyroid carcinoma with high-grade features versus poorly differentiated thyroid carcinoma: an analysis of clinicopathologic and molecular features and outcome. Thyroid 2021;31(6):933–40.
13. Baloch ZW, LiVolsi VA. Special types of thyroid carcinoma. Histopathology 2018;72(1):40–52.
14. Nath MC, Erickson LA. Aggressive variants of papillary thyroid carcinoma: hobnail, tall cell, columnar, and solid. Adv Anat Pathol 2018;25(3):172–9.
15. Xu B, David J, Dogan S, et al. Primary high-grade non-anaplastic thyroid carcinoma: a retrospective study of 364 cases. Histopathology 2022;80(2): 322–37.
16. Bai S, Baloch ZW, Samulski TD, et al. Poorly differentiated oncocytic (hürthle cell) follicular carcinoma: an institutional experience. Endocr Pathol 2015; 26(2):164–9.
17. Dettmer M, Schmitt A, Steinert H, et al. Poorly differentiated oncocytic thyroid carcinoma–diagnostic implications and outcome. Histopathology 2012;60(7): 1045–51.
18. Lukovic J, Petrovic I, Liu Z, et al. Oncocytic papillary thyroid carcinoma and oncocytic poorly differentiated thyroid carcinoma: clinical features, uptake, and response to radioactive iodine therapy, and outcome. Front Endocrinol (Lausanne) 2021;12: 795184.
19. Cancer Genome Atlas Research Network. Integrated genomic characterization of papillary thyroid carcinoma. Cell 2014;159(3):676–90.
20. Volante M, Lam AK, Papotti M, et al. Molecular pathology of poorly differentiated and anaplastic thyroid cancer: what do pathologists need to know? Endocr Pathol 2021;32(1):63–76.
21. Landa I, Ibrahimpasic T, Boucai L, et al. Genomic and transcriptomic hallmarks of poorly differentiated and anaplastic thyroid cancers. J Clin Invest 2016; 126(3):1052–66.

22. Haroon Al Rasheed MR, Xu B. Molecular Alterations in Thyroid Carcinoma. Surg Pathol Clin 2019;12(4): 921–30.
23. Ibrahimpasic T, Ghossein R, Shah JP, et al. Poorly differentiated carcinoma of the thyroid gland: current status and future prospects. Thyroid 2019; 29(3):311–21.
24. Huang J, Sun W, Zhang Q, et al. Clinicopathological characteristics and prognosis of poorly differentiated thyroid carcinoma diagnosed according to the turin criteria. Endocr Pract 2021;27(5): 401–7.
25. Haugen BR, Alexander EK, Bible KC, et al. 2015 American Thyroid Association Management Guidelines for Adult Patients with Thyroid Nodules and Differentiated Thyroid Cancer: The American Thyroid Association Guidelines Task Force on Thyroid Nodules and Differentiated Thyroid Cancer. Thyroid 2016;26(1):1–133.
26. Papotti M, Torchio B, Grassi L, et al. Poorly differentiated oxyphilic (Hurthle cell) carcinomas of the thyroid. Am J Surg Pathol 1996;20(6):686–94.
27. Rivera M, Ghossein RA, Schoder H, et al. Histopathologic characterization of radioactive iodine-refractory fluorodeoxyglucose-positron emission tomography-positive thyroid carcinoma. Cancer 2008;113(1):48–56.
28. Xu B, Ghossein R. Evolution of the histologic classification of thyroid neoplasms and its impact on clinical management. Eur J Surg Oncol 2018;44(3): 338–47.
29. Dettmer MS, Schmitt A, Komminoth P, et al. Poorly differentiated thyroid carcinoma : An underdiagnosed entity. Gering differenzierte Schilddrüsenkarzinome : Eine unterdiagnostizierte Entität. Pathologe 2020;41(Suppl 1): 1–8.
30. Dettmer M, Schmitt A, Steinert H, et al. Poorly differentiated thyroid carcinomas: how much poorly differentiated is needed? Am J Surg Pathol 2011;35(12): 1866–72.
31. Xu B, Ibrahimpasic T, Wang L, et al. Clinicopathologic Features of Fatal Non-Anaplastic Follicular Cell-Derived Thyroid Carcinomas. Thyroid 2016; 26(11):1588–97.
32. Patel KN, Shaha AR. Poorly differentiated thyroid cancer. Curr Opin Otolaryngol Head Neck Surg 2014;22(2):121–6.
33. Chernock RD, Rivera B, Borrelli N, et al. Poorly differentiated thyroid carcinoma of childhood and adolescence: a distinct entity characterized by DICER1 mutations. Mod Pathol 2020;33(7):1264–74.
34. Wasserman JD, Sabbaghian N, Fahiminiya S, et al. DICER1 Mutations Are Frequent in Adolescent-Onset Papillary Thyroid Carcinoma. J Clin Endocrinol Metab 2018;103(5):2009–15, [published correction appears in J Clin Endocrinol Metab. 2018 Aug 1;103(8):3114].
35. Ghossein CA, Dogan S, Farhat N, et al. Expanding the spectrum of thyroid carcinoma with somatic DICER1 mutation: a survey of 829 thyroid carcinomas using MSK-IMPACT next-generation sequencing platform. Virchows Arch 2022;480(2):293–302.

This is Your Thyroid on Drugs
Targetable Mutations and Fusions in Thyroid Carcinoma

Ying-Hsia Chu, MD

KEYWORDS

• Kinase fusion • *BRAF* V600 E • *NTRK* • *RET* • Inhibitor • Resistance

Key points

- Activating alterations of receptor tyrosine kinases and downstream effectors in the mitogen-activated protein kinase (MAPK) and PI3K pathways are the main drivers of thyroid carcinogenesis.

- *BRAF* V600 E mutation and rearrangements of *RET* and *NTRK* are the most common actionable targets in thyroid cancer with the United States Food and Drug Administration (FDA)-approved inhibitor therapy.

- Rearrangements of other kinases (eg, *ALK*, *MET*, *ROS1*, and *BRAF*), deregulation of the PI3K/Akt/mTOR pathway, microsatellite instability status, and tumor mutation burden are emerging biomarkers of therapeutic actionability under active research.

ABSTRACT

This review aims to provide an overview of the molecular pathogenesis thyroid carcinomas, emphasizing genetic alterations that are therapeutically actionable. The main pathways in thyroid carcinogenesis are the MAPK and PI3K pathways. Point mutations and gene rearrangements affecting the pathway effectors and receptor tyrosine kinases are well-known drivers of thyroid cancer. Research over the past few decades has successfully introduced highly effective treatments for unresectable thyroid cancer, evolving from multi-kinase inhibitors to structurally selective agents, with constantly improving toxicity profiles and coverage of resistance mechanisms. The pros and cons of major laboratory techniques for therapeutic target identification are discussed.

OVERVIEW

The overall incidence of thyroid cancer has been steadily increasing in the United States over the past few decades.[1,2] Rising incidences are seen across different histologic subtypes, in microcarcinomas and large (>4 cm) tumors, in thyroid-confined and metastatic cases.[1,2] Although most patients with thyroid cancer have a surgically manageable disease, postoperative persistent and recurrent tumors cause significant morbidity and mortality in 10% to 30% of differentiated thyroid carcinoma (DTC) and the majority of medullary and anaplastic carcinoma patients. To treat DTC, radioactive iodine (RAI) has long been used to ablate remnant thyroid tissue and control residual and recurrent disease.[3] However, de novo and acquired RAI refractoriness, although controversially defined,[3] is a well-recognized clinical conundrum associated with adverse prognosis, with only 10% of such patients reaching 10-year survival.[4] Virtually all poorly differentiated and anaplastic carcinomas are RAI-refractory and respond poorly to conventional chemoradiation, with a five-year disease-specific survival of 50% to 60% and almost none, respectively.[5,6] This underscores a growing need for systemic therapy with genomics-guided precision to improve patient

The author declares no conflict of interest.

Department of Pathology, Chang Gung Memorial Hospital and Chang Gung University, No. 5, Fuxing Street, Guishan District, Taoyuan City 333, Taiwan

E-mail address: yinghsia.c@gmail.com

Surgical Pathology 16 (2023) 57–73

https://doi.org/10.1016/j.path.2022.09.007

outcomes. This review presents an overview of the genetic underpinnings of thyroid cancer, focusing on recent advances in targeted therapy.

MOLECULAR LANDSCAPE OF FOLLICULAR-DERIVED THYROID CARCINOMA

WELL-DIFFERENTIATED THYROID CARCINOMAS

Activating alterations of receptor tyrosine kinases (RTKs) and the downstream mitogen-activated protein kinase (MAPK) pathway are the main drivers for well-differentiated thyroid carcinomas (Fig. 1). The Cancer Genome Atlas (TCGA) program analyzed 496 papillary thyroid carcinomas (PTC), composed mainly of classic (69%), follicular (21%), and tall cell (7.5%) types, and was able to divide the cohort into $BRAF^{V600E}$-like (BVL) and RAS-like (RL) tumors using a $BRAF^{V600E}$-RAS score (BRS) derived from a 71-gene expression signature.[7] $BRAF$ V600 E mutation (47% of all cases), $BRAF$ fusions (2%), and RET fusions (5%) were the main drivers in the BVL group, which was characterized by decreased thyroid differentiation and a predominance of classic, tall cell, and infiltrative follicular variant histology. In contrast,

the RL group consists mainly of highly differentiated, follicular variant PTC driven by $N/H/KRAS$ (11%), $EIF1AX$ (1%), non-V600 E $BRAF$ (1%) mutations, and $PAX8::PPARG$ fusion (1%).

Yoo and colleagues[8] subsequently performed a transcriptomic analysis of a large cohort of follicular-patterned neoplasms including follicular adenoma (FA), follicular thyroid carcinomas (FTC), follicular variant PTC, and a comparison group of classic PTC. In addition to affirming the key genetic onco-drivers of the BVL and RL molecular subtypes observed by TCGA, the study identified a new non-BRAF-non-RAS (NBNR) subtype associated with mutations in $IDH1$, $DICER1$, $EIF1AX$, $PTEN$, $SPOP$, $SOS1$, and $PAX8::PPARG$ rearrangement. Similar to the RL samples, the NBNR group was characterized by highly differentiated tumors with preserved expression of genes involved in thyroid function and metabolism. All the FA and FTC samples clustered into the RL and NBNR categories, as did most encapsulated follicular variant PTC. Infiltrative follicular variant PTCs, in contrast, had variable transcriptomic profiles that were distributed roughly equally to the BVL and RL groups.

Kinase fusions have a predilection for pediatric and radiation-associated PTCs, at 56% and 41%

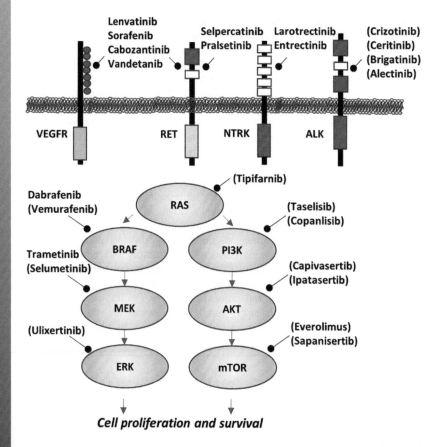

Fig. 1. Intracellular signaling pathways in thyroid carcinogenesis. Genetic alterations of the MAPK and PI3K pathways are the most common druggable drivers. Targeted inhibitors are listed, with investigational therapies that have not received FDA approval for thyroid cancer placed in parentheses.

prevalence, respectively,[9,10] and have also been reported in up to 25% of adult PTC.[11] In all the three patient populations, *RET* is the most commonly rearranged kinase gene (approximately 28%, 17%, 14% in pediatric, post-radiation, and adult PTC, respectively), followed by *NTRK* (15%, 11%, and 8%).[9–11] Other kinase fusions involving *BRAF*, *ALK*, *ROS1*, and *MET* also rarely occur.[11] In RTK gene fusions, the partner genes typically provide dimerization domains, such as the coiled coil domains in *CCDC6*, *NCOA4*, *PPL*, *TPR*, *TPM3*, the WD domain in *EML4*, the PNT domain in *ETV6*, the zinc finger domain in *IRF2BP2*, the PB1 domains in *TFG* and *SQSTM1*, and the RNA recognition motif of *RBPMS*, which enables the kinase domain to undergo ligand-independent dimerization and activation. Fusions involving the RAF family serine/threonine kinase genes such as *BRAF*, in contrast, cause aberrant activation by replacing the 5′ autoinhibitory domain-encoding sequence with a partner gene sequence that may not contain a dimerization domain. In a recent analysis of 100 *BRAF* fusion-positive melanocytic tumors, only 55% of the partner sequences were found to contain dimerization domains, in keeping the idea that the loss of auto-inhibition plays a major oncogenic role. In the pre-treatment setting, kinase fusions are mutually exclusive with the *BRAF* V600 E and *RAS* mutations, but have been found concurrent with mutations in *TP53*, *SMARCA4*, *VHL*, *PIK3R1*, *GNAQ*, *CDH1*, *AKT2*, *FBXW7*, *JAK2*, *GNA11*, *IDH1*, *MEN1*, *SETD2*, *IGF2R*, *SDHA*, *CDKN2A*, *MSH6*, and the *TERT* promoter.[11,12] Interestingly, in the TCGA study, *NTRK* (2%) and *ALK* (1%) fusion cases tended to show intermediate BRS and a neutral transcriptional profile in the BVL-RL spectrum.[7]

Several recent studies have reported distinct clinicopathologic features of kinase fusion-driven PTC. In fine needle aspiration specimens, *NTRK* and *ALK* fusion tumors have been noted to frequently show indeterminate cytology with most cases in The Bethesda System for Reporting Thyroid Cytopathology (TBS) categories III and IV.[13,14] Higher percentages of categories V to VI have been reported by other studies,[15,16] reflecting possible confounding by inter-observer variability and a need for further research. Histology-wise, commonly observed features included multinodular growth, intratumoral fibrosis, and lymphovascular spread (Fig. 2).[9,11,17] *RET* fusions have long been associated with the diffuse sclerosing type of PTC, characterized by extensive lymphovascular involvement, stromal fibrosis, lymphocytic inflammation, and squamous metaplasia (see Fig. 2A–

B). *ALK* fusion tumors are frequently follicular-patterned (see **Fig. 2**C).[14] An intriguing finding of glomeruloid papillary formation has been described in *NTRK* fusion cases (see **Fig. 2**D).[11] In addition to PTC, primary thyroid secretory carcinomas represent a rare phenotype of *ETV6::NTRK3* fusion thyroid carcinoma.[18] Histologically, these tumors may show microcystic, tubular, and solid growth with production of eosinophilic secretions (see **Fig. 2**E–F). The nuclei are vacuolar with well-visible nucleoli (see **Fig. 2**F inset) and may show grooves and rare pseudoinclusions. Most studies reported a tendency for aggressive behavior for fusion-positive tumors. Over 50% of fusion-positive PTC presented as T3 or T4 disease in pediatric, post-radiation, and adult settings, and up to 81%, 39%, and 75%, respectively, had lymph node metastases at the time of diagnosis.[9–11]

POORLY DIFFERENTIATED AND ANAPLASTIC CARCINOMAS

Progression of well-differentiated thyroid carcinoma to poorly differentiated thyroid carcinoma (PDTC) and anaplastic thyroid carcinoma (ATC) is accompanied by increasing mutation burden.[19,20] In addition to retaining the tumor-initiating *BRAF/RAS* mutations and kinase fusions, PDTC and ATC frequently harbor mutations in *TP53*, *TERT* promoter, mediators of the PI3K/Akt/mTOR pathway (*PIK3CA*, *PTEN*, *AKT*, *TSC1/2*, *MTOR*), SWI/SNF chromatin-remodeling complexes (*ARID1A/1 B/2/5B*, *SMARCB1*, *PBRM1*, *ATRX*), histone-modifying enzymes (*KMT2A/2 C/2D* and *SETD2*), and mismatch repair proteins (*MSH2*, *MSH6*, *MLH1*) genes.[19–22] Copy number alterations (CNAs) affecting cell cycle regulation (deletion of *CDKN2A/2B*, amplification of *CCNE1*), RTKs (*KDR*, *KIT*, *PDGFRA*), and immune evasion-related genes have also been associated with high-grade non-anaplastic and anaplastic carcinomas.[20,22]

ONCOCYTIC CARCINOMAS

Hurthle cell (oncocytic) carcinomas, as defined by voluminous eosinophilic cytoplasm of the neoplastic cells as a result of mitochondrial hyperplasia, characteristically harbor mitochondrial DNA (mtDNA) mutations and CNAs.[23–26] Nonsilent mtDNA mutations, found in 71% of oncocytic carcinomas, most commonly affect genes that encode subunits of the complex I (67%) of the electron transport chain, followed by complexes IV (9%), III (4%), and V (3%).[24] Approximately 14% of mutations occur in mitochondrial transfer RNA and ribosomal RNA.[24] Pro-oncogenic

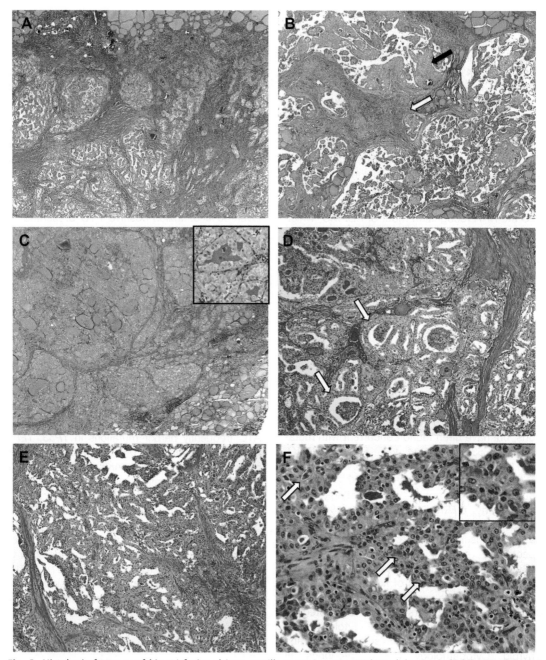

Fig. 2. Histologic features of kinase fusion-driven papillary carcinomas. Multinodular growth (*A*), intratumoral fibrosis (*A*), and lymphovascular spread are frequently seen with various kinase fusions. *RET* fusions are associated with the diffuse sclerosing variant with additional features of lymphocytic inflammation (*B, white arrow*) and squamous metaplasia (*B, black arrow*). *ALK* fusion tumors are often follicular-patterned (*C*, magnified in inset). Glomeruloid papillary formation has been described in *NTRK* fusion tumors (*D, white arrows*). Primary thyroid secretory carcinoma is a rare phenotype of *NTRK*-rearranged thyroid carcinoma, typically carrying *ETV6::NTRK3* fusions. These tumors are characterized by microcystic architecture (*E*) and intracellular and extracellular globules of eosinophilic secretions (*F, white arrows*, also seen in inset). The nuclei are low grade-appearing with well-visible nucleoli (*F*, inset).

cytophysiologic deregulations in oncocytic carcinomas have been shown *in vitro*, including a shift from oxidative phosphorylation to aerobic glycolysis and increased reactive oxygen species genesis.[23] Another oncogenic force comes from frequent whole chromosome duplications (WCDs) of chromosomes 5, 7, and 12 in approximately 55% of oncocytic carcinomas.[23–26] WCDs lead to amplification and overexpression of several MAPK and PI3K pathway effectors, including *RICTOR* and *GOLPH3* on chromosome 5, *MET*, *CDK6*, and *BRAF* on chromosome 7, *KRAS*, *CDK4*, and *MDM2* on chromosome 12. Approximately 54% of oncocytic carcinomas show widespread chromosomal losses in a near-haploid tumor genome, often with concurrent WCD of the remaining chromosomes 5, 7, and 12 leading to extensive loss of heterozygosity (LOH), an adverse prognosticator for oncocytic carcinoma.[24,25] In addition, somatic mutations in the RAS/RAF/MAPK and PI3K/AKT/mTOR pathways (55%), DNA damage and repair machineries (38%), epigenetic modifying enzymes (59%), and the *TERT* promoter (22% to 32%) have been reported.[23–26]

TARGETED THERAPY FOR FOLLICULAR-DERIVED CARCINOMAS

Currently, kinase fusions and the *BRAF* V600 E mutation are the main druggable genetic alterations in thyroid cancer. Although *RAS* mutations account for most FTC and many follicular-patterned PTC, the development of RAS inhibitors has been hindered by the lack of drug-binding pocket.[27] Although two covalent inhibitors of the *KRAS* G12 C mutant, sotorasib and adagrasib, have recently become available,[28] *KRAS* G12 C is extremely rare in thyroid cancer. Instead, most *RAS* mutations in follicular-derived carcinomas occur at the Q61 locus, which is currently undruggable. Nevertheless, thyroid cancer overall harbors the highest frequency of kinase fusions of all solid tumors.[29] Selective kinase inhibitors have become the first-choice treatment for clinically significant, radioactive iodine-refractory (RAIR) kinase fusion-positive tumors. For fusion-negative RAIR DTC, multi-kinase inhibitors represent the current standard of care based on well-established survival benefits from two pivotal phase III trials (**Table 1**). MAPK pathway blockade, through directly targeting the BRAF V600 E mutant or inducing tumor redifferentiation, has also shown clinical efficacy.

MULTI-KINASE INHIBITORS

Sorafenib and lenvatinib are the current first-line kinase inhibitor therapy for clinically significant RAIR DTC. These agents exert anti-tumoral effects mainly through targeting the vascular endothelial growth factor receptors (VEGFRs) and suppressing tumor-induced angiogenesis. In the SELECT trial, 392 patients were randomized to receive lenvatinib versus placebo.[30] Median progression-free survival (PFS) was significantly improved in the lenvatinib group (18.3 months vs 3.6 months).[30]

Survival benefits were also observed for sorafenib in the DECISION trial, with a median PFS of 10.8 months versus 5.8 months in the placebo group.[31] Despite their inhibitory activities against multiple additional kinases including RET, repurposing MKI for direct RET targeting has shown significant off-target toxicities and inferior pharmacokinetics compared with selective RET inhibitors.[32] Most adverse effects of MKI are related to impaired vascular repair and vasomotor regulation leading to hypertension and mucocutaneous inflammation. Toxicities frequently led to dose interruptions, reductions, and discontinuations in 66.2%, 64.3%, and 18.8% of subjects in the DECISION trial and 82.4%, 67.8%, and 14.2% in the SELECT trial,[30,31] respectively. As many patients with RAIR DTC can have slowly progressive disease, deciding when to initiate MKI therapy require careful clinical evaluation to balance between life quality and tumor control.

MITOGEN-ACTIVATED PROTEIN KINASE PATHWAY BLOCKERS

Direct BRAF inhibition has been evaluated in *BRAF* V600E-mutated thyroid carcinoma in two open-label phase II trials.[33–35] Brose and colleagues[33] investigated the use of vemurafenib in 51 patients with RAIR PTC, including 26 patients without (cohort 1) and 25 with prior MKI treatment (cohort 2). In cohort 1, over a median follow-up of 18·8 months, partial response was achieved in 38.5%, and the median PFS was 18.2 months. In cohort 2, over a median follow-up of 12.0 months, partial response was achieved in 27.3%, and the median PFS was 8.9 months. It was noteworthy that cutaneous squamous cell carcinoma (SCC) was the most common serious adverse effect in the trial, developing in 27% of cohort 1 and 20% of cohort 2. BRAF inhibitor-associated SCC is believed to result from paradoxical RAF activation in BRAF-wildtype cells, and its occurrence can be effectively reduced with combination therapy of BRAF and MEK inhibitors.[36,37] Indeed, in the ROAR trial by Subbiah and colleagues[34,35] on treating 36 patients with BRAF V600E-mutated ATC with dabrafenib and trametinib combination therapy, no secondary SCC was noted. The ROAR trial showed an objective response rate (ORR) of 56% and a median PFS of 6.7 months, leading to the United States Food and Drug Administration (FDA) approval of dabrafenib and trametinib for the treatment of ATC in 2018 followed by accelerated histology-agnostic approval for BRAF V600E-positive solid tumors in 2022.[34,35] Despite the protective effect of co-administered MEK inhibitor against MAPK pathway reactivation,

Table 1
FDA-approved targeted therapy for thyroid cancer

Agent	Target(s)	Approved Thyroid Indication(s)	Registrational Trial	Design	Tumor Histology (Case no.)	ORR	Median PFS
Lenvatinib	VEGFR1/2/3, FGFR1/2/3/4, PDGFRα, RET, KIT	RAI-refractory thyroid cancer	SELECT[30]	Phase III	PTC (200), FTC (75), HCC (70), PDTC (47)	64.8%	18.3 months (lenvatinib) vs 3.6 months (placebo)
Sorafenib	VEGFR1/2/3, RET, RAF, PDGFRβ, KIT	RAI-refractory thyroid cancer	DECISION[31]	Phase III	PTC (237), FTC (106), PDTC (40), WDC (3)	12.2%	10.8 months (sorafenib) vs 5.8 months (placebo)
Cabozantinib	VEGFR1/2/3, RET, MET, FLT3, KIT	DTC failing prior anti-VEGF therapy	COSMIC-311[76]	Phase III	PTC (102), FTC (90)	15%	Not reached (cabozantinib) vs 1.9 months (placebo)
		MTC	EXAM[75]	Phase III	MTC (330)	28%	11.2 months (cabozantinib) vs 4.0 months (placebo)
Vandetanib	VEGFR1/2/3, RET, EGFR	MTC	ZETA[74]	Phase III	MTC (331)	45%	Not reached (vandetanib) vs 19.3 months (placebo)
Dabrafenib, trametinib	BRAF (dabrafenib), MEK (trametinib)	BRAF V600E-mutant solid tumors[b]	ROAR/ BRF117019[35]	Phase II	ATC (36)	56%	6.7 months
Selpercatinib	RET	RET fusion + solid tumors[b]	LIBRETTO-001[42]	Phase I/II	PTC (13), PDTC (3), ATC (2), HCC (1)	79%	20.1 months
		RET-mutant MTC	LIBRETTO-001[42]	Phase I/II	MTC (55 with and 88 without prior MKI treatment)	69%, 73%[a]	Not reached (previously treated with MKI); 23.6 months (MKI-naïve)

Pralsetinib	RET	RET fusion + thyroid cancer	ARROW[43]	Phase I/II	RET fusion-positive thyroid cancer (11)	89%	Not reached
		RET-mutant MTC	ARROW[43]	Phase I/II	55 with and 21 without prior MKI treatment	60%, 71%[a]	Not reached
Larotrectinib	NTRK1/2/3	NTRK fusion + solid tumors[b]	NAVIGATE, SCOUT, LOXO-TRK-14001[46]	Phase I/II	PTC (20), ATC (7), FTC (2)	71%	2.2 months for ATC; not reached for other histologic types
Entrectinib	NTRK1/2/3, ROS1, ALK	NTRK fusion + solid tumors[b]	ALKA-372–001, STARTRK-1, STARTRK-2[47]	Phase I/II	NTRK fusion-positive thyroid cancer (5)	20%	-

Abbreviations: ATC, anaplastic thyroid carcinoma; DTC, differentiated thyroid carcinoma; FTC, follicular thyroid carcinoma; HCC, Hurthle cell carcinoma; MKI, multikinase inhibitors vandetanib and cabozantinib; MTC, medullary thyroid carcinoma; ORR, objective response rate; PDTC, poorly differentiated thyroid carcinoma; PFS, progression-free survival; PTC, papillary thyroid carcinoma; RAI, radioactive iodine; WDC, well-differentiated carcinoma.

[a] See text for details.

[b] Histology-agnostic approval.

resistance has since still emerged due to acquired *RAS* mutations.[38] BRAF and/or MEK inhibitors have also attracted significant research interest in inducing tumor redifferentiation and restoring RAI sensitivity in RAIR DTC,[39–41] which is outside the scope of this review.

SELECTIVE RET INHIBITORS

Pralsetinib and selpercatinib are selective RET inhibitors with significantly improved antitumoral activity and tolerability compared with MKI. Selpercatinib received FDA approval in 2020 for treating *RET* fusion-positive advanced or metastatic thyroid cancer followed by histology-agnostic approval in 2022 based on the efficacy data from the phase 1-2 trial LIBRETTO-001 (see **Table 1**).[42] The trial evaluated a total of 19 non-medullary thyroid cancer patients, including 13 PTC, 1 oncocytic carcinoma, 3 PDTC, and 2 ATC. The ORR was 79% including 1 complete response and 14 partial responses, whereas the remaining patients all showed stable disease.[42] The median duration of response was not reached, and the median PFS was 20.1 months.[42] Overall, toxicities led to dose reductions in 30% of the patients and treatment termination in 2% due to abnormal liver function and hypersensitivity.[42] Pralsetinib was granted accelerated FDA approval in 2020 for thyroid cancer based on the ARROW trial (see **Table 1**).[43] This phase 1/2 trial evaluated 11 *RET* fusion-positive thyroid cancer patients with an ORR of 89% and a disease control rate of 100%.[43] Acquired resistance to selective RET inhibition has been emerging in *RET* fusion-positive thyroid cancer, including one ATC that developed *EGFR* amplification as a bypassing mechanism that caused selpercatinib resistance.[11]

NTRK INHIBITORS

Larotrectinib and entrectinib are the first TRK inhibitors approved by the FDA for the treatment of adult and pediatric *NTRK*-rearranged solid tumors. Oncogenic *NTRK* rearrangements are rare drivers of thyroid, breast, lung, pancreatic, and colonic carcinomas, melanomas, gliomas, and sarcomas, while being pathognomonic in several unusual tumor types (eg, secretory carcinomas, infantile fibrosarcomas, and congenital mesoblastic nephromas). The body-wide distribution of *NTRK*-rearranged tumors inspired the histology-agnostic design of clinical trials[44–47] (see **Table 1**). Combining three phase 1/2 trials in 159 patients, larotrectinib showed an ORR of 79% across various solid tumors, with complete response in 16%.[44] By mid-2020, the trials included a total of 29 thyroid

carcinoma cases (20 PTC, 7 ATC, 2 FTC), with an ORR of 71%.[46] As for entrectinib, three phase 1/2 trials reported an ORR of 57% among all enrolled subjects and 20% among thyroid cancer cases.[47] Both larotrectinib and entrectinib were well tolerated. Less than 5% of the trial subjects discontinued treatment due to toxicities. Only 8% (larotrectinib) and 30% (entrectinib) required dose reductions due to anemia, elevated blood creatinine, hepatic or pancreatic enzymes, fatigue, and nausea.[44,47] On-target resistance-mediating mutations have been reported in multiple tumor types (colonic, thyroid, pancreatic, pulmonary, salivary gland carcinomas, cholangiocarcinoma, gastrointestinal stromal tumor, sarcomas)[48–50] at the solvent front (*NTRK1* G595 R, *NTRK3* G623 R) and gatekeeper (*NTRK1* F589 L, *NTRK3* F617 L) positions as well as in the xDFG motif (*NTRK1* G667 C/S, *NTRK3* G696 A).[48–51] Fortunately, next-generation NTRK inhibitors selitrectinib and repotrectinib have shown great promise in restoring tumor response in resistant cases.[52,53]

ALK inhibitors

ALK fusions are rarely found in thyroid cancer, with only scattered case reports in PTC,[54] oncocytic carcinoma,[55] PDTC,[11] ATC,[56,57] and MTC.[58] Crizotinib is a first-generation ALK inhibitor with concurrent inhibitory activities against ROS1 and MET. Originally approved by the FDA in 2011 for treating *ALK*-rearranged lung cancer, crizotinib has since shown therapeutic success in various organs including in thyroid cancer. However, resistance inevitably develops 1 to 2 years into treatment due to acquired kinase domain mutations[59] and, less commonly, through activating mutations or amplifications of genes involved in bypassing pathways such as *EGFR*, *KRAS*, and *MET*.[60] Among the five reported cases of *ALK*-rearranged thyroid carcinomas treated with crizotinib (**Table 2**), initial crizotinib response was noted to last for 6 to 36 months.[11,54–56,58] One patient with ATC was able to switch to second-generation inhibitors ceritinib and brigatinib but eventually succumbed to progressive disease.[56] None of the reported cases underwent post-treatment sequencing, and their resistance mechanisms remained uncharacterized.

PI3K/AKT/mTOR inhibition

The targeting of the PI3K/AKT/mTOR pathway has thus far shown limited success in thyroid cancer. Everolimus, an mTOR inhibitor, has been evaluated by several recent phase II trials.[61–63] Schneider and colleagues[63] studied 28 patients with RAIR DTC and 7 ATC with daily treatment of 10 mg everolimus

Table 2
Reported cases of thyroid carcinomas receiving ALK inhibitor therapy

Reference	Histology	Molecular Abnormalities	ALK Inhibitor	Best Response, Duration	Side Effects
[54]	PTC	*EML4::ALK;* mutations in 55 genes	Crizotinib	SD, over 6 months to the end of study	Fatigue, cough
[55]	OC	*ALK* fusion with unknown partner	Crizotinib	CR, 6 months	Constipation
[11]	PDTC	*STRN::ALK; TP53* c.772 G > C	Crizotinib	SD, 11 months	Fatigue
[56]	ATC	*STRN::ALK*	Crizotinib, switched to ceritinib and then brigatinib for resistance	CR, 36 months (crizotinib); PR, 16 months (ceritinib); PR, 8 months (brigatinib)	–
[58]	MTC	*CCDC6::ALK*	Crizotinib, switched to alectinib for tolerance	PR, over 280 days to the end of the study	Myalgia

Abbreviations: ATC, anaplastic thyroid carcinoma; CR, complete response; MTC, medullary thyroid carcinoma; OC, oncocytic carcinoma; PDTC, poorly differentiated thyroid carcinoma; PR, partial response; PTC, papillary thyroid carcinoma; SD, stable disease.

10 mg orally. At a median follow-up of 38 months, 65% achieved stable disease, whereas partial or complete response was not observed. Hanna and colleagues[62] evaluated 33 RAIR DTC, 10 MTC, and 7 ATC patients with the same everolimus regimen for a median follow-up of 31.8 months. The ORR was 3%, 10%, and 14% in DTC, MTC, and ATC, whereas 82%, 80%, and 28% achieved stable disease, respectively.[62] Although both studies performed genetic analysis and found *PI3K/AKT/mTOR* pathway mutations in subsets of patients, a solid correlation between tumor genotype and everolimus response has not been made with the small cohort sizes. This remains to be resolved by several ongoing clinical trials at the time of this writing.

MEDULLARY THYROID CARCINOMA

Medullary thyroid carcinomas (MTC) are neuroendocrine tumors showing differentiation towards the parafollicular cells of thyroid gland. Despite their uncommonness (approximately 5% of all thyroid cancers), most patients present with advanced disease (50% to 70% with regional and 105 to 15% with distant metastases) which is not amenable to RAI therapy.[64,65] For patients with advanced, recurrent, or metastatic disease beyond surgical control, the current American Thyroid Association guidelines recommend the use of external beam radiotherapy radiation and systemic therapy with MKI or selective RET inhibitors.[66] MTC is known to have low response rate to conventional cytotoxic chemotherapeutic agents, which are therefore not recommended for the first-line setting.

RET

Activating alterations of *RET* serve as the key genetic drivers for nearly all hereditary and approximately 40% of sporadic MTC. The *RET* proto-oncogene encodes a transmembrane RTK composed of four extracellular cadherin-like domains, a cysteine-rich region, a transmembrane domain, and an intracellular part that contains the kinase domain. Various point mutations can cause aberrant kinase activation, and, in the hereditary setting, interesting genotype-phenotype correlations have been characterized. Multiple endocrine neoplasia (MEN) syndrome type 2A presents with MTC, pheochromocytomas, hyperparathyroidism, and cutaneous lichen amyloidosis (CLM). Over 90% of MEN-2A cases result from mutations in cysteine codons 611, 618, 620, and 634. These mutations are thought to promote intermolecular disulfide bone formation, leading to aberrant RET dimerization and activation. In contrast, the MEN type 2B syndrome arises from a kinase domain mutation M918 T, which leads to increased ATP-binding affinity, loss of autoinhibition, and ultimately ligand-independent monomeric and dimeric autophosphorylation and activation.[67] Unlike those affected by MEN-2A, patients with the MEN-2B syndrome tend not to develop hyperparathyroidism and CLM, but instead present with mucosal and intestinal neuromas and a marfanoid appearance. Among sporadic MTC, the most common RET mutation is M918 T (in 69%) followed by codon 634 mutations (11%).[68] The M918 T mutation has been associated with more aggressive tumor behavior in both hereditary and sporadic settings.[69,70] RET fusions are exceptionally rare in MTC.[71] Fusions involving other kinases, such as ALK and BRAF, have been reported in isolated cases with notable response to targeted therapy.[58,72,73]

Inhibition of RET signaling can be achieved through MKI and selective RET inhibitors.[74–76] Among MKI, vandetanib and cabozantinib have both been approved by the FDA for treating MTC (see **Table 1**). In the registrational ZETA trial, vandetanib led to a superior median PFS of 30.5 months compared with 19.3 months in the placebo group.[74] Patients receiving cabozantinib also showed a clear survival benefit, with a median PFS of 11.2 months compared with 4.0 months in those receiving placebo.[75] To overcome MKI's frequent toxicities and to tackle MKI-resistant mutations such as V804 L/M, selective RET inhibitors have been developed with excellent efficacy and tolerability (see **Table 1**). In the LIBRETTO-001 trial, selpercatinib showed durable partial to complete response in 69% of those with preceding MKI treatment and 73% of MKI-naïve patients.[42] More recently, pralsetinib showed similarly impressive clinical benefits, with an ORR of 60% and 71% among subjects with and without prior MKI exposure, respectively.[43] Based on the trial results, both selpercatinib and pralsetinib have received the FDA approval for treating advanced or metastatic RET-altered MTC. However, acquired resistance to selpercatinib has since emerged due to solvent front mutations G810 C/S and hinge region mutations Y806 C/N.[77,78] These mutations are also predicted to confer resistance to pralsetinib.[78] Fortunately, next-generation RET inhibitors such as TPX-0046 have shown potent *in vitro* and *in vivo* activity against a broad range of RET alterations including resistance-mediating solvent front mutations.[79]

RAS

Among RET-wildtype MTC, up to 68% harbor hotspot RAS mutations, most commonly in HRAS (56%) and occasionally in KRAS (12%) and NRAS (rare).[80] Uncommonly, HRAS may be co-mutated along with RET in the same tumor.[80] Various mutations in codons 12, 13, and 61 have been reported in the Catalogue Of Somatic Mutations In Cancer (COSMIC) database,[81] such as G12 V/R, G13 V/R, and Q61 K/L/R. However, KRAS G12 C, the primary target of sotorasib and adagrasib, has been vanishingly rare. Other RAS-targeting strategies being developed include mutant-specific T cell receptor-engineered T cell therapy, cancer vaccines, and inhibition of post-transcriptional RAS processing.[82] Multiple post-transcriptional enzymatic steps are required for RAS proteins to become functional, including pre-nylation by farnesyltransferase or geranylgeranyl-transferase. Unlike KRAS and NRAS, HRAS can only be prenylated by farnesyltransferase and is therefore vulnerable to farnesyltransferase inhibition. Tipifarnib is a farnesyltransferase inhibitor that has been studied in a combination therapy with sorafenib in a phase II trial that included 13 MTC patients.[83] The trial observed an ORR of 38%, whereas 31% had stable disease as the best response.[83] As the study did not analyze RAS mutation status in the MTC cases, the relationship between tumor genotype and therapeutic sensitivity was unclear.

LABORATORY IDENTIFICATION OF THERAPEUTIC TARGETS

IMMUNOHISTOCHEMISTRY

Immunohistochemical assays (IHCs) have been developed for detecting BRAF V600 E[84,85] and RAS Q61 R[86,87] mutations and for rearrangements of NTRK (pan-TRK),[88,89] ALK,[90,91] RET,[92] and ROS1.[93] IHC are advantageous for its short turn-around time, low tissue input and the ability to visualize biomarker expression within histologic context. Recent studies have reported reasonable performance for BRAF V600 E (clone VE1, sensitivity 89–100%; specificity 62–100%[85]) and RAS Q61 R[86] (clone SP174, sensitivity 90.6%, specificity 92.3%) mutant-directed IHC. The VE1 antibody does not label BRAF V600 K or K601 E mutations or BRAF fusions.[85] The performance of kinase-based IHC in detecting gene fusions may be partner gene-dependent. For pan-TRK IHC, Solomon and colleagues[88] reported a sensitivity of 81.1% and a specificity of 99.9% in 87 NTRK fusion tumors. The sensitivity was higher in NTRK1 (96%) and NTRK2 (100%) fusions compared with NTRK3-rearranged samples (79%).[88,94] It is noteworthy that tumors with neural and smooth muscle differentiation can show positive TRK staining in the absence of *NTRK* rearrangement.[89] Also partner-dependent was RET-directed IHC, for which Yang and colleagues[92] reported a sensitivity of 100% for *KIF5B-RET*, 88.9% for *CCDC6-RET* cases, and 50% for *NCOA4-RET*; the specificity was approximately 82%. Unlike ALK IHC which has nearly 100% sensitivity and specificity for ALK fusions, ROS1 IHC may show high background staining that limits its clinical application.[93]

FLUORESCENCE IN SITU HYBRIDIZATION

For a long time, fluorescence in situ hybridization (FISH) has been the mainstay method for detecting gene rearrangements. Break-apart FISH probe design allows for fusion detection without knowledge about partner gene identity and breakpoint location. However, FISH has limited multiplexing capability and cannot provide therapeutically relevant functional details such as the reading frame and the preservation of drug-binding domain (eg, the kinase domain in kinase fusions). As a result, biologically nonproductive fusions have led to treatment failure in up to 40% of ALK FISH-positive lung cancer.[95] Moreover, fusions secondary to short-segment inversions, such as the *NCOA4-RET* fusion commonly encountered in thyroid carcinomas, may not produce visually discernible probe separation resulting in false negative results.[92]

CONVENTIONAL POLYMERASE CHAIN REACTION-BASED ASSAYS

Single-gene polymerase chain reaction (PCR)-based assays are widely performed in clinical laboratories due to their technical versatility. Point mutations, such as *BRAF* V600 E, can be detected at the DNA level using Sanger sequencing, restriction enzyme processing, and allele-specific amplification methods. Gene fusions are generally queried at the RNA level using revere-transcription PCR as post-transcriptional splicing circumvents several technical challenges caused by intronic breakpoints, as discussed in the next section. Fusion-specific (FS) detection and expression imbalance (EI) quantification are the two main assay design strategies used to detect gene fusions.[96] FS detection requires knowing the identity of both partner genes and the breakpoint location for designing opposing primers (**Fig. 3**C), which precludes detection of novel fusions. In contrast, EI-based detection only analyzes one target gene and quantifies the expression levels of the 3′ and 5′ regions using separate amplicons (**Fig. 3**E). As oncogenic

fusions are overexpressed, the sequence incorporated by the fusion transcript (eg, the 3′ part of *NTRK3*) is detected at a much higher level compared with the unincorporated part (eg, the 5′ part of *NTRK3*).[96] EI-based detection has been used by several rapid testing platforms, including quantitative PCR,[97] digital droplet PCR,[98] hybridization-based transcript enumeration,[99,100] matrix-assisted laser desorption/ionization time-of-flight analysis[100] as well as next-generation sequencing (NGS) (discussed below) with variable performance. EI-based detection can be significantly hindered by endogenous expression of the wildtype gene. For example, *ROS1* have a high physiologic expression in pneumocytes, which has been shown to obscure EI in *ROS1*-rearranged tumors and reduce fusion detection sensitivity.[96,99]

NEXT-GENERATION SEQUENCING

Over the past decade, NGS has significantly improved the efficiency of therapeutic target identification through expanded throughput and drastically reduced per-gene analytic time and cost. Although detection of point mutations and small indels has been well-validated in most platforms, several challenges persist for NGS-based fusion detection. Fusion breakpoints are often intronic and can be analyzed through hybrid capture or amplicon-based enrichment (**Fig. 3**). However, extensive intronic tiling can cause inefficient consumption of sequencing capacity. Furthermore, intronic repetitive sequences and complex rearrangement events can render bioinformatic mapping challenging and error-prone with short-read sequencing. For this reason, instead of direct DNA sequencing, fusion detection is often performed using tumor-derived complementary DNA (cDNA), in which introns have been spliced out, and the analysis can focus on the exons. One additional advantage of cDNA sequencing is that oncogenic fusions are highly expressed, which aids in detection in low tumor purity samples. Complementary DNA sequencing can also characterize oncogenic splice variants such as the *BRAF* splice variants in PTC and ATC[101] as well as the *NTRK1* splice variants deltaTRKA and TRKAIII.[102] The main limitation of cDNA sequencing is RNA degradation. Molecular pathologists play an important role in ensuring the validity of sequencing results by thoroughly evaluating quality metrics and verifying each fusion call based on the alignment quality, the predicted reading frame, and literature support of biological relevance.

Very recently, the American Head and Neck Society (AHNS) Endocrine Surgery Section and

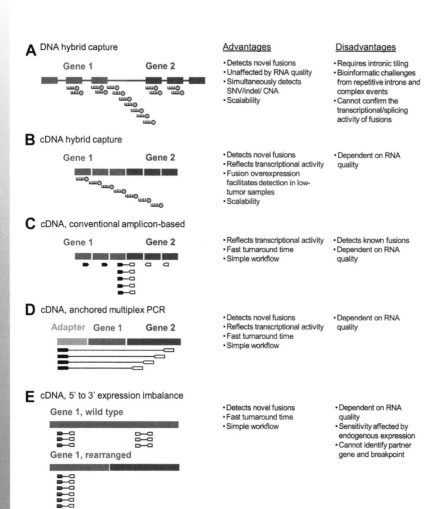

A DNA hybrid capture

<u>Advantages</u>
- Detects novel fusions
- Unaffected by RNA quality
- Simultaneously detects SNV/indel/ CNA
- Scalability

<u>Disadvantages</u>
- Requires intronic tiling
- Bioinformatic challenges from repetitive introns and complex events
- Cannot confirm the transcriptional/splicing activity of fusions

B cDNA hybrid capture

- Detects novel fusions
- Reflects transcriptional activity
- Fusion overexpression facilitates detection in low-tumor samples
- Scalability

- Dependent on RNA quality

C cDNA, conventional amplicon-based

- Reflects transcriptional activity
- Fast turnaround time
- Simple workflow

- Detects known fusions
- Dependent on RNA quality

D cDNA, anchored multiplex PCR

- Detects novel fusions
- Reflects transcriptional activity
- Fast turnaround time
- Simple workflow

- Dependent on RNA quality

E cDNA, 5' to 3' expression imbalance

- Detects novel fusions
- Fast turnaround time
- Simple workflow

- Dependent on RNA quality
- Sensitivity affected by endogenous expression
- Cannot identify partner gene and breakpoint

Fig. 3. Common NGS-based assay designs for gene fusion detection. Fusion breakpoints are often intronic. Genes are depicted with exons in wide bands and introns in thin lines. Detection at the DNA level (*A*) requires intronic bait tiling that can be costly. Furthermore, repetitive sequences and complex rearrangement events can be difficult to resolve with short-read sequencing. RNA (cDNA) sequencing detects transcriptionally active fusions. Target enrichment can be achieved through hybrid capture (*B*), opposing primer amplicons (*C*), anchored multiplex PCR (*D*), and 5' to 3' imbalance (*E*). Hybrid capture is highly scalable without the limitation of primer multiplexibility such as primer dimer formation. Amplicon-based methods have been believed to be more sensitive in low-input and low-purity specimens compared with hybrid capture. However, this could be variable with constantly optimized and diversified assay designs in recent literature. The main downside of conventional opposing primer amplicons is inability to cover novel fusions (*C*). Anchored multiplex PCR (AMP) amplifies a fusion sequence using gene-specific primer on one side and adapter-based primer on the other side, allowing detection without the identity of the partner gene (*D*). Expression imbalance has been used by several non-NGS and NGS platforms such as the Oncomine panels. In fusion-negative tumors (*E*, upper part), there will be approximately equal expressions of the 3' and 5' amplicons. In fusion-positive tumors (*E*, lower part), the 5' region, which is incorporated by the fusion, is overrepresented in tumor transcriptome compared with the 3' region. In tissues with high endogenous expression of the wildtype gene, expression imbalance may be obscured leading to suboptimal sensitivity.

International Thyroid Oncology Group published a consensus document on molecular testing in thyroid cancer.[103] The expert panel recommends applying either upfront use of comprehensive NGS or a multi-step approach in identifying therapeutic targets in advanced DTC. The advantages of multi-step testing, starting with a screening test for the *BRAF* V600 E mutation followed by fusion testing using NGS or FISH in *BRAF*-negative cases, may include lower cost and faster turn-around time compared with NGS, given that *BRAF* V600 E accounts for the majority of PTC and is mutually exclusive with kinase fusions in the pretreatment setting. The advantage of upfront use of NGS may include workflow acceleration for rapidly progressive tumors such as ATC and tissue conservation for small biopsies and cytologic samples. For characterizing acquired therapy resistance, a comprehensive panel analysis will be the most ideal for exploring various on-target and bypassing mechanisms.

SUMMARY

Despite the remarkable advances in targeted therapy for thyroid cancer in recent years, several areas remain to be elucidated by future research. Firstly, although tumors driven by *ALK* and *ROS1* fusions have standard targeted therapy in the pulmonary setting, those of thyroid origin are not currently FDA-approved indications of *ALK* and *ROS1* inhibitors. *MET* fusions are even rarer and also in need of evidence-based therapy. Secondly, microsatellite instability (MSI) status and tumor mutation burden (TMB) are increasingly recognized predictors of immunotherapy response. However, MSI have only been reported in a small number of thyroid carcinomas with limited data on their clinical behavior.[19,41,104,105] TMB, when assessed using targeted panels instead of whole-exome sequencing, is well known to be affected by sequencing panel design and preanalytical factors such as tumor purity and tissue quality. Standardization of TMB assessment is an ongoing effort in the field to provide solid guidance for clinical decision-making. Lastly, several intracellular pathways implicated in the high-grade transformation of thyroid carcinoma, such as the PI3K/Akt/mTOR pathway, SWI/SNF chromatin-remodeling complexes, and histone-modifying enzymes, are the targets of a rapidly growing armamentarium of novel therapeutics, which stand great promises as new treatment options in the near future.

ACKNOWLEDGMENT

Dr. Chu prepared Figure 2 with materials from Massachusetts General Hospital in Boston, Massachusetts, United States from a study mentored by Dr. Peter M. Sadow.

REFERENCES

1. Megwalu UC, Moon PK. Thyroid cancer incidence and mortality trends in the United States: 2000-2018. Thyroid 2022;32(5):560–70.
2. Lim H, Devesa SS, Sosa JA, et al. Trends in Thyroid Cancer Incidence and Mortality in the United States, 1974-2013. JAMA 2017;317(13):1338–48.
3. Tuttle RM, Ahuja S, Avram AM, et al. Controversies, consensus, and collaboration in the use of (131)i therapy in differentiated thyroid cancer: a joint statement from the american thyroid association, the european association of nuclear medicine, the society of nuclear medicine and molecular imaging, and the european thyroid association. Thyroid 2019;29(4):461–70.
4. Durante C, Haddy N, Baudin E, et al. Long-term outcome of 444 patients with distant metastases from papillary and follicular thyroid carcinoma: benefits and limits of radioiodine therapy. J Clin Endocrinol Metab 2006;91(8):2892–9.
5. Wong KS, Dong F, Telatar M, et al. Papillary thyroid carcinoma with high-grade features versus poorly differentiated thyroid carcinoma: an analysis of clinicopathologic and molecular features and outcome. Thyroid 2021;31(6):933–40.
6. Ibrahimpasic T, Ghossein R, Carlson DL, et al. Outcomes in patients with poorly differentiated thyroid carcinoma. J Clin Endocrinol Metab 2014;99(4):1245–52.
7. The Cancer Genome Atlas Research Network. Integrated genomic characterization of papillary thyroid carcinoma. Cell 2014;159(3):676–90.
8. Yoo SK, Lee S, Kim SJ, et al. Comprehensive Analysis of the Transcriptional and Mutational Landscape of Follicular and Papillary Thyroid Cancers. PLoS Genet 2016;12(8):e1006239.
9. Pekova B, Sykorova V, Dvorakova S, et al. RET, NTRK, ALK, BRAF, and MET Fusions in a large cohort of pediatric papillary thyroid carcinomas. Thyroid 2020;30(12):1771–80.
10. Morton LM, Karyadi DM, Stewart C, et al. Radiation-related genomic profile of papillary thyroid carcinoma after the Chernobyl accident. Science 2021;372(6543):eabg2538–725.
11. Chu YH, Wirth LJ, Farahani AA, et al. Clinicopathologic features of kinase fusion-related thyroid carcinomas: an integrative analysis with molecular characterization. Mod Pathol 2020;33(12):2458–72.
12. Vanden Borre P, Schrock AB, Anderson PM, et al. pediatric, adolescent, and young adult thyroid carcinoma harbors frequent and diverse targetable genomic alterations, including kinase fusions. Oncologist 2017;22(3):255–63.
13. Lee YC, Hsu CY, Lai CR, et al. NTRK-rearranged papillary thyroid carcinoma demonstrates frequent subtle nuclear features and indeterminate cytologic diagnoses. Cancer Cytopathol 2022;130(2):136–43.
14. Panebianco F, Nikitski AV, Nikiforova MN, et al. Characterization of thyroid cancer driven by known and novel ALK fusions. Endocr Relat Cancer 2019;26(11):803–14.
15. Viswanathan K, Chu YH, Faquin WC, et al. Cytomorphologic features of NTRK-rearranged thyroid carcinoma. Cancer Cytopathol 2020;128(11):812–27.
16. Abi-Raad R, Prasad ML, Adeniran AJ, et al. Fine-needle aspiration cytomorphology of papillary thyroid carcinoma with NTRK gene rearrangement from a case series with predominantly indeterminate cytology. Cancer Cytopathol 2020;128(11):803–11.
17. Prasad ML, Vyas M, Horne MJ, et al. NTRK fusion oncogenes in pediatric papillary thyroid carcinoma in northeast United States. Cancer 2016;122(7):1097–107.
18. Desai MA, Mehrad M, Ely KA, et al. secretory carcinoma of the thyroid gland: report of a highly

aggressive case clinically mimicking undifferentiated carcinoma and review of the literature. Head Neck Pathol 2019;13(4):562–72.

19. Landa I, Ibrahimpasic T, Boucai L, et al. Genomic and transcriptomic hallmarks of poorly differentiated and anaplastic thyroid cancers. J Clin Invest 2016;126(3):1052–66.

20. Pozdeyev N, Gay LM, Sokol ES, et al. Genetic analysis of 779 advanced differentiated and anaplastic thyroid cancers. Clin Cancer Res 2018;24(13): 3059–68.

21. Kunstman JW, Juhlin CC, Goh G, et al. Characterization of the mutational landscape of anaplastic thyroid cancer via whole-exome sequencing. Hum Mol Genet 2015;24(8):2318–29.

22. Xu B, David J, Dogan S, et al. Primary high-grade non-anaplastic thyroid carcinoma: a retrospective study of 364 cases. Histopathology 2022;80(2): 322–37.

23. Kumari S, Adewale R, Klubo-Gwiezdzinska J. The molecular landscape of hürthle cell thyroid cancer is associated with altered mitochondrial function-a comprehensive review. Cells 2020;9(7):1570.

24. Ganly I, Makarov V, Deraje S, et al. Integrated genomic analysis of hürthle cell cancer reveals oncogenic drivers, recurrent mitochondrial mutations, and unique chromosomal landscapes. Cancer Cell 2018;34(2):256–70.e255.

25. Gopal RK, Kübler K, Calvo SE, et al. Widespread chromosomal losses and mitochondrial DNA alterations as genetic drivers in hürthle cell carcinoma. Cancer Cell 2018;34(2):242–55.e245.

26. Gasparre G, Porcelli AM, Bonora E, et al. Disruptive mitochondrial DNA mutations in complex I subunits are markers of oncocytic phenotype in thyroid tumors. Proc Natl Acad Sci U S A 2007;104(21): 9001–6.

27. Cruz-Migoni A, Canning P, Quevedo CE, et al. Structure-based development of new RAS-effector inhibitors from a combination of active and inactive RAS-binding compounds. Proc Natl Acad Sci U S A 2019;116(7):2545–50.

28. Liu J, Kang R, Tang D. The KRAS-G12C inhibitor: activity and resistance. Cancer Gene Ther 2022; 29(7):875–8.

29. Stransky N, Cerami E, Schalm S, et al. The landscape of kinase fusions in cancer. Nat Commun 2014;5:4846.

30. Schlumberger M, Tahara M, Wirth LJ, et al. Lenvatinib versus placebo in radioiodine-refractory thyroid cancer. N Engl J Med 2015;372(7): 621–30.

31. Brose MS, Nutting CM, Jarzab B, et al. Sorafenib in radioactive iodine-refractory, locally advanced or metastatic differentiated thyroid cancer: a randomised, double-blind, phase 3 trial. Lancet 2014; 384(9940):319–28.

32. Subbiah V, Cote GJ. Advances in targeting RET-dependent cancers. Cancer Discov 2020;10(4): 498–505.

33. Brose MS, Cabanillas ME, Cohen EE, et al. Vemurafenib in patients with BRAF(V600E)-positive metastatic or unresectable papillary thyroid cancer refractory to radioactive iodine: a non-randomised, multicentre, open-label, phase 2 trial. Lancet Oncol 2016;17(9):1272–82.

34. Subbiah V, Kreitman RJ, Wainberg ZA, et al. Dabrafenib and trametinib treatment in patients with locally advanced or metastatic BRAF V600-mutant anaplastic thyroid cancer. J Clin Oncol 2018; 36(1):7–13.

35. Subbiah V, Kreitman RJ, Wainberg ZA, et al. Dabrafenib plus trametinib in patients with BRAF V600E-mutant anaplastic thyroid cancer: updated analysis from the phase II ROAR basket study. Ann Oncol 2022;33(4):406–15.

36. Poulikakos PI, Zhang C, Bollag G, et al. RAF inhibitors transactivate RAF dimers and ERK signalling in cells with wild-type BRAF. Nature 2010; 464(7287):427–30.

37. Purdie KJ, Proby CM, Rizvi H, et al. The Role of Human Papillomaviruses and Polyomaviruses in BRAF-Inhibitor Induced Cutaneous Squamous Cell Carcinoma and Benign Squamoproliferative Lesions. Front Microbiol 2018;9:1806.

38. Cabanillas ME, Dadu R, Iyer P, et al. Acquired secondary RAS mutation in BRAF(V600E)-mutated thyroid cancer patients treated with BRAF inhibitors. Thyroid 2020;30(9):1288–96.

39. Ho AL, Grewal RK, Leboeuf R, et al. Selumetinib-enhanced radioiodine uptake in advanced thyroid cancer. N Engl J Med 2013;368(7):623–32.

40. Tchekmedyian V, Dunn L, Sherman E, et al. Enhancing radioiodine incorporation in BRAF-mutant, radioiodine-refractory thyroid cancers with vemurafenib and the anti-ErbB3 monoclonal antibody CDX-3379: results of a pilot clinical trial. Thyroid 2022;32(3):273–82.

41. Qiao PP, Tian KS, Han LT, et al. Correlation of mismatch repair deficiency with clinicopathological features and programmed death-ligand 1 expression in thyroid carcinoma. Endocrine 2022;76(3):660–70.

42. Wirth LJ, Sherman E, Robinson B, et al. Efficacy of selpercatinib in RET-altered thyroid cancers. N Engl J Med 2020;383(9):825–35.

43. Subbiah V, Hu MI, Wirth LJ, et al. Pralsetinib for patients with advanced or metastatic RET-altered thyroid cancer (ARROW): a multi-cohort, open-label, registrational, phase 1/2 study. Lancet Diabetes Endocrinol 2021;9(8):491–501.

44. Hong DS, DuBois SG, Kummar S, et al. Larotrectinib in patients with TRK fusion-positive solid tumours: a pooled analysis of three phase 1/2 clinical trials. Lancet Oncol 2020;21(4):531–40.

45. Laetsch TW, DuBois SG, Mascarenhas L, et al. Larotrectinib for paediatric solid tumours harbouring NTRK gene fusions: phase 1 results from a multicentre, open-label, phase 1/2 study. Lancet Oncol 2018;19(5):705–14.

46. Waguespack SG, Drilon A, Lin JJ, et al. Efficacy and safety of larotrectinib in patients with TRK fusion-positive thyroid carcinoma. Eur J Endocrinol 2022;186(6):631–43.

47. Doebele RC, Drilon A, Paz-Ares L, et al. Entrectinib in patients with advanced or metastatic NTRK fusion-positive solid tumours: integrated analysis of three phase 1-2 trials. Lancet Oncol 2020; 21(2):271–82.

48. Drilon A, Li G, Dogan S, et al. What hides behind the MASC: clinical response and acquired resistance to entrectinib after ETV6-NTRK3 identification in a mammary analogue secretory carcinoma (MASC). Ann Oncol 2016;27(5):920–6.

49. Drilon A, Laetsch TW, Kummar S, et al. Efficacy of larotrectinib in TRK fusion-positive cancers in adults and children. N Engl J Med 2018;378(8): 731–9.

50. Russo M, Misale S, Wei G, et al. Acquired resistance to the TRK inhibitor entrectinib in colorectal cancer. Cancer Discov 2016;6(1):36–44.

51. Hong DS, Bauer TM, Lee JJ, et al. Larotrectinib in adult patients with solid tumours: a multi-centre, open-label, phase I dose-escalation study. Ann Oncol 2019;30(2):325–31.

52. Florou V, Nevala-Plagemann C, Whisenant J, et al. clinical activity of selitrectinib in a patient with mammary analogue secretory carcinoma of the parotid gland with secondary resistance to entrectinib. J Natl Compr Canc Netw 2021;19(5):478–82.

53. Murray BW, Rogers E, Zhai D, et al. Molecular characteristics of repotrectinib that enable potent inhibition of TRK fusion proteins and resistant mutations. Mol Cancer Ther 2021;20(12):2446–56.

54. Demeure MJ, Aziz M, Rosenberg R, et al. Whole-genome sequencing of an aggressive BRAF wild-type papillary thyroid cancer identified EML4-ALK translocation as a therapeutic target. World J Surg 2014;38(6):1296–305.

55. de Salins V, Loganadane G, Joly C, et al. Complete response in anaplastic lymphoma kinase-rearranged oncocytic thyroid cancer: a case report and review of literature. World J Clin Oncol 2020; 11(7):495–503.

56. Leroy L, Bonhomme B, Le Moulec S, et al. Remarkable response to ceritinib and brigatinib in an anaplastic lymphoma kinase-rearranged anaplastic thyroid carcinoma previously treated with crizotinib. Thyroid 2020;30(2):343–4.

57. Godbert Y, Henriques de Figueiredo B, Bonichon F, et al. Remarkable response to crizotinib in woman with anaplastic lymphoma kinase-rearranged anaplastic thyroid carcinoma. J Clin Oncol 2015; 33(20):e84–7.

58. Hillier K, Hughes A, Shamberger RC, et al. A novel ALK fusion in pediatric medullary thyroid carcinoma. Thyroid 2019;29(11):1704–7.

59. Dagogo-Jack I, Rooney M, Lin JJ, et al. Treatment with next-generation ALK inhibitors fuels plasma ALK mutation diversity. Clin Cancer Res 2019; 25(22):6662–70.

60. Toyokawa G, Seto T. Updated evidence on the mechanisms of resistance to ALK inhibitors and strategies to overcome such resistance: clinical and preclinical data. Oncol Res Treat 2015;38(6):291–8.

61. Lim SM, Chang H, Yoon MJ, et al. A multicenter, phase II trial of everolimus in locally advanced or metastatic thyroid cancer of all histologic subtypes. Ann Oncol 2013;24(12):3089–94.

62. Hanna GJ, Busaidy NL, Chau NG, et al. Genomic correlates of response to everolimus in aggressive radioiodine-refractory thyroid cancer: a phase II study. Clin Cancer Res 2018;24(7):1546–53.

63. Schneider TC, de Wit D, Links TP, et al. Everolimus in patients with advanced follicular-derived thyroid cancer: results of a phase II clinical trial. J Clin Endocrinol Metab 2017;102(2):698–707.

64. Roman S, Lin R, Sosa JA. Prognosis of medullary thyroid carcinoma: demographic, clinical, and pathologic predictors of survival in 1252 cases. Cancer 2006;107(9):2134–42.

65. Stamatakos M, Paraskeva P, Stefanaki C, et al. Medullary thyroid carcinoma: The third most common thyroid cancer reviewed. Oncol Lett 2011; 2(1):49–53.

66. Wells SA Jr, Asa SL, Dralle H, et al. Revised american thyroid association guidelines for the management of medullary thyroid carcinoma. Thyroid 2015; 25(6):567–610.

67. Gujral TS, Singh VK, Jia Z, et al. Molecular mechanisms of RET receptor-mediated oncogenesis in multiple endocrine neoplasia 2B. Cancer Res 2006;66(22):10741–9.

68. Chu YH, Lloyd RV. Medullary thyroid carcinoma: recent advances including MicroRNA expression. Endocr Pathol 2016;27(4):312–24.

69. Leboulleux S, Travagli JP, Caillou B, et al. Medullary thyroid carcinoma as part of a multiple endocrine neoplasia type 2B syndrome: influence of the stage on the clinical course. Cancer 2002;94(1):44–50.

70. Moura MM, Cavaco BM, Pinto AE, et al. Correlation of RET somatic mutations with clinicopathological features in sporadic medullary thyroid carcinomas. Br J Cancer 2009;100(11):1777–83.

71. Grubbs EG, Ng PK, Bui J, et al. RET fusion as a novel driver of medullary thyroid carcinoma. J Clin Endocrinol Metab 2015;100(3):788–93.

72. Kasaian K, Wiseman SM, Walker BA, et al. Putative BRAF activating fusion in a medullary thyroid

cancer. Cold Spring Harb Mol Case Stud 2016; 2(2):a000729.

73. Ji JH, Oh YL, Hong M, et al. Identification of driving ALK fusion genes and genomic landscape of medullary thyroid cancer. PLoS Genet 2015;11(8): e1005467.

74. Jr SAW, Robinson BG, Gagel RF, et al. Vandetanib in patients with locally advanced or metastatic medullary thyroid cancer: a randomized, double-blind phase III trial. J Clin Oncol 2012;30(2): 134–41.

75. Elisei R, Schlumberger MJ, Müller SP, et al. Cabozantinib in progressive medullary thyroid cancer. J Clin Oncol 2013;31(29):3639–46.

76. Brose MS, Robinson B, Sherman SI, et al. Cabozantinib for radioiodine-refractory differentiated thyroid cancer (COSMIC-311): a randomised, double-blind, placebo-controlled, phase 3 trial. Lancet Oncol 2021;22(8):1126–38.

77. Solomon BJ, Tan L, Lin JJ, et al. RET Solvent Front Mutations Mediate Acquired Resistance to Selective RET Inhibition in RET-Driven Malignancies. J Thorac Oncol 2020;15(4):541–9.

78. Subbiah V, Shen T, Terzyan SS, et al. Structural basis of acquired resistance to selpercatinib and pralsetinib mediated by non-gatekeeper RET mutations. Ann Oncol 2021;32(2):261–8.

79. Drilon AE, Zhai D, Rogers E, et al. The next-generation RET inhibitor TPX-0046 is active in drug-resistant and naïve RET-driven cancer models. J Clin Oncol 2020;38(15_suppl):3616.

80. Moura MM, Cavaco BM, Pinto AE, et al. High prevalence of RAS mutations in RET-negative sporadic medullary thyroid carcinomas. J Clin Endocrinol Metab 2011;96(5):E863–8.

81. Tate JG, Bamford S, Jubb HC, et al. COSMIC: the catalogue of somatic mutations in cancer. Nucleic Acids Res 2019;47(D1):D941–7.

82. Moore AR, Rosenberg SC, McCormick F, et al. RAS-targeted therapies: is the undruggable drugged? Nat Rev Drug Discov 2020;19(8): 533–52.

83. Hong DS, Cabanillas ME, Wheler J, et al. Inhibition of the Ras/Raf/MEK/ERK and RET kinase pathways with the combination of the multikinase inhibitor sorafenib and the farnesyltransferase inhibitor tipifarnib in medullary and differentiated thyroid malignancies. J Clin Endocrinol Metab 2011; 96(4):997–1005.

84. Loo E, Khalili P, Beuhler K, et al. BRAF V600E mutation across multiple tumor types: correlation between DNA-based sequencing and mutation-specific immunohistochemistry. Appl Immunohistochem Mol Morphol 2018;26(10):709–13.

85. Ritterhouse LL, Barletta JA. BRAF V600E mutation-specific antibody: a review. Semin Diagn Pathol 2015;32(5):400–8.

86. Saliba M, Katabi N, Dogan S, et al. NRAS Q61R immunohistochemical staining in thyroid pathology: sensitivity, specificity and utility. Histopathology 2021;79(4):650–60.

87. Crescenzi A, Fulciniti F, Bongiovanni M, et al. Detecting N-RAS Q61R Mutated Thyroid Neoplasias by Immunohistochemistry. Endocr Pathol 2017; 28(1):71–4.

88. Solomon JP, Linkov I, Rosado A, et al. NTRK fusion detection across multiple assays and 33,997 cases: diagnostic implications and pitfalls. Mod Pathol 2020;33(1):38–46.

89. Solomon JP, Hechtman JF. Detection of NTRK fusions: merits and limitations of current diagnostic platforms. Cancer Res 2019;79(13):3163–8.

90. Park G, Kim TH, Lee HO, et al. Standard immunohistochemistry efficiently screens for anaplastic lymphoma kinase rearrangements in differentiated thyroid cancer. Endocr Relat Cancer 2015;22(1): 55–63.

91. Chou A, Fraser S, Toon CW, et al. A detailed clinicopathologic study of ALK-translocated papillary thyroid carcinoma. Am J Surg Pathol 2015;39(5): 652–9.

92. Yang SR, Aypar U, Rosen EY, et al. A performance comparison of commonly used assays to detect RET fusions. Clin Cancer Res 2021;27(5):1316–28.

93. Nozaki Y, Yamamoto H, Iwasaki T, et al. Clinicopathological features and immunohistochemical utility of NTRK-, ALK-, and ROS1-rearranged papillary thyroid carcinomas and anaplastic thyroid carcinomas. Hum Pathol 2020;106:82–92.

94. Lee YC, Chen JY, Huang CJ, et al. Detection of NTRK1/3 rearrangements in papillary thyroid carcinoma using immunohistochemistry, fluorescent in situ hybridization, and next-generation sequencing. Endocr Pathol 2020;31(4):348–58.

95. Rosenbaum JN, Bloom R, Forys JT, et al. Genomic heterogeneity of ALK fusion breakpoints in non-small-cell lung cancer. Mod Pathol 2018;31(5): 791–808.

96. Chu YH, Barbee J, Yang SR, et al. Clinical utility and performance of an ultrarapid multiplex RNA-based assay for detection of ALK, ROS1, RET, and NTRK1/2/3 rearrangements and MET exon 14 skipping alterations. J Mol Diagn 2022;24(6): 642–54.

97. Tong Y, Zhao Z, Liu B, et al. 5′/3′ imbalance strategy to detect ALK fusion genes in circulating tumor RNA from patients with non-small cell lung cancer. J Exp Clin Cancer Res 2018;37(1):68.

98. Liu Y, Wu S, Shi X, et al. Clinical evaluation of the effectiveness of fusion-induced asymmetric transcription assay-based reverse transcription droplet digital PCR for ALK detection in formalin-fixed paraffin-embedded samples from lung cancer. Thorac Cancer 2020;11(8):2252–61.

99. Lira ME, Choi YL, Lim SM, et al. A single-tube multiplexed assay for detecting ALK, ROS1, and RET fusions in lung cancer. J Mol Diagn 2014;16(2): 229–43.

100. Rogers TM, Arnau GM, Ryland GL, et al. Multiplexed transcriptome analysis to detect ALK, ROS1 and RET rearrangements in lung cancer. Sci Rep 2017;7:42259.

101. Baitei EY, Zou M, Al-Mohanna F, et al. Aberrant BRAF splicing as an alternative mechanism for oncogenic B-Raf activation in thyroid carcinoma. J Pathol 2009;217(5):707–15.

102. Cocco E, Scaltriti M, Drilon A. NTRK fusion-positive cancers and TRK inhibitor therapy. Nat Rev Clin Oncol 2018;15(12):731–47.

103. Shonka DC Jr, Ho A, Chintakuntlawar AV, et al. american head and neck society endocrine surgery section and international thyroid oncology group consensus statement on mutational testing in thyroid cancer: defining advanced thyroid cancer and its targeted treatment. Head Neck 2022;44(6):1277–300.

104. Wong KS, Lorch JH, Alexander EK, et al. Clinicopathologic features of mismatch repair-deficient anaplastic thyroid carcinomas. Thyroid 2019; 29(5):666–73.

105. Genutis LK, Tomsic J, Bundschuh RA, et al. Microsatellite instability occurs in a subset of follicular thyroid cancers. Thyroid 2019;29(4):523–9.

FURTHER READING

1. Subbiah Vivek, Wolf Jürgen, Konda Bhavana, et al. Tumour-agnostic efficacy and safety of selpercatinib in patients with RET fusion-positive solid tumours other than lung or thyroid tumours (LIBRETTO-001): a phase 1/2, open-label, basket trial. Lancet Oncology 2022;23(10):1261–73. https://doi.org/10.1016/S1470-2045(22)00541-1. In this issue.

It Does Exist! Diagnosis and Management of Thyroid Carcinomas Originating in Struma Ovarii

Lynelle P. Smith, MD[a], Lindsay W. Brubaker, MD[b],
Rebecca J. Wolsky, MD[a],*

KEYWORDS

- Struma ovarii • Ovary • Teratoma • Papillary thyroid carcinoma (PTC)
- Follicular variant papillary thyroid carcinoma (FVPTC) • Follicular thyroid carcinoma (FTC)
- Highly differentiated follicular carcinoma arising from struma ovarii (HDFCO)

Key points

- Although rare, thyroid carcinoma can originate in struma ovarii.
- The most common type of thyroid carcinoma found in struma ovarii is papillary thyroid carcinoma.
- The cytologic features of thyroid carcinomas originating in struma ovarii can be bland and subtle.
- The diagnosis of highly differentiated follicular carcinoma arising from struma ovarii (HDFCO) should be considered in the event of extraovarian spread, including tumor morphologically resembling normal or hyperplastic thyroid tissue.

ABSTRACT

Thyroid carcinoma originating in struma ovarii comprises a small minority of all cases of struma ovarii. Given the rarity of this diagnosis, literature to guide evaluation and management is limited. The most common carcinoma originating from struma ovarii is papillary thyroid carcinoma. Treatment includes surgery, including a fertility sparing approach if disease is confined to the ovary, with consideration of total thyroidectomy and radioactive iodine ablation for high-risk pathologic features or disease spread beyond the ovary. This review discusses the histopathologic findings, molecular pathology, clinical implications and management, and prognosis of thyroid carcinomas originating in struma ovarii.

OVERVIEW

Teratomas are the most common ovarian germ cell tumor accounting for approximately 20% of all ovarian tumors.[1,2] A teratoma is a neoplasm composed of tissues derived from the 3 embryological germ cell layers (endoderm, mesoderm, and ectoderm); teratomas can be broadly subdivided into mature teratomas and immature teratomas.[1] Mature teratomas are comprised exclusively of mature adult-type tissues not native to the ovary, commonly including hair, skin, teeth, bone, and thyroid tissues, and follow a benign course with specific exceptions of malignant tumors originating within mature teratoma.[2] In some cases, teratomas can be composed predominantly or exclusively of one tissue type, termed a monodermal or specialized teratoma.[1]

---

[a] Department of Pathology, University of Colorado School of Medicine, 12605 East 16th Avenue, Mail Stop F768, Aurora, CO 80045, USA; [b] Department of Obstetrics and Gynecology, Division of Gynecologic Oncology, University of Colorado School of Medicine, Academic Office 1 12631 East 17th Avenue, B198-6, Aurora, CO 80045, USA
* Corresponding author.
E-mail address: rebecca.wolsky@cuanschutz.edu

Surgical Pathology 16 (2023) 75–86
https://doi.org/10.1016/j.path.2022.09.008
1875-9181/23/© 2022 Elsevier Inc. All rights reserved.

Teratomas containing any amount of mature thyroid tissue make up approximately 20% of all ovarian teratomas.[3–5] Struma ovarii is a type of mature teratoma composed predominantly (≥50%) or exclusively of thyroid tissue, accounting for approximately 5% of all ovarian teratomas.[5,6] The thyroid tissue present in ovarian teratomas can be histologically similar to normal, hyperplastic/adenomatous, or carcinomatous thyroid tissue, alone or in combination.[7]

A rare finding is a malignancy originating within struma ovarii. In the past, the term "malignant struma ovarii" was favored. However, this term has been applied to 2 distinct scenarios: (1) histologic carcinoma originating within struma ovarii and (2) ovarian surface involvement, extraovarian spread, and/or metastases (biological malignancy) of otherwise benign-appearing or proliferative struma ovarii. Owing to this ambiguity, this diagnosis of "malignant struma ovarii" is no longer recommended.[8] Rather, the preferred terminology is more specifically thyroid carcinoma originating in struma ovarii.[2] This most commonly occurs in women in their fourth or fifth decade of life.[6] The true incidence of thyroid carcinoma originating in struma ovarii is difficult to determine; however, it has been estimated to represent 0.5% to 10% of all struma ovarii.[2] The most common carcinoma to originate from struma ovarii is papillary thyroid carcinoma (PTCSO); less frequently, the malignant component is follicular variant papillary thyroid carcinoma (FVPTCSO) or follicular thyroid carcinoma (FTCSO).[3,4,9] Anaplastic thyroid carcinoma and medullary thyroid carcinoma originating in struma ovarii have been reported in single case studies.[9] It is important to note that thyroid-type carcinomas can be found in the ovary outside of the context of struma ovarii. This includes thyroid carcinoma originating in a strumal carcinoid and metastasis to the ovary from a primary thyroid carcinoma.[2,10]

Due to the rare nature of this tumor, clinical management is not standardized and is largely based on available information from published case studies. The presence of recurrent molecular mutations in thyroid carcinomas originating in struma ovarii has become increasingly recognized and may have implications for the identification of malignant components of struma ovarii and treatment modalities.

CLINICAL FINDINGS/PRESENTATION

As with most teratomas, all forms of struma ovarii are typically found incidentally on imaging studies but may present with symptoms related to a pelvic mass such as lower abdominal pain, palpable mass, or abnormal vaginal bleeding.[2–4,9,11] Occasionally, patients may be found to have ascites, pleural effusion, and hyperthyroidism with radioactive iodine uptake localizing to the pelvis.[1,3,4,11] Features that are concerning for malignancy in a struma ovarii at the time of surgery include ovarian surface involvement, multifocal adhesions, peritoneal fluid (≥1L), serosal tear in the struma ovarii, and hemorrhagic ascites.[2,3,12] Often though, there is no indication of malignancy until microscopic review of the tumor. Metastasis has been documented in approximately 5% to 23% of thyroid carcinomas originating in struma ovarii.[13] The most common sites of metastatic disease include ascitic fluid, pelvic peritoneum, and other pelvic structures.[2,13] Less common sites of metastasis include abdominal peritoneum, lung, chest, omentum, bone, liver, rectum, and pelvic lymph nodes.[2,13] Follicular carcinoma shows a predilection for metastasis to the lung, liver, and central nervous system while papillary carcinoma favors the abdominal cavity, lymph nodes, and liver metastasis.[13] Metastatic disease most often presents as disease recurrence years after initial diagnosis with a median interval of approximately 14 years.[6]

Tumor markers such as CA125 have not been shown to be increased in cases of struma ovarii and, therefore, have no role in diagnosis.[4] Imaging studies, including ultrasound, computed tomography (CT), and MRI, do not show any distinctive features. Radiographically, struma ovarii are miscategorized in up to 98.2% of cases, most commonly as a dermoid cyst.[4]

Cases of previously unknown synchronous primary thyroid carcinoma and thyroid carcinoma originating in struma ovarii have been reported. The majority of reported synchronous thyroid carcinomas are papillary thyroid carcinoma (PTC).[2] Although there are no standardized guidelines to clinical monitoring and follow-up in patients with thyroid carcinoma originating in struma ovarii, clinical assessment of the thyroid for a previously undetected synchronous thyroid carcinoma is strongly encouraged.[2]

GROSS FEATURES

Struma ovarii is most often unilateral but can be bilateral or associated with a mature teratoma of the contralateral ovary containing no thyroid tissue.[1] Tumors have an average size of 12 ± 5 cm in greatest dimension.[1,3,4] Larger tumors as well as tumors with a larger proportion of struma ovarii are more likely to be associated with malignant transformation.[3] The tumors are predominantly solid but may have multiloculated or uniloculated cystic components. The cystic component, if present, contains mucinous/colloid type material.[1] On cut surface, the strumal component is beefy red-brown resembling normal thyroid tissue; the cystic components resemble follicular nodular disease of the native thyroid gland. Foci of malignancy tend to recapitulate findings of carcinoma in the native thyroid gland. Grossly, nodules are discrete and ill-defined, with color ranging from white to tan-brown as well as being described as having a green-brown tinge.[3,13] Surface adhesions, particularly when dense and numerous, are more associated with malignant tumors than with benign tumors.[3] It is important to note that malignant foci may be microscopic and thus undetectable on gross examination. Thus, thorough sampling of struma ovarii for microscopic review is always recommended.

MICROSCOPIC FEATURES AND DIAGNOSIS

Struma ovarii is composed of thyroid follicles of varying size that are lined by low cuboidal to columnar cells with pale eosinophilic cytoplasm (Fig. 1). Macrofollicular patterns are typically predominant but solid, microfollicular, trabecular, and pseudotrabecular patterns can be seen.[1] The nuclei are small, round to oval with evenly dispersed chromatin without crowding. The follicles are filled with brightly eosinophilic, homogenous colloid material that may contain the birefringent calcium oxalate monohydrate crystals

seen in normal thyroid colloid.[1,3] Struma ovarii histologically resembling normal, nonproliferative (nonadenomatous) thyroid gland tissue, without extraovarian spread, including lacking ovarian surface involvement, will almost always behave in a benign fashion. Rare case reports have described normal struma ovarii with malignant behavior, defined as extraovarian spread but adequate, thorough evaluation of the original ovarian tumors could not be confirmed on later review.[3]

The histopathologic criteria for thyroid carcinoma originating in struma ovarii mirror those in primary thyroid carcinoma (Fig. 2). Features of PTC include true papillary formation with a central fibrovascular core lined by cuboidal to columnar epithelial cells. The neoplastic epithelial cells show an increased nuclear to cytoplasmic ratio with nuclear crowding; nuclei are round to oval with powdery to optically clear chromatin and irregular nuclear membranes resulting in nuclear grooves and pseudoinclusions.[13,14] These nuclear features of PTC are considered diagnostic of malignancy in PTCSO.[14] The finding of psammoma bodies is highly supportive of the diagnosis of malignancy in this setting and, when present, is less likely to represent a benign proliferative lesion.[3,13,14]

FVPTCSO displays the characteristic cytologic features of PTC but, by definition, lacks papillary architecture, instead demonstrating a follicular pattern of growth comprising at least 99% of the tumor[14] (Fig. 3). In the native thyroid gland proper, follicular variant papillary thyroid carcinoma

Fig. 1. Benign struma ovarii with normal appearing thyroid follicles of varying size lined by low cuboidal cells containing pale eosinophilic cytoplasm and small round nuclei with even chromatin. The nuclear to cytoplasmic ratio is maintained, and there is no nuclear crowding or atypia. The follicles contain bright, eosinophilic, homogenous colloid material (400×).

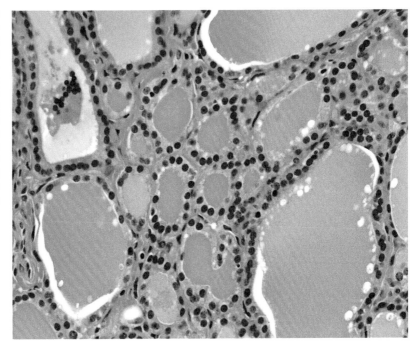

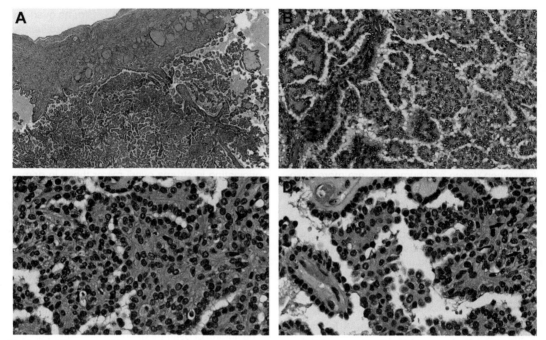

Fig. 2. Papillary thyroid carcinoma originating in struma ovarii. (*A*) Low-power image showing papillary thyroid carcinoma (bottom) adjacent to thyroid follicles of benign struma ovarii (top) (20×). (*B*) PTC with true papillae lined by cuboidal to columnar epithelial cells with increased nuclear to cytoplasmic ratio. The nuclei are oval with significant crowding, irregular nuclear membranes, and powdery to optically clear chromatin (100×). (*C*) Prominent nuclear membrane irregularity with nuclear grooves, occasional pseudoinclusions, and rare mitotic figures (*arrowhead*) (200×). (*D*) Nuclear pseudoinclusions (*arrows*) (200×).

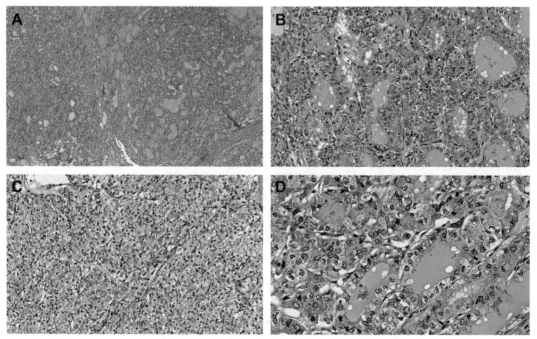

Fig. 3. Follicular variant papillary thyroid carcinoma originating in struma ovarii. (*A*) Low-power image showing both microfollicular and macrofollicular growth patterns lacking the formation of true papillae (20×). (*B*) The follicles are lined by cuboidal to columnar cells with nuclear crowding (100×). (*C*) Areas of microfollicular to solid trabecular growth pattern (100×). (*D*) The nuclei are round to oval and demonstrate optically clear to powdery chromatin and nuclear membrane irregularity including grooves (200×).

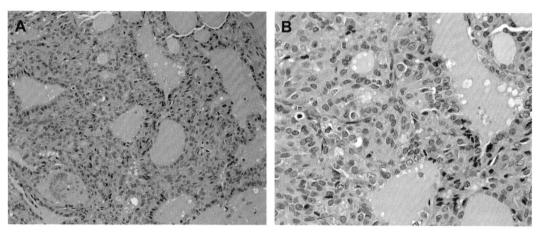

Fig. 4. Subtle features of PTC in struma ovarii. (A) A case of struma ovarii that is composed predominantly of benign thyroid follicles with evenly spaced nuclei, smooth nuclear borders and even chromatin (200×) *(B)* Focally there is nuclear crowding, irregular nuclear membranes with occasional grooves but lacking pseudoinculsions and characteristic powdery to optically clear chromatin (400×).

(FVPTC) is distinguished from the more recently described neoplastic entity, noninvasive follicular thyroid neoplasm with papillary-like nuclear features (NIFTP). This neoplasm with low biological potential for aggressive behavior is similar to circumscribed FVPTC that lacks invasion. NIFTP by name has not been reported in the struma ovarii literature, to our knowledge, although this is not surprising given that the majority of thyroid carcinomas and adenomatous lesions in struma ovarii lack distinct capsules.

Subtle features of PTC that are easily overlooked, or initially judged as not reaching the threshold for carcinoma in the native thyroid, have been described in patients with subsequent metastatic disease (Fig. 4). These bland yet key features can be focal and include nuclear enlargement, crowding, and chromatin clearing without classical nuclear pseudoinclusions or grooves.[2,14] Thorough sampling for microscopic review with attention to nuclear detail is warranted. In one such case (Patient #2 in Garg and colleagues[14]), cytologic features within the struma ovarii were limited to subtle foci of irregular nuclei, whereas the recurrence was unequivocally diagnostic of PTCSO. In another example, focally angulated, overlapping nuclei with fine powdery chromatin and nuclear grooves were concerning for PTCSO but the lack of nuclear pseudoinclusions, as well as papillary or infiltrative growth, ultimately resulted in a descriptive diagnosis of struma ovarii with atypical features. This descriptive diagnosis was sufficient to prompt referral to endocrinology and thyroid ultrasound revealed a 4-cm heterogenous nodule diagnosed as PTC on fine needle aspiration. In a review of 195 patients with "malignant struma ovarii," synchronous thyroid carcinoma in struma ovarii and the thyroid gland were reported in 6.2% of cases.[2]

Similar to subtle PTCSO, FTCSO originating in struma ovarii can be difficult to definitively diagnose, particularly well-differentiated FTCSO.[13] In the thyroid, histological identification of definitive capsular invasion or vascular invasion is necessary to be classified as follicular carcinoma. In struma ovarii, follicular lesions are typically unencapsulated and the ovarian surface should not be considered a capsule. The lack of a capsule makes the identification of invasion incumbent on invasion into surrounding normal ovarian tissue, vascular invasion, or inferred by evidence of malignant behavior.[3,13,15] In order to differentiate from artifact, definitive vascular invasion requires sculpting to the vascular contours and/or adherence to the vessel wall, as well as involvement of numerous vessels.[3] Neoplastic cells in this category can be arranged in trabeculae, microfollicles, macrofollicles, or even grow as solid sheets, with varying amounts of colloid present. Cytologically, the neoplastic cells show an increased nuclear to cytoplasmic ratio, various degrees of nuclear pleomorphism, and nuclear hyperchromasia.[14] Nuclear membrane irregularities typical of PTC (grooves, pseudoinclusions) are not seen in FTCSO.[14] Without evidence of malignancy by invasion, many of these lesions are categorized as proliferative struma ovarii (adenoma or hyperplasia). In some series, such cases have only declared themselves as malignant at disease recurrence.[3,4,13,14] It has been recommended that cases of struma ovarii with foci of borderline nuclear atypia and a follicular growth pattern should be reviewed by at least 2 pathologists to prevent overdiagnosis or underdiagnosis of thyroid carcinoma in struma ovarii.[14] More poorly differentiated follicular carcinomas are easier to identify histologically due to definitive architectural abnormalities, more significant nuclear atypia, and increased mitotic activity, all of which indicate a malignant diagnosis.[1,12,13,15,16]

Thyroid tissue with hyperplastic and adenomatous changes may be identified in struma ovarii, so called proliferative struma ovarii.[17] Architecturally, proliferative struma lesions are distinct from background thyroid tissue with the majority exhibiting a predominantly microfollicular or macrofollicular growth pattern, although the features of proliferative struma can be limited to hypercellularity or compact follicles exceeding normal. Rarely, proliferative struma may be composed exclusively of oxyphilic cells or with pseudopapillae. Proliferative/adenomatous lesions should lack features that are otherwise diagnostic of malignancy in the native thyroid gland.[3] In practice, strict histologic criteria for proliferative struma are difficult to define and an inevitable degree of subjectivity must be acknowledged. Importantly, recurrence and biologically malignant behavior has been documented, although rarely. Therefore, it has been suggested that proliferative struma should be considered to have low-grade malignant potential.[3]

Histologically benign-appearing extraovarian implants of thyroidal tissue in patients with struma ovarii have previously been described as "strumosis" but the term is now discouraged due to the implication of benignity.[3] Rather, peritoneal dissemination of well-differentiated thyroid tissue, including tissue histologically indistinguishable from normal thyroid, is favored to represent metastasis from a highly differentiated follicular carcinoma originating from struma ovarii (HDFCO).[1,8,15] One difficulty, not unique to this particular endocrine neoplasm, is that HDFCO cannot be diagnosed until extraovarian spread is discovered (**Fig. 5**). Furthermore, the interval from ovarian tumor to extraovarian dissemination has been reported as ranging from a few years to up to 48 years.[15] HDFCO may histologically resemble normal thyroid tissue or proliferative/adenomatous struma. In one illustrative example (case #3, Roth and colleagues[15] 2021), a patient in her early 20s underwent right ovarian cystectomy revealing histologically bland nodular struma ovarii with moderate variation in follicular size. Subsequently, she had local recurrence 3.5 years later and abdominal recurrences at 6 and 9 years postcystectomy. Thyroidectomy revealed only a benign colloid nodule, and the patient underwent I-131 therapy. At her last reported follow-up, 12 years after initial diagnosis, she was alive with disease. All lesions examined microscopically showed hypercellularity and adenomatous change but lacked features of carcinoma.

MOLECULAR PATHOLOGY FEATURES

Primary PTCs harbor a variety of well-known recurrent pathogenic molecular alterations such as *BRAF* V600 E mutation, *RET*, *NTRK*, *ALK*, or *BRAF* rearrangements,[13,18] whereas primary follicular thyroid carcinomas (FTCs) tend to have *RAS* mutations or *PPARg* rearrangements.[19] The molecular mutations present in primary thyroid carcinomas have been shown to predict clinical outcomes. The presence of similar recurrent molecular mutations in thyroid carcinomas originating in struma ovarii has been explored in several case reports and case series.[5,19–22]

The identification of recurrent molecular alterations of significance in struma ovarii is most frequently seen in cases of PTCSO and FVPTCSO. In one series, *BRAF* mutations were identified in 4 of 6 cases, 2 of which were PTCSO with *BRAF* V600 E mutations; the remaining 2 cases were FVPTCSO and harbored non-V600 E *BRAF* mutations.[20] Importantly, this same series showed that none of the 9 benign struma ovarii cases tested showed a mutation in *BRAF*.[20] A separate case series assessed 13 cases and found that 7 of the 10 cases with features of FVPTCSO exhibited a *RET* rearrangement.[22] These findings suggest that there is a similar carcinogenesis between primary thyroidal PTC/FVPTC and PTC/FVPTC originating in struma ovarii. The utility of molecular testing is of particular interest in determining if synchronous primary thyroid carcinomas and thyroid carcinomas originating in struma ovarii are mutationally related or independent primary tumors. One such case study reported that a patient with synchronous primary thyroid PTC and PTCSO indeed represented 2 separate primary tumors by molecular analysis.[23] Both tumors demonstrated *RAS* mutations; however, the primary thyroidal PTC had an *HRAS* Q61 R mutation; and the PTC in struma ovarii harbored an *NRAS* Q61 R mutation. These distinct point mutations in the well-known *RAS* oncogene were interpreted as evidence that the 2 tumors developed independently.[23]

Recurrent molecular alterations have not been as readily identified in FTCSO. Few case studies have been published assessing these tumors for molecular alterations of significance. One such study notes that the lack of significant recurrent molecular alterations typical of FTC is similar to the findings in pediatric FTC, which is usually negative for the common mutations in *RAS* and fusion transcripts with *PPARg*.[19]

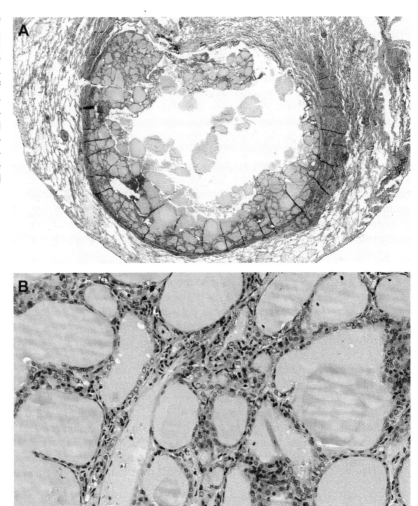

Fig. 5. Metastatic HDFCO in a patient with a known history of struma ovarii and no evidence of primary thyroid carcinoma. (*A*) Pulmonary metastasis of highly differentiated thyroid tissue. (*B*) The metastatic deposit is composed of well-differentiated thyroid follicles that are histologically indistinguishable from normal thyroid (100×).

The few struma ovarii and HDFCO that have been subject to testing lack the typical oncogenic driver molecular alterations typically seen in papillary or FTCSOs. Henderson and colleagues[24] reported struma ovarii and associated extraovarian spread as having identical mutations: segmental, and less commonly, complete whole genome homozygosity, attributed to errors in meiosis.

PROGNOSIS AND TREATMENT

Although the rare nature of these tumors makes it difficult to definitively assess prognosis, in general, thyroid carcinomas originating in struma ovarii, including HDFCO, seem to have a favorable prognosis.[15] Robboy and colleagues[3] found the overall survival for patients with thyroid carcinoma originating in struma ovarii at 10 and 25 years to be high at 81%, and 60%, respectively. Goffredo and colleagues[25] reported the overall survival of their cohort at 5, 10, and 20 years to be 96.7%,

94.3%, and 84.9%, respectively. The reported recurrence rates are varied from as low as 7.5% up to 35%.[6] Factors that have been suggested to portend poorer prognosis with associated rapid disease progression and even death include tumor size greater than 10 cm, larger strumal component (>80%), and extensive high-grade papillary carcinoma.[3,4,6,12]

Due to the favorable prognosis of thyroid carcinomas in struma ovarii, the treatment of such tumors should be highly individualized based on the patient characteristics and features of the tumor.[6] The surgical approaches reported in the literature include ovarian cystectomy, unilateral salpingo-oophorectomy, bilateral salpingo-oophorectomy, total abdominal hysterectomy and bilateral salpingo-oophorectomy, and debulking procedures in the cases of extraovarian spread. The aggressiveness of the surgical procedure relates to disease extent, patient age, and fertility status, with older, postmenopausal women more likely to undergo more extensive procedures than younger patients desiring preserved fertility.[6,12]

In addition to primary surgery, if malignant transformation is noted within a struma ovarii, a staging CT scan and ultrasound evaluation of the thyroid are recommended given risk of metastases or synchronous primary.[2,25,26] In a case series of 195 patient cases, identified through review of 104 individual studies, 25.1% of patients had metastatic disease at diagnosis and 6.2% had a synchronous primary carcinoma in the thyroid.[2] Given this risk, the evaluation and treatment of these patients should be performed in a multidisciplinary fashion, wherever possible, in close collaboration with head and neck surgery and endocrine specialists.[4]

Approaches to adjuvant treatment of carcinoma originating in struma ovarii vary. Some groups recommend thyroidectomy followed by ^{131}I ablation because it is thought to optimize survival and reduce recurrence risk.[27] The argument for thyroidectomy is 2-fold: it allows for thorough evaluation of the thyroid and the possibility of diagnosing microscopic disease, either metastasis or synchronous primary, as well as potentiation of ^{131}I ablation.[27] The resection of all normal thyroid tissue allows radioactive iodine to preferentially target metastatic thyroid carcinoma. In a case series of 24 cases, 4 patients received adjuvant therapy including both thyroidectomy and iodine radio-ablation, and none of these patients

experienced recurrence. Those that did recur in this series were treated with a combination of secondary debulking, thyroidectomy, and radioactive iodine, and most patients were alive without disease at follow-up.[27] However, other groups recommend thyroid ultrasound for all patients with malignant transformation, and low threshold for fine need aspiration, and ultimately risk stratification based on pathologic findings and extent of disease.[26,28]

In 2021, Addley and colleagues published an algorithm for adjuvant management of carcinoma in struma ovarii based on one institution's experience during 10 years. They describe high-risk histopathologic criteria as close surgical margins, greater than 10 mm PTCSO, lymphovascular invasion, aggressive histopathologic features, and *BRAF/RAS* mutations.[4] For early-stage disease based on intraoperative findings and CT scan, and low-risk pathologic features, they recommend completion unilateral salpingo-oophorectomy if cystectomy was performed, thyroid ultrasound with biopsy if indicated, and thyroid suppression to normal levels with levothyroxine with serum monitoring. For a patient with early-stage disease and high-risk pathologic features, they recommend completion unilateral salpingo-oophorectomy in the setting of initial cystectomy, consideration of total thyroidectomy with radioactive iodine ablation, and thyroid suppression to below normal levels with levothyroxine with serum monitoring. If there is concern for disease outside

---

Table 1
Differential diagnosis for struma ovarii and carcinoma arising in struma ovarii

Diagnosis	Distinguishing Morphologic and Immunohistochemical Features	Image
Serous cystadenoma	• Low cuboidal to columnar cells • Larger cystic spaces with increased variation in cyst size • Overall, lower cellularity • TTF1 negative • Can be particularly problematic at intraoperative frozen section	[See Fig. 6]
Granulosa cell tumor	• Nuclear grooves, without nuclear pseudoinclusions • Call-Exner bodies may mimic thyroid follicles but the lining cells show nuclei occupying more of the cell, rather than the basally oriented nuclei of thyroid tissue • TTF1 negative • FOXL2, SF-1 positive	[See Fig. 7]
Strumal carcinoid	• Synaptophysin/chromogranin positive	[See Fig. 8]
Primary thyroid carcinoma metastatic to ovary	• Distinction is based on history and absence of background struma ovarii/teratoma	

Fig. *6.* Serous cystadenoma 200×.

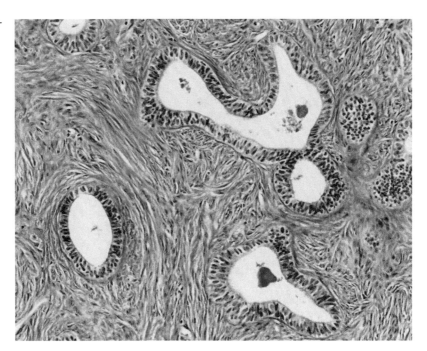

of the ovary, completion staging procedure is recommended, including total abdominal hysterectomy, bilateral salpingo-oophorectomy, and omentectomy; consideration of total thyroidectomy with radioactive iodine ablation; and thyroid suppression with levothyroxine with serum monitoring.[4] In other words, if the disease seems confined to the ovary, a fertility sparing approach is indicated; however, a complete oophorectomy is recommended. The utility of thyroid-directed therapy, including both thyroidectomy and ^{131}I ablation, can be considered if high-risk pathologic features are found, or if there is concern for disease outside of the ovary. For any patients who undergo thyroidectomy and ^{131}I ablation, the goal is to achieve undetectable thyroglobulin levels by 6 to 12 months posttreatment.[4]

Fig. 7. Granulosa cell tumor 40×.

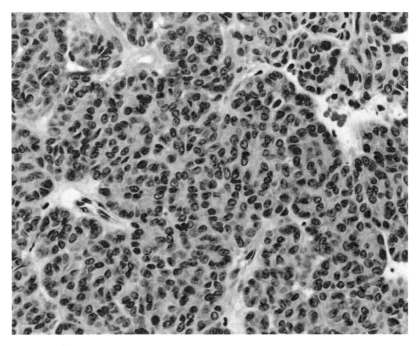

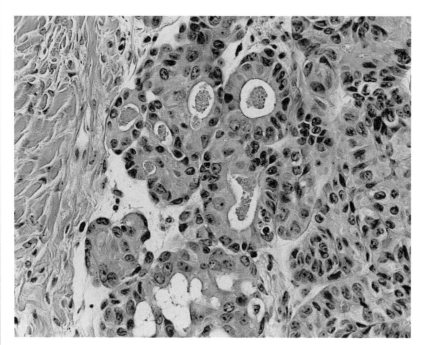

Fig. 8. Carcinoid 40×.

Recommended follow-up for patients with carcinoma originating in struma ovarii include annual serum thyroid function tests and thyroglobulin levels for 10 years posttreatment.[4,29] It is important to note that serum thyroglobulin is most sensitive in patients who have undergone total thyroidectomy and ^{131}I ablation.[4,28] Decision-making around adjuvant therapy, thyroid management, goal suppression levels, and follow-up are best made in close collaboration with endocrine specialists.

DIFFERENTIAL DIAGNOSIS

Although the diagnosis of struma ovarii, and malignancy originating in struma ovarii, is often straightforward, a few entities may cause diagnostic difficulty, in particular on intraoperative frozen section or in small samples. In well-differentiated thyroid tissue, including struma ovarii, as well as many thyroid carcinomas (PTC and FTC), immunohistochemical stains TTF-1, and thyroglobulin are typically positive. Rare cases of primary thyroid carcinoma that is metastatic to the ovary have been reported and require a detailed history and examination[2,4,13] (Table 1).

SUMMARY

Struma ovarii is defined as an ovarian teratoma comprising at least 50% thyroid stroma. Frank carcinoma resembling native thyroid carcinoma, such as PTC, rarely originates within struma

ovarii. These malignant tumors have the capacity for extraovarian spread and metastasis but with an overall favorable prognosis. Struma ovarii with histologic changes limited to subtle features suggestive of PTC has been described in patients with subsequent recurrent disease. Therefore, extensive sampling and careful histologic review of any struma ovarii case is recommended. The suggested terminology for benign-appearing struma ovarii with extension to the ovarian surface and spread beyond the ovary is HDFCO, and use of the term "strumosis" is discouraged. Proliferative struma describes adenomatous or hyperplastic struma ovarii. Any diagnosis other than normal struma ovarii confined to the ovary should warrant clinical attention. Carcinoma originating in struma ovarii should prompt imaging in order to evaluate for metastatic disease or synchronous primary of the thyroid gland; multidisciplinary review, including endocrinology, where available, and consideration for management including ^{131}I ablation, thyroid suppression, and surgical staging.

CLINICS CARE POINTS

- Extensive sampling of struma ovarii for microscopic review is recommended.

- In addition to surgery, management considerations for carcinoma arising in struma ovarii should include ^{131}I ablation, radiographic staging, and ultrasound evaluation of the thyroid due to the risk of metastases and/or a synchronous primary in the thyroid.

- Wherever possible, evaluation and treatment should be done in a multidisciplinary fashion, in close collaboration with head and neck/endocrine specialists.

ACKNOWLEDGMENTS

The authors thank Dr Joseph T. Rabban (University of California, San Francisco), Dr Cynthia Gasper (University of California, San Francisco), Dr Amy Joehlin-Price (Cleveland Clinic), and Dr Natalie Banet (Cleveland Clinic) for providing several of the Figures. Dr Lindsay Brubaker would like to acknowledge the financial support of the Ovarian Cancer Research Alliance through The Liz Tilberis Early Career Award.

REFERENCES

1. Shaco-Levy R, M F, Stewart CJR. WHO Classification of Female Genital Tumors: Struma ovarii. 5th ed. Lyon: World Health Organization; 2020, 132–22.
2. Siegel MR, Wolsky RJ, Alvarez EA, et al. Struma ovarii with atypical features and synchronous primary thyroid cancer: a case report and review of the literature. Arch Gynecol Obstet 2019;300(6): 1693–707.
3. Robboy SJ, Shaco-Levy R, Peng RY, et al. Malignant struma ovarii: an analysis of 88 cases, including 27 with extraovarian spread. Int J Gynecol Pathol 2009;28(5):405–22.
4. Addley S, Mihai R, Alazzam M, et al. Malignant struma ovarii: surgical, histopathological and survival outcomes for thyroid-type carcinoma of struma ovarii with recommendations for standardising multi-modal management. A retrospective case series sharing the experience of a single institution over 10 years. Arch Gynecol Obstet 2021;303(4): 863–70.
5. Tan A, Stewart CJ, Garrett KL, et al. Novel BRAF and KRAS mutations in papillary thyroid carcinoma arising in struma ovarii. Endocr Pathol 2015;26(4): 296–301.
6. Li S, Yang T, Xiang Y, et al. Clinical characteristics and survival outcomes of malignant struma ovarii confined to the ovary. BMC Cancer 2021;21(1):383.
7. Khunamornpong S, Settakorn J, Sukpan K, et al. Poorly differentiated thyroid carcinoma arising in struma ovarii. Case Rep Pathol 2015;2015: 826978.
8. Roth LM, Karseladze AI. Highly differentiated follicular carcinoma arising from struma ovarii: a report of 3 cases, a review of the literature, and a reassessment of so-called peritoneal strumosis. Int J Gynecol Pathol 2008;27(2):213–22.
9. Cui Y, Yao J, Wang S, et al. The clinical and pathological characteristics of malignant struma ovarii: an analysis of 144 published patients. Front Oncol 2021;11:645156.
10. Young RH, Jackson A, Wells M. Ovarian metastasis from thyroid carcinoma 12 years after partial thyroidectomy mimicking struma ovarii: report of a case. Int J Gynecol Pathol 1994;13(2):181–5.
11. Yoo SC, Chang KH, Lyu MO, et al. Clinical characteristics of struma ovarii. J Gynecol Oncol 2008;19(2): 135–8.
12. Shaco-Levy R, Bean SM, Bentley RC, et al. Natural history of biologically malignant struma ovarii: analysis of 27 cases with extraovarian spread. Int J Gynecol Pathol 2010;29(3):212–27.
13. Zhang X, Axiotis C. Thyroid-type carcinoma of struma ovarii. Arch Pathol Lab Med 2010;134(5):786–91.
14. Garg K, Soslow RA, Rivera M, et al. Histologically bland "extremely well differentiated" thyroid carcinomas arising in struma ovarii can recur and metastasize. Int J Gynecol Pathol 2009;28(3):222–30.
15. Roth LM, Czernobilsky B, Roth DJ, et al. Highly differentiated follicular thyroid-type carcinoma of the ovary reconsidered. J Clin Pathol 2021;74(9): 553–7.
16. Shaco-Levy R, Peng RY, Snyder MJ, et al. Malignant struma ovarii: a blinded study of 86 cases assessing which histologic features correlate with aggressive clinical behavior. Arch Pathol Lab Med 2012; 136(2):172–8.
17. Devaney K, Snyder R, Norris HJ, et al. Proliferative and histologically malignant struma ovarii: a clinicopathologic study of 54 cases. Int J Gynecol Pathol 1993;12(4):333–43.
18. Cancer Genome Atlas Research N. Integrated genomic characterization of papillary thyroid carcinoma. Cell 2014;159(3):676–90.
19. Tsukada T, Yoshida H, Ishikawa M, et al. Malignant struma ovarii presenting with follicular carcinoma: A case report with molecular analysis. Gynecol Oncol Rep 2019;30:100498.
20. Schmidt J, Derr V, Heinrich MC, et al. BRAF in papillary thyroid carcinoma of ovary (struma ovarii). Am J Surg Pathol 2007;31(9):1337–43.
21. Poli R, Scatolini M, Grosso E, et al. Malignant struma ovarii: next-generation sequencing of six cases revealed Nras, Braf, and Jak3 mutations. Endocrine 2021;71(1):216–24.
22. Boutross-Tadross O, Saleh R, Asa SL. Follicular variant papillary thyroid carcinoma arising in struma ovarii. Endocr Pathol 2007;18(3):182–6.
23. Gomes-Lima CJ, Nikiforov YE, Lee W, et al. Synchronous independent papillary thyroid carcinomas in struma ovarii and the thyroid gland with different RAS mutations. J Endocr Soc 2018;2(8):944–8.

24. Henderson BB, Chaubey A, Roth LM, et al. Whole-genome and segmental homozygosity confirm errors in meiosis as etiology of struma ovarii. Cytogenet Genome Res 2020;160(1):2–10.

25. Goffredo P, Sawka AM, Pura J, et al. Malignant struma ovarii: a population-level analysis of a large series of 68 patients. Thyroid 2015;25(2):211–5.

26. Leong A, Roche PJ, Paliouras M, et al. Coexistence of malignant struma ovarii and cervical papillary thyroid carcinoma. J Clin Endocrinol Metab 2013; 98(12):4599–605.

27. DeSimone CP, Lele SM, Modesitt SC. Malignant struma ovarii: a case report and analysis of cases reported in the literature with focus on survival and I131 therapy. Gynecol Oncol 2003;89(3):543–8.

28. Yassa L, Sadow P, Marqusee E. Malignant struma ovarii. Nat Clin Pract Endocrinol Metab 2008;4(8): 469–72.

29. Rose PG, Arafah B, Abdul-Karim FW. Malignant struma ovarii: recurrence and response to treatment monitored by thyroglobulin levels. Gynecol Oncol 1998;70(3):425–7.

Preoperative, Intraoperative, and Postoperative Parathyroid Pathology
Clinical Pathologic Collaboration for Optimal Patient Management

Hailey L. Gosnell, MD[a], Peter M. Sadow, MD, PhD[b],*

KEYWORDS
- Parathyroid • Frozen section • Parathyroid hyperplasia • Oil red O • Parathyroid adenoma • ioPTH

Key points

- Intraoperative frozen section of parathyroids should be to confirm parathyroid origin.
- Intraoperative consult does not replace a thorough preoperative parathyroid function work up.
- Atypical parathyroid tumors are of uncertain biological potential.
- Malignancy in parathyroid neoplasia should be viewed skeptically, in clinical context, and with molecular data.

ABSTRACT

Parathyroid disease typically presents with parathyroid hyperfunction as result of neoplasia or a consequence of non-neoplastic systemic disease. Given the parathyroid gland is a hormonally active organ with broad physiologic implications and serologically accessible markers for monitoring, the diagnosis of parathyroid disease is predominantly a clinical pathologic correlation. We provide the current pathological correlates of parathyroid disease and discuss preoperative, intraoperative, and postoperative pathology consultative practice for optimal patient care.

INTRODUCTION

Primary hyperparathyroidism, or inappropriate parathyroid hormone secretion in the setting of hypercalcemia, is a common disease process that can result in skeletal and renal complications in severe, untreated cases.[1] Solitary parathyroid adenoma is, by far, the most common cause of primary hyperparathyroidism (affecting approximately 80% of cases), followed by multiglandular disease (multiple adenomas or hyperplasia), attributable to approximately 15% of cases.[2,3] Less common causes of primary hyperparathyroidism include atypical parathyroid tumors and parathyroid carcinoma (affecting 1% to 3% and less than 1% of primary hyperparathyroidism cases, respectively).[3,4] Though nonoperative surveillance or medical management may be utilized for a subset of patients with mild disease, surgery is the only definitive treatment for primary hyperparathyroidism.[5–7]

Pathologist consultation for the assessment of parathyroid disease has evolved over time but continues to be fraught with controversy, particularly regarding intraoperative consultation for

---

[a] Department of Pathology, Cleveland Clinic, 9500 Euclid Avenue, Mail Code L25, Cleveland, OH 44195, USA;
[b] Department of Pathology, Pathology Service, Massachusetts General Hospital, Harvard Medical School, WRN219, 55 Fruit Street, Boston, MA 02114, USA
* Corresponding author.
E-mail address: psadow@mgh.harvard.edu

Surgical Pathology 16 (2023) 87–96
https://doi.org/10.1016/j.path.2022.10.001
1875-9181/23/© 2022 Elsevier Inc. All rights reserved.

patient management. Intraoperative assessment of surgically excised tissue by the pathologist has evolved from attempting to render the specific etiology of parathyroid pathology to solely confirming the presence of parathyroid tissue.[8,9] This change was prompted by the advent of intraoperative parathyroid hormone (ioPTH) assays, a modality that has been shown in remote and recent studies to be a superior determinant of successful lesional excision over intraoperative histologic analysis despite its drawbacks.[10–13] However, in many hospitals, despite the utilization of ioPTH testing modalities, there is still the expectation, including by subspecialist endocrine surgeons, for an assessment of parathyroid pathology in addition to simple identification of the gland.

Permanent histologic evaluation of parathyroid specimens that may include immunohistochemical and molecular studies, in addition to preoperative, intraoperative, and postoperative clinical evaluation, may solidify a clinical pathologic diagnosis for etiologic purposes. However, even in this context, long-term clinical follow-up, with pathologic interpretation as a basis, is a crucial component of any individual diagnosis. Clinical correlation is challenging to execute intraoperatively or even immediately postoperatively without a detailed history defining the etiology of hyperparathyroidism such as a genetic syndrome or end-stage kidney disease. This review explores the literature surrounding current best practices for utilization of intraoperative (frozen) consultation and permanent histologic evaluation of parathyroid lesions in the context of recent trends shaping the field.

INTRAOPERATIVE ASSESSMENT OF PARATHYROID LESIONS

THE HISTORIC APPROACH TO EVALUATING PARATHYROID LESIONS

The recommended intraoperative pathology consultation approach to parathyroid lesion assessment and its influence on the patient's intraoperative course has changed dramatically over the last several decades. Historically, intraoperative diagnosis of parathyroid lesions was rendered according to weight, gross examination, and histologic appearance.[14] Often, the primary task of the pathologist had been to discern a parathyroid adenoma from normal parathyroid tissue. An enlarged (>300 mg) red-brown, well-circumscribed gland with or without foci of hemorrhage and cystic degeneration was grossly consistent with parathyroid adenoma. Chief cell hyperplasia, nuclear atypia, a normocellular rim, and a paucity

of fat met the criteria for diagnosis as an adenoma microscopically.[14–21] A hypercellular gland without other adenomatous features necessitated comparison with a biopsy of an additional gland. A higher intracellular fat content and lower parenchymal cell-to-fat ratio in the biopsy supported a diagnosis of adenoma in the first gland (**Fig. 1**).[20–22] Rapid toluidine blue or oil red o stains were routinely utilized to discern fat content in normal versus hypercellular or adenomatous glands.[23–25] Measurement of parathyroid activity by scintigraphy was also useful to corroborate single glandular disease in cases of prominent adenoma or allude to multiglandular disease in ambiguous instances.[26]

Differentiating parathyroid adenoma from primary parathyroid hyperplasia proved a common diagnostic challenge, such that the pathologist's gross and histologic examination were the only determinants of the patient's intraoperative course. Histologically, chief, oxyphilic, or transitional cell hyperplasia with a decreased intra- and intercellular fat content was observed in both entities.[27,28] Although a normocellular rim was not usually noted in hyperplastic glands, this phenomenon had limited diagnostic utility because it proved to be absent in up to half of adenomas.[12,29] Thus, the surgeon's intraoperative impression of glandular size discrepancies was vital in cases of histologic ambiguity.

The diagnosis of atypical parathyroid adenomas (now designated as atypical parathyroid tumors)[30] and parathyroid carcinomas as lesional entities on frozen section was often more definitive in comparison to their lower grade counterparts. Grossly, the majority of parathyroid carcinomas were noted to be large (weighing an average of 12 grams), displaying obvious invasion of surrounding tissue preoperatively.[29,30] Atypical parathyroid adenomas were usually less pronounced in size but could be adherent to surrounding tissues (without overt signs of invasion).[31] Microscopically, a diagnosis of atypical parathyroid adenoma was rendered with the observance of worrisome features including mitoses, desmoplastic reaction, nuclear atypia, necrosis, monotonous sheet-like or trabecular growth, fibrosis, and tumor cells in the capsule.[4,30–35] Histologic signs of invasion (perineural, intravascular, lymphatic, or pericapsular) or metastasis upgraded the diagnosis to a parathyroid carcinoma.[30]

The bulk of primary hyperparathyroidism cases (approximately 85%) were known to be caused by single glandular disease (conventional adenoma, atypical adenoma, or parathyroid carcinoma) and these cases were often histologically diagnostic and easily detected with preoperative

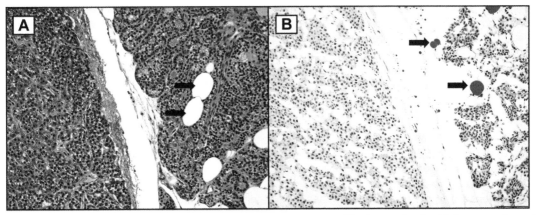

Fig. 1. Intraoperative evaluation of parathyroid tissue at 200× magnification, stained with hematoxylin and eosin (*A*) or Oil Red O vital stain (*B*). The images are serial sections of the same tissue, showing more cellular parathyroid tissue (*left side of image*) with some preservation of stromal fat (*arrows*). Oil Red O stain highlights the large red globules of stromal fat (*arrows*) and retained intracellular fat (*dot-like red globules*), which is slightly increased in the cells on the right side of the field. Diagnostically, this difference is of limited utility.

scintigraphy.[26] However, cases of multiglandular disease (hyperplasia or multiple adenomas) were often more difficult to identify on imaging and posed a challenging histologic workup.[2,16,36] The advent of ioPTH dramatically changed the role of the pathologist in the workup of both single and multiglandular parathyroid disease.

THE INTRAOPERATIVE PARATHYROID HORMONE ASSAY

The introduction of ioPTH in the 1990s altered the frozen section analysis of parathyroid lesions. The short half-life of parathyroid hormone (3 to 5 min) enabled a quick resulting time for an intraoperative assay of the hormone (both pre- and post-parathyroid gland excision), making it a clinically useful tool for surgeons to use as part of a parathyroidectomy.[37–39] Following the standard criteria for permissible ioPTH decline during the procedure (>50% decrease in PTH concentration from pre- to post-glandular excision values at 5 to 15 min) resulted in a high cure rate (>97%).[40–42]

ioPTH usage largely replaced frozen section histologic diagnosis as a determinant of successful parathyroid lesion resection.[8,9,11] Utilization of ioPTH was found to be associated with a lower disease recurrence rate (3%) in comparison to intraoperative frozen section (approximately 5%).[43–45] Implementation of this tool was also associated with a shorter hospital stay, reduced incidence of postoperative hypocalcemia, and decreased risk of recurrent laryngeal nerve injury as it enabled the usage of a minimally invasive parathyroidectomy procedure in place of the standard bilateral neck exploration.[44,46] This method was noted to be particularly useful in solitary adenomas with discordant preoperative imaging and multiglandular disease amenable to a minimally invasive surgical approach.[8,12,47]

A NEW ROLE FOR THE PATHOLOGIST

Although ioPTH usage has become a fixture in the therapeutic intervention of primary hyperparathyroidism, there are clinical contexts in which intraoperative histologic analysis, albeit at a smaller scale, is still warranted. Frozen section evaluation is a useful adjunct to ioPTH in patients presenting with normal PTH and hypercalcemia or those whose lesions do not localize preoperatively.[42,48] However, instead of providing a histologic diagnosis or attempting to predict surgical cure, the recommended role of the pathologist is to discern normal parathyroid from thyroid, lymph node, or adipose tissue.[8] Reporting successful excision of parathyroid tissue in cases of hypercalcemia with normal parathyroid hormone levels and in patients with lesions that cannot be localized on preoperative imaging can provide valuable information to the surgeon with an incredibly high accuracy rate (approximately 99.2%).[49–51]

Despite the preponderance in the literature advising against intraoperative and even postoperative (final) pathological confirmation of disease etiology, there is still an expectation in many routine clinical surgical practices for this etiologic affirmation.[12] Along with this expectation, some pathology practices still use Oil Red O stain to investigate the presence of intracellular and stromal fat content to discern adenoma from hyperplasia, as reported in prior reports.[20–22] However, this concept has been largely debunked.[12,27,28]

Discerning normal parathyroid tissue from the thyroid can be challenging in the context of adenomatous lesions with prominent follicular structures.[30] However, the follicular structures in parathyroid tissue are devoid of colloid and lack bi-refringent calcium-oxalate crystals. Additionally, parathyroid cells are smaller than thyrocytes, contain more rounded nuclei with denser chromatin, have an intracellular fat component, and are enveloped by more distinct membranes, one possible argument for the retention of Oil Red O in the frozen section laboratory.[30]

SUMMARY

The pathologist's intraoperative evaluation of primary hyperparathyroidism has pivoted from rendering a histologic diagnosis and determining a surgical cure in every therapeutic intervention to ascertaining excision of normal parathyroid tissue in a subset of cases where this finding is pertinent. Although the scope of frozen section histologic evaluation of entities associated with primary hyperparathyroidism has diminished over time, the importance of clinicopathologic correlation in cases requiring histologic assessment has not. Pathologists must collaborate with surgical colleagues, given years of evidence and follow-up data, for optimal use of intraoperative consultation in parathyroid disease.

PERMANENT SECTION EVALUATION OF PARATHYROID LESIONS

IN GENERAL

Permanent section remains a more definitive setting for ascertaining both the diagnosis and etiology of parathyroid lesions given the superior visibility of these entities on hematoxylin and eosin (H&E) stain and the array of immunohistochemical and molecular studies available. Even so, the clinicopathologic correlation remains an essential part of the diagnostic workup.

PARATHYROID ADENOMAS

Histology

Parathyroid adenomas are well-circumscribed lesions displaying proliferation of chief, oncocytic, transitional, or water-clear cells.[52] Chief cells have scant cytoplasm and small, regular nuclei that lack nucleoli. Palisades of chief cells surround an intricate network of capillaries. Follicular

structures are often identified, resembling thyroid tissue.[30] Oncocytic parathyroid adenomas consist of >75% of oncocytic cells.[53] These cells possess a granular, pink cytoplasm and nuclei with varying degrees of pleomorphism. Oncocytic lesions are larger than their chief cell counterparts and are more easily picked up by scintigraphy.[53,54] True to their name, water-clear cell adenomas are comprised of cells with hyperchromatic, basally oriented nuclei and dilated, vacuolated cytoplasms, and distinct cell borders.[54–56] These lesions, being rarest and the largest subclassification of parathyroid adenomas, are difficult to localize via scintigraphy.[57] As in the historic intraoperative workup of parathyroid adenomas, a normocellular rim, a paucity of intracellular fat, and a high parenchymal cell-to-fat ratio are also helpful in rendering the diagnosis.[14–21,52]

Immunohistochemistry

Immunohistochemical stains can be beneficial in identifying parathyroid adenomas and discerning these entities from thyroid tissue in cases of histologic ambiguity. Parathyroid adenomas are positive for PTH, GATA3, chromogranin, and synaptophysin (in some circumstances).[58–61] Cells that comprise these lesions, unlike thyroid cells, are negative for TTF1, PAX8, and thyroglobulin.[62,63]

Molecular Genetic Implications

Multiple somatic and germline mutations are associated with parathyroid adenoma, conferring various degrees of clinical significance. Overexpression of cyclin D1, a protooncogene encoded by the gene *CCND1* is noted in a substantial portion of parathyroid adenomas.[64] This process is often caused by methylation of cyclin-dependent kinase inhibitors, but may also occur due to an inversion in chromosome 11, resulting in regulation of the *CCND1* gene by the PTH gene promoter.[65] The prognostic significance of this genetic aberration has not been described, nor has its utility in diagnostic workup or therapeutic intervention of parathyroid adenomas. Somatic genetic defects in *POT1*, *EZH2*, and B-catenin (*CTNNB1*) have also been implicated in the development of parathyroid adenoma, but the nature and extent of their contribution remains unknown.[29,66]

Although parafibromin deficiency is noted in a small fraction of typical parathyroid adenomas, this etiology is important to recognize because it can have profound clinical implications. Parafibromin deficiency is caused by inactivation of *CDC73* (formerly *HRPT2*), a nuclear tumor suppressor protein with multiple functions including modulating transcription and promoting cell cycle arrest to regulate cell proliferation.[67–70] Germline inactivation of *CDC73* is associated with hyperparathyroidism jaw tumor syndrome (HPT-JT), a familial condition associated with ossifying fibromas of the mandible and maxilla, uterine tumors, renal hamartomas, and cystic kidney disease, in addition to parathyroid neoplasms.[71–73] Somatic *CDC73* gene mutations are not associated with the same syndromic features as their germline counterparts, but they are histologically identical. Both somatic and germline aberrant *CDC73* tumor cells have eosinophilic cytoplasm displaying perinuclear clearing and nuclear enlargement (but preserved nuclear to cytoplasmic ratios). The architecture of these entities is sheet-like and binucleate or multinucleate cells are interspersed throughout the lesion.[30]

As parafibromin deficiency of somatic and germline etiologies has the same microscopic features, immunohistochemistry should be performed in individuals suspected to have parafibromin-deficient parathyroid adenoma on histology (**Fig. 2**). A loss of nuclear parafibromin staining is considered abnormal and requires molecular sequencing of *CDC73* to discern germline or somatic causation.[74,75] Although parafibromin deficiency is more commonplace in atypical parathyroid tumors and most frequently noted in parathyroid carcinomas, parathyroid adenomas with histologic features suggestive of *CDC73* aberrancy should still be evaluated so that those with germline mutations can obtain appropriate clinical follow-up.[30,76]

ATYPICAL PARATHYROID TUMORS

Histology and Immunohistochemistry

Atypical parathyroid tumors (recently designated by the 2022 WHO Classification of Parathyroid Tumors) show histologic features concerning for parathyroid carcinoma including trabecular growth, increased mitotic activity, adherence to adjacent structures without gross invasion, cellular atypia, and tumor cells extending into the capsule. However, these tumors do not show evidence of invasion or metastasis.[4,33] Calcium levels of patients with atypical parathyroid tumors are elevated, usually measuring between the average value for patients with parathyroid adenoma and those with parathyroid carcinoma.[33] The immunohistochemical profile of atypical parathyroid tumors mirrors that of parathyroid adenomas. These lesions are also positive for GATA3, chromogranin, and TTF1.[58–61]

Molecular Genetic Implications

Immunohistochemical and molecular testing for parafibromin deficiency is essential in atypical parathyroid tumors. Somatic and germline *CDC73* mutations in atypical parathyroid tumors are associated with a poorer prognosis than their wildtype counterparts.[77,78] Patients with these neoplasms are at higher risk of tumor recurrence in the affected gland as well as metachronous development of additional lesions in the other parathyroid glands.[30] Thus, atypical parathyroid tumors with histology concerning for parafibromin deficiency should undergo parafibromin immunohistochemistry and molecular testing, even if the immunohistochemistry is wildtype. Abnormal

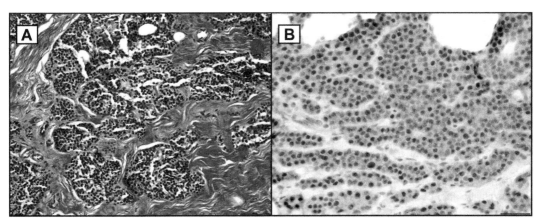

Fig. 2. Atypical parathyroid tumor. Hematoxylin and eosin stain at 200× magnification (*A*) shows tight clusters of cells with an absence of stromal fat (see **Fig. 1**) and clusters separated by dense fibrosis. At higher magnification (400×, *B*), parafibromin shows an intact nuclear stain consistent with a functional *CDC73* (*HRPT2*) gene.

parafibromin expression is defined as diffuse nuclear or nucleolar loss of parafibromin in lesional cells, with retention in internal control (stromal) cells. Although a wildtype parafibromin immunostaining pattern would rule out germ-line aberrancy, the point mutations that cause *CDC73* deficiency of somatic etiology might not cause a loss in parafibromin staining.[30]

CARCINOMAS

Histology

As previously stated, parathyroid carcinomas display the same worrisome histologic features noted in atypical parathyroid tumors. However, the diagnosis is characterized by evidence of full-thickness capsular invasion, perineural invasion (affecting at least the epineurium), lymphovascular invasion, or metastasis.[30] Often, invasion is appreciable on gross examination. These tumors are large, weighing an average of 12 g (weight of normal and weight of adenoma). They are also associated with elevated calcium values (surpassing those of an atypical parathyroid tumor).[33]

Differential Diagnosis

There are several entities that can mimic parathyroid carcinoma histologically. These include parathyromatosis (microscopic foci of ectopic parathyroid tissue as a result of a prior procedure), a benign parathyroid lesion with prior biopsy site changes, and irregular parathyroid contour resulting from chronic secondary or tertiary hyperparathyroidism.[30,79–81] Clinicopathologic correlation is essential in this context.

Immunohistochemistry

Immunohistochemical staining can attempt to discern parathyroid carcinomas from other parathyroid tumors and can highlight areas of invasion that would otherwise be inconspicuous. Parathyroid carcinoma is more likely to be positive for PGP9.5 and Galectin-3, negative for APC, and often shows parafibromin loss. However, no single immunostain or panel of stains is definitively diagnostic of carcinoma, and variable expression of these markers is noted in atypical parathyroid tumors.[57,61,82,83] The Ki67 labeling index is also noted to be much higher (>5%) in parathyroid carcinomas relative to parathyroid adenomas (usually 1% or less).[31,84,85] Parathyroid carcinomas also may display loss of mdm2, bcl-2, p27, E-cadherin, and positivity for p53, pTERT, and galectin-3.[51,60,82,83,86–88] However, most laboratories do not routinely use this entire series of immunohistochemical markers, and a more limited panel combined with morphologic features, surgical features, and serologies will be most helpful in formulating this diagnosis.

GATA3 and PTH highlight tumor cells at the edge of the lesion such that invasion can be assessed in histologically ambiguous cases.[30] CD31 or D2-40 stains may be useful in the discernment of vascular or lymphatic invasion in these lesions. However, as these tumors are typically quite vascular, particular attention should be paid to not overinterpret invasion. A fibrin-thrombus component of the invasion can be highlighted with CD61 or Martius-Scarlet blue staining.[30]

Molecular Implications

Numerous somatic and germline mutations are associated with the development of parathyroid carcinoma. Most parathyroid carcinomas are parafibromin deficient (approximately 60%).[89] Thus, pursuing an immunohistochemical and molecular workup for germline and somatic *CDC73* mutations is highly recommended.[78,79] As is the case for atypical parathyroid tumors, patients diagnosed with parafibromin deficient parathyroid carcinoma have a poorer prognosis than their wildtype counterparts, although cases of parathyroid carcinoma, in general, are limited, and this differential prognosis may be somewhat anecdotal.

Mutations in *PI3K*, *TP53*, *pTERT*, *DICER1*, phosphate and tensin homolog *(PTEN)*, and neurofibromatosis 1 (NF1) related pathways are also linked to the development of parathyroid carcinoma.[90,91] Therapeutic interventions targeted to *PIK3CA*, *PTEN*, and *NF1* are already available. Thus, in parathyroid carcinoma patients resistant to conventional therapy, molecular testing for these entities may prove clinically useful.[91]

MULTIGLANDULAR DISEASE

Multiglandular causes of primary hyperparathyroidism include parathyroid hyperplasia and multiple parathyroid adenomas. Primary enlargement of all four glands was previously thought to be a hyperplastic process.[2–4,29] However, most instances of multiglandular parathyroid disease have been recognized to represent multiple parathyroid adenomas, and characterization as such is supported by the 2022 WHO. Affected glands are round and red-brown on gross examination, but present with variable size and weight.[28,51] Histologically, chief, oncocytic, or transitional cell proliferation with decreased inter and intracellular fat content is noted.[12,27–29] Nuclear atypia and pleomorphism of varying degrees may also be observed. As was the case in the context of intraoperative evaluation, clinicopathologic correlation is essential in rendering a diagnosis of primary parathyroid adenomas versus secondary hyperplasia on permanent section.

Summary: Morphologic diagnosis of parathyroid lesions should take into account clinical findings, including serology, imaging, and surgical findings. The final diagnosis is often clinical pathologic with all ancillary testing, including intraoperative evaluation (histology and ioPTH), immunohistochemistry, and possible genetic testing supporting the ultimate follow-up and treatment plan.

CLINICS CARE POINTS

- Providing an etiology for hypercellular parathyroid tissue assessed at frozen section should be avoided given the typically limited clinical information at the time of consultation.

- Oil Red O stain is not of routine utility for intraoperative consultation to differentiated between parathyroid adenoma and parathyroid hyperplasia but may bear rare utility in identification of parathyroids.

- Parafibromin immunostain may be used as a screen for CDC73 genetic anomalies that should be followed, if expression of parafibromin is lost, by genetic studies if possible.

- Parathyroid carcinoma is an exceptionally rare diagnosis, and many of the histologically diagnostic features are subjective, save for distant metastasis. Care should be taken when rendering the diagnosis given the emotional and clinical consequences of a cancer diagnosis currently lacking effective, non-surgical therapies.

DISCLOSURE

The authors have no commercial interests to disclose. Dr P.M. Sadow has funding from the National Cancer Institute of the National Institutes of Health, 5P01CA240239-4.

REFERENCES

1. Bilezikian JP, Bandeira L, Khan A, et al. Hyperparathyroidism. Lancet 2018;391(10116):168–78. ISSN 0140-6736.
2. Barczyński M, Bränström R, Dionigi G, et al. Sporadic multiple parathyroid gland disease–a consensus report of the European Society of Endocrine Surgeons (ESES). Langenbeck's Arch Surg 2015;400(8):887–905.
3. Insogna KL. Primary Hyperparathyroidism. N Engl J Med 2018;379(11):1050–9.
4. Galani A, Morandi R, Dimko M, et al. Atypical parathyroid adenoma: clinical and anatomical pathologic features. World J Surg Oncol 2021;19(1):19.
5. Walker MD, Silverberg SJ. Primary hyperparathyroidism. Nat Rev Endocrinol 2018;14(2):115–25.
6. Pappachan JM, Elnaggar MN, Sodi R, et al. Primary hyperparathyroidism: findings from the retrospective evaluation of cases over a 6-year period from a regional UK centre. Endocrine 2018;62(1):174–81.
7. Bilezikian JP, Luisa Brandi M, Eastell R, et al. Claudio Marcocci, John T. Potts, Jr, Guidelines for the Management of Asymptomatic Primary Hyperparathyroidism: Summary Statement from the Fourth International Workshop. J Clin Endocrinol Metab 2014;99(10):3561–9.
8. Wilhelm SM, Wang TS, Ruan DT, et al. The American Association of Endocrine Surgeons Guidelines for Definitive Management of Primary Hyperparathyroidism. JAMA Surg 2016;151(10):959–68.
9. Elliott DD, Monroe DP, Perrier ND. Parathyroid histopathology: is it of any value today? J Am Coll Surg 2006;203:758e65.
10. Starr FL, DeCresce R, Prinz RA. Use of intraoperative parathyroid hormone measurement does not improve success of bilateral neck exploration for hyperparathyroidism. Arch Surg 2001;136:536–42.
11. Perrier ND, Ituarte P, Kikuchi S, et al. Intraoperative parathyroid aspiration and parathyroid hormone assay as an alternative to frozen section for tissue identification. World J Surg 2000;24:1319–22.
12. Cipriani NA, Glomski K, Sadow PM. Intraoperative assessment of parathyroid pathology in sporadic primary hyperparathyroidism: an institutional experience. Hum Pathol 2022;123:40–5.
13. McCoy KL, Yip L, Dhir M, et al. Histologic hypercellularity in a biopsied normal parathyroid gland does not correlate with hyperfunction in primary hyperparathyroidism. Surgery 2021;169(3):524–7.
14. Castleman B, Mallory TB. The Pathology of the Parathyroid Gland in Hyperparathyroidism: A Study of 25 Cases. Am J Pathol 1935;11(1):1–72.
15. Nazikawa H, Rosen P, Lane N, et al. Frozen section experience in 3000 cases. Accuracy, limitations, and value in residency training. Am J Clin Pathol 1968;49(1):41–51.
16. Roth SI, Sadow PM, Belsley Johnson N, et al. Parathryoid. In: Mills SE, editor. *Histopathology for Pathologists*. 4th Edition. Philadelphia, PA: Wolters Kuwer Lippincott Williams & Wilkins. 2012. pp. 1209-1230.
17. Dehner LP, Rosai J. Frozen section examination in surgical pathology: a retrospective study of one year experience, comprising 778 cases. Minn Med 1977;60(2):83–94.

18. Mcgarity WC, Mathews WH, Fulenwider JT, et al. The surgical management of primary hyperparathyroidism: a personal series. Ann Surg 1981;193(6):794–804.

19. Dankawa EK, Davies JD. Frozen section diagnosis: an audit. J Clin Pathol 1985;38(11):1235–40.

20. Baloch ZW, LiVolsi VA. Intraoperative assessment of thyroid and parathyroid lesions. Semn Diagn Pathol 2002;19(4):219–26.

21. Dewan AK, Kapadia SB, Hollenbeack CS, et al. Is routine frozen section necessary for parathyroid surgery? Otolaryngol Head Neck Surg 2005;133(6):857–62.

22. Faquin WC, Roth SI. Frozen section of thyroid and parathyroid specimens. Arch Pathol Lab Med 2006;130(9):1260.

23. Singleton AO, Allums J. Identification of Parathyroid Glands by Toluidine Blue Staining. Arch Surg 1970;100(4):372–5.

24. Rosen IB, Bohnen DR, Walfish PG. The use of toluidine blue in locating abnormal parathyroid tissue at operation. Can Med Assoc J 1974;110(4):393–6.

25. Monchik JM, Farrugia R, Teplitz C, et al. Parathyroid surgery: the role of chief cell intracellular fat staining with osmium carmine in the intraoperative management of patients with primary hyperparathyroidism. Surgery 1983;94(6):877–86.

26. Taillefer R, Boucher Y, Potvin C, et al. Detection and localization of parathyroid adenomas in patients with hyperparathyroidism using a single radionuclide imaging procedure with technetium-99m-sestamibi (double-phase study). J Nucl Med 1992;33:1801–7.

27. Penner CR, Thompson LD. Primary parathyroid hyperplasia. Ear Nose Throat J 2003;82(5):363.

28. Takahashi F, Denda M, Finch JL, et al. Hyperplasia of the parathyroid gland without secondary hyperparathyroidism. Kidney Int 2002;61(4):1332–8.

29. Guilmette J, Sadow PM. Parathyroid Pathology. Surg Pathol Clin 2019;12(4):1007–19.

30. Erickson LA, Mete O, Juhlin CC, et al. Overview of the 2022 WHO Classification of Parathyroid Tumors. Endocr Pathol 2022;33(1):64–89.

31. Cetani F, Marcocci C, Torregrossa L, et al. Atypical parathyroid adenomas: challenging lesions in the differential diagnosis of endocrine tumors. Endocrine-Related Cancer 2019;26(7):R441–64. Retrieved Apr 7, 2022.

32. Persson S, Hansson G, Hedman I, et al. Primary parathyroid hyperplasia of water-clear cell type. Transformation of water-clear cell type. Acta Pathol Microbiol Immunol Scand A 1986;94(6):391–5.

33. Fernandez-Ranvier GG, Khanafshar E, Jensen K, et al. Parathyroid carcinoma, atypical parathyroid adenoma, or parathyromatosis? Cancer 2007;110(2):255–64.

34. Wani S, Hao Z. Atypical cystic adenoma of the parathyroid gland: case report and review of the literature. Endocr practices 2005;11(6):389–93.

35. Bergenfelz A, Tennvall J, Valdermarsson S, et al. Sestamibi versus thallium subtraction scintigraphy in parathyroid localization: a prospective comparative study in patients with predominantly mild primary hyperparathyroidism. Surgery 1997;121:601–5.

36. Leiker AJ, Yen TW, Eastwood DC, et al. Factors that influence parathyroid hormone half-life: determining if new intraoperative criteria are needed. JAMA Surg 2013;148(7):602–6.

37. Sokoll LJ, Drew H, Udelsman R. Intraoperative parathyroid hormone analysis: A study of 200 consecutive cases. Clin Chem 2000 Oct;46(10):1662–8.

38. Calò PG, Pisano G, Loi G, et al. Intraoperative parathyroid hormone assay during focused parathyroidectomy: the importance of 20 minutes measurement. BMC Surg 2013;13:36.

39. Mak NTJJ, Li J, Vasilyeva E, et al. Intraoperative parathyroid hormone measurement during parathyroidectomy for treatment of primary hyperparathyroidism: When should you end the operation? Am J Surg 2020;219(5):785–9.

40. Richards ML, Thompson GB, Farley DR, et al. An Optimal Algorithm for Intraoperative Parathyroid Hormone Monitoring. Arch Surg 2011;146(3):280–5.

41. Iacobone M, Scarpa M, Lumachi F, et al. Are frozen sections useful and cost-effective in the era of intraoperative qPTH assays? Surgery 2005;138(6):1159–64, [discussion: 1164-5].

42. Low RA, Katz AD. Parathyroidectomy via bilateral cervical exploration: a retrospective review of 866 cases. Head Neck 1998;20(7):583–7.

43. Quinn AJ, Ryan ÉJ, Garry S, et al. Use of Intraoperative Parathyroid Hormone in Minimally Invasive Parathyroidectomy for Primary Hyperparathyroidism: A Systematic Review and Meta-analysis. JAMA Otolaryngol Head Neck Surg 2021;147(2):135–43.

44. Medas F, Cappellacci F, Canu GL, et al. The role of Rapid Intraoperative Parathyroid Hormone (ioPTH) assay in determining outcome of parathyroidectomy in primary hyperparathyroidism: A systematic review and meta-analysis. Int J Surg 2021;92:106042.

45. Chen H, Pruhs Z, Starling JR, et al. Intraoperative parathyroid hormone testing improves cure rates in patients undergoing minimally invasive parathyroidectomy. Surgery 2005;138(4):583–7.

46. Barczynski M, Konturek A, Cichon S, et al. Intraoperative parathyroid hormone assay improves outcomes of minimally invasive parathyroidectomy mainly in patients with a presumed solitary parathyroid adenoma and missing concordance of

preoperative imaging. Clin Endocrinol (Oxf) 2007; 66(6):878–85.

47. Li J, Vasilyeva E, Hiebert J, et al. Limited clinical utility of intraoperative frozen section during parathyroidectomy for treatment of primary hyperparathyroidism. Am J Surg 2019;217(5):893–8.

48. Westra WH, Pritchett DD, Udelsman R. Intraoperative confirmation of parathyroid tissue during parathyroid exploration: a retrospective evaluation of the frozen section. Am J Surg Pathol 1998;22: 538–44.

49. Anton RC, Wheeler TM. Frozen section of thyroid and parathyroid specimens. Arch Pathol Lab Med 2005;129(12):1575–84.

50. Chan RK, Ibrahim SI, Pil P, et al. Validation of a Method to Replace Frozen Section During Parathyroid Exploration by Using the Rapid Parathyroid Hormone Assay on Parathyroid Aspirates. Arch Surg 2005;140(4):371–3.

51. DeLellis R. Parathyroid tumors and related disorders. Mod Pathol 2011;24:S78–93.

52. Howson P, Kruijff S, Aniss A, et al. Oxyphil Cell Parathyroid Adenomas Causing Primary Hyperparathyroidism: a Clinico-Pathological Correlation. Endocr Pathol 2015 Sep;26(3):250–4.

53. Bleier BS, LiVolsi VA, Chalian AA, et al. Technetium Tc 99m Sestamibi Sensitivity in Oxyphil Cell–Dominant Parathyroid Adenomas. Arch Otolaryngol Head Neck Surg 2006;132(7):779–82.

54. Erickson LA, Jin L, Papotti M, et al. Oxyphil Parathyroid Carcinomas. The Am J Surg Pathol March 2002; 26(3):344–9.

55. Bai S, LiVolsi VA, Fraker DL, et al. Water-Clear Parathyroid Adenoma: Report of Two Cases and Literature Review. Endocr Pathol 2012;23: 196–200.

56. Juhlin CC, Nilsson IL, Falhammar H, et al. Institutional characterisation of water clear cell parathyroid adenoma: a rare entity often unrecognised by TC-99m-sestamibi scintigraphy. Pathology 2021;53(7): 852–9.

57. Schmid KW, Hittmair A, Ladurner D, et al. Chromogranin A and B in parathyroid tissue of cases of primary hyperparathyroidism: an immunohistochemical study. Virchows Arch A Pathol Anat Histopathol 1991;418(4):295–9.

58. Ordóñez NG. Value of GATA3 immunostaining in the diagnosis of parathyroid tumors. Appl Immunohistochem Mol Morphol 2014;22(10):756–61.

59. Takada N, Hirokawa M, Suzuki A, et al. Diagnostic value of GATA-3 in cytological identification of parathyroid tissues. Endocr J 2016;63(7):621–6.

60. Erickson LA, Mete O. Immunohistochemistry in Diagnostic Parathyroid Pathology. Endocr Pathol 2018;29(2):113–29.

61. Cameselle-Teijeiro JM, Eloy C, Sobrinho-Simões, et al. Challenging Thyroid Tumors: Emphasis on Differential Diagnosis and Ancillary Biomarkers. Endocr Pathol 2020;31:197–217.

62. Cimino-Mathews A, Sharma R, Netto GJ. Diagnostic use of PAX8, CAIX, TTF-1, and TGB in metastatic renal cell carcinoma of the thyroid. Am J Surg Pathol 2011;35(5):757–61.

63. Hsi ED, Zukerberg LR, Yang WI, et al. Cyclin D1/PRAD1 expression in parathyroid adenomas: an immunohistochemical study. J Clin Endocrinol Metab 1996;81(5):1736–9.

64. Arnold A, Kim HG, Gaz RD, et al. Molecular cloning and chromosomal mapping of DNA rearranged with the parathyroid hormone gene in a parathyroid adenoma. J Clin Invest 1989;83:2034–40.

65. Costa-Guda J, Arnold A. Genetic and epigenetic changes in sporadic endocrine tumors: parathyroid tumors. Mol Cell Endocrinol 2014;386(1–2):46–54.

66. Masi G, Barzon L, Iacobone M, et al. Clinical, genetic, and histopathologic investigation of CDC73-related familial hyperparathyroidism. Endocrine-Related Cancer 2008;15(4):1115–26.

67. Woodard GE, Lin L, Zhang JH, et al. Parafibromin, product of the hyperparathyroidism–jaw tumor syndrome gene HRPT2, regulates cyclin D1/PRAD1 expression. Oncogene 2005;24:1272–6.

68. Zhang C, Kong D, Tan MH, et al. Parafibromin inhibits cancer cell growth and causes G1 phase arrest. Biochem Biophys Res Commun 2006;350:17–24.

69. Yart A, Gstaiger M, Wirbelauer C, et al. The HRPT2 tumor suppressor gene promin associated with human PAF1 and RNA polymerase II. Mol Cell Biol 2005;25:5052–60.

70. Caroling T, Udelsman R. Parathyroid surgery in familial hyperparathyroid disorders. J Intern Med 2005;257(1):27–37.

71. Bradley KJ, Hobbs MR, Buley ID, et al. Uterin tumors are a phenotypic manifestation of the hyperparathyroidism-jaw tumor syndrome. J Intern Med 2005;257(1):18–26.

72. Teh BT, Farnebo F, Kristoffersson U, et al. Autosomal dominant primary hyperparathyroidism and jaw tumor syndrome associated with renal hamartomas and cystic kidney disease: linkage to 1q21-q32 and loss of the wild type allele in renal hamartomas. J Clin Endocrinol Metab 1996;81(12):4204–11.

73. Gill AJ, Lim G, Cheung V, et al. Parafibromin-deficient (HPT-JT Type, CDC73 Mutated) Parathyroid Tumors Demonstrate Distinctive Morphologic Features. Am J Surg Pathol 2019;43(1):35–46.

74. Cetani F, Banti C, Pardi E, et al. CDC73 mutational status and loss of parafibromin in the outcome of parathyroid cancer. Endocr Connections 2013;2(4): 186–95.

75. Carpten JD, Robbins CM, Villablanca A, et al. HRPT2, encoding parafibromin, is mutated in hyperparathyroidism-jaw tumor syndrome. Nat Genet 2002;32(4):676–80.

76. Kruijff S, Sidhu SB, Sywak MS, et al. Negative parafibromin staining predicts malignant behavior in atypical parathyroid adenomas. Ann Surg Oncol 2014 Feb;21(2):426–33.

77. Pyo JS, Cho WJ. Diagnostic and prognostic implications of parafibromin immunohistochemistry in parathyroid carcinoma. Biosci Rep 2019;39(4). BSR20181778.

78. Wei CH, Harari A. Parathyroid carcinoma: update and guidelines for management. Curr Treat Options Oncol 2012;13(1):11–23.

79. Schulte JJ, Pease G, Taxy JB, et al. Distinguishing parathyromatosis, atypical parathyroid adenomas, and parathyroid carcinomas utilizing histologic and clinical features. Head Neck Pathol 2021;15:727–36.

80. Hirokawa M, Suzuki A, Higuchi M, et al. Histological alterations following fine-needle aspiration for parathyroid adenoma: incidnce and diagnostic problems. Pathol Int 2021;71:400–5.

81. Hosny Mohammed K, Siddiqui MT, Willis BC, et al. Parafibromin, APC, and MIB-1 Are Useful Markers for Distinguishing Parathyroid Carcinomas from Adenomas. Appl Immunohistochem Mol Morphol 2017; 25(10):731–5.

82. Gill AJ, Clarkson A, Gimm O, et al. Loss of nuclear expression of parafibromin distinguishes parathyroid carcinomas and hyperparathyroidism-jaw tumor (HPT-JT) syndrome-related adenomas from sporadic parathyroid adenomas and hyperplasias. Am J Surg Pathol 2006;30(9):1140–9.

83. Abbona GC, Papotti M, Gasparri G, et al. Proliferative activity in parathyroid tumors as detected by Ki-67 immunostaining. Hum Pathol 1995;26(2):135–8.

84. Lloyd RV, Carney JA, Ferreiro JA, et al. Immunohistochemical Analysis of the Cell Cycle-Associated Antigens Ki-67 and Retinoblastoma Protein in Parathyroid Carcinomas and Adenomas. Endocr Pathol 1995;6(4):279–87.

85. Erovic BM, Harris L, Jamali M, et al. Biomarkers of parathyroid carcinoma. Endocr Pathol 2012;23(4): 221–31.

86. Bergero N, De Pompa R, Sacerdote C, et al. Galectin-3 expression in parathyroid carcinoma: immunohistochemical study of 26 cases. Hum Pathol 2005 Aug;36(8):908–14.

87. Howell VM, Gill A, Clarkson A, et al. Accuracy of combined protein gene product 9.5 and parafibromin markers for immunohistochemical diagnosis of parathyroid carcinoma. J Clin Endocrinol Metab 2009;94(2):434–41.

88. Osawa N, Onoda N, Kawajiri H, et al. Diagnosis of parathyroid carcinoma using immunohistochemical staining against hTERT. Int J Mol Med 2009;24(6): 733–41.

89. Guarnieri V, Battista C, Muscarella LA, et al. CDC73 mutations and parafibromin immunohistochemistry in parathyroid tumors: clinical correlations in a single-centre patient cohort. Cell Oncol 2012;35:411–22.

90. Kutahyalioglu M, Nguyen HT, Kwatampora L, et al. Genetic profiling as a clinical tool in advanced parathyroid carcinoma. J Cancer Res Clin Oncol 2019; 145(8):1977–86.

91. Kang H, Pettinga D, Schubert AD, et al. Genomic Profiling of Parathyroid Carcinoma Reveals Genomic Alterations Suggesting Benefit from Therapy. Oncologist 2019;24(6):791–7.

Para This, Fibromin That
The Role of CDC73 in Parathyroid Tumors and Familial Tumor Syndromes

Emad Ababneh, MD[a,b], Vania Nosé, MD, PhD[a],*

KEYWORDS

- Parathyroid • Hyperparathyroidism • HPT-JT syndrome • CDC73 • Parafibromin
- Parathyroid carcinoma • Parafibromin-deficient parathyroid tumor

---

Key points

- *CDC73* alterations are defining for hyperparathyroidism-jaw tumor (HPT-JT) syndrome-associated adenomas and are associated with most sporadic parathyroid carcinomas.
- The loss of nuclear parafibromin expression is a good surrogate marker for *CDC73* alterations.
- Parafibromin-deficient parathyroid tumors show cystic spaces, abundant eosinophilic cytoplasm, and perinuclear clearing.
- The loss of nuclear parafibromin expression can be used in clinical practice to stratify atypical parathyroid tumors in the absence of histologic features of malignancy as well as screen for association with HPT-JT syndrome.

ABSTRACT

CDC73 alterations are associated with three main parathyroid lesions according to the World Health Organization (WHO) classification of tumors of the endocrine system. These include hyperparathyroidism-jaw tumor (HPT-JT) syndrome-associated adenomas, atypical parathyroid tumors (APTs), and parathyroid carcinomas (PCs). The loss of nuclear parafibromin expression, which serves as a surrogate marker for the underlying CDC73 alteration, encompasses these tumors under the term parafibromin-deficient parathyroid tumors. They have distinct morphologic features of more abundant eosinophilic cytoplasm with perinuclear clearing surrounding a large nucleus as well as prominent dilated branching "hemangiopericytoma-like" vasculature and a thick capsule as well as variably sized cystic spaces. These tumors include cases that show unequivocal histologic features fulfilling the criteria for PCs with growing data indicating a higher rate of recurrence or metastasis compared with parafibromin intact PCs. More importantly, the loss of parafibromin expression can be used in clinical practice to recognize APTs that fall short of a conclusive diagnosis of PCs, but clinically behave akin to them. Moreover, recognizing these tumors can lead to an underlying germline mutation and a diagnosis of HPT-JT, which impacts long-term treatment and surveillance for patients and close family.

OVERVIEW

Carcinomas of the parathyroid gland are very rare and represent a very small fraction of human cancers.[1,2] Nevertheless, like their benign counterpart, they are frequently encountered as a part of tumor syndromes, namely, hyperparathyroidism-jaw tumor (HPT-JT) syndrome.[1–3] Diagnosing parathyroid carcinomas (PCs) prospectively on histologic grounds can be very challenging and depends on finding a constellation of evidence

---

[a] Department of Pathology, Warren 214, Massachusetts General Hospital, 55 Fruit street, Boston, MA 02114, USA; [b] Pathology and Laboratory medicine Institute, L25, Cleveland Clinic foundation, 9500 Euclid ave, Cleveland, OH 44118, USA
* Corresponding author.
E-mail address: vnose@mgh.harvard.edu

Surgical Pathology 16 (2023) 97–105
https://doi.org/10.1016/j.path.2022.09.009
1875-9181/23/© 2022 Elsevier Inc. All rights reserved.

for invasive behavior.[4,5] Often, the diagnosis of PCs is made only after evidence of more aggressive behavior such as recurrence and distant metastasis,[6,7] when conclusive morphologic evidence is lacking. Pathologic evidence of metastatic disease or local invasion is required for diagnosis, and they are not seen in all cases, this includes capsular, vascular, perineural, or soft tissue invasion. Other features associated with malignancy in other organs, such as pleomorphism, increased mitoses, and fibrous bands, can be seen in parathyroid adenomas (PA) and atypical parathyroid tumors (APTs), and thus not pathognomonic.[4,5] According to the most recent edition of the World Health Organization (WHO) classification of endocrine system tumors, there are three types of parathyroid lesions/diseases involved by CDC73 alterations and subsequent loss of parafibromin protein expression. These lesions are HPT-JT-associated parathyroid adenomas (HPT-JT-PAs), PCs, and sporadic parafibromin-deficient parathyroid tumors (PDPTs).[4,5]

1. HPT-JT syndrome is one of the rarest hereditary causes of primary hyperparathyroidism. It is associated with PA with distinct morphology as well as with a high lifetime risk of PC, approximately 15%.[4,6,8] As the name implies, HPT-JT is also associated with jaw tumors, mainly ossifying fibromas (OFs).[9,10] Case reports also describe renal tumors as well as some uterine pathologies in association.[4,9] The molecular basis of HPT-JT was described in 2002. Carpten and colleagues described heterozygous, germline, inactivating mutation in CDC73 (previously known as HRPT2) in 14 families with HPT-JT. CDC73 gene is present on chromosome 1 and encodes parafibromin, which plays a role in chromatin remodeling, and is a part of polymerase-associated factor-1 (PAF1) complex interacting with RNA polymerase II, as well as cell cycle remodeling through its interaction with P53.[11–13]

2. PCs, even in the sporadic settings, are associated with CDC73 alteration with approximately 80% of clinically aggressive PCs harboring these alterations in some reports.[14–17] Indeed, it is rare for PC to develop outside the setting of germline or somatic inactivating mutations/deletions of CDC73.[3,6,18]

3. PDPTs are recently recognized distinct subset of parathyroid tumors associated with CDC73 alterations. They are mostly included morphologically under the category of APTs.[4] Typical, recurrence-free sporadic PAs are only rarely associated with CDC73 alterations.[4,19]

Many reports and meta-analyses explored the role of CDC73 alterations and parafibromin expression in the diagnosis of various parathyroid tumors and their prognostic value.[6–8,16,20–24] This is a brief and practical overview of parafibromin-deficient/CDC73 altered parathyroid tumors with emphasis on a pragmatic approach to their diagnosis in daily surgical pathology practice.

PARAFIBROMIN AS A SURROGATE FOR CDC73 ALTERATIONS AND PARATHYROID CARCINOMAS

Tan and colleagues[25] were the first to study the loss of parafibromin expression as an adjunct tool for the diagnosis of PCs, on the basis that it is a surrogate for an underlying CDC73 alteration. They reported that loss of nuclear parafibromin immunoreactivity has high sensitivity and specificity for the diagnosis of PCs with a negative predictive value approaching 100% (given the low prevalence of PCs). They also described that most HPT-JT syndrome adenomas also showed loss of nuclear parafibromin expression. These findings were mostly validated by multiple subsequent studies.[8,21,22,26–28]

The loss of parafibromin nuclear immunoreactivity is a good surrogate for CDC73 alterations, yet multiple reports in the literature show inconsistencies between the rate of loss of parafibromin expression and the rate of underlying CDC73 alterations. These inconsistencies go in both directions, but more often show that many cases of loss of parafibromin expression fail to show either somatic or germline CDC73 alterations.[6,16,20,24,27] Of course, this discrepancy can have some technical and biological reasons such as epigenetic mutations or promotor site mutations not detected by testing methods used in these studies.[26,29,30] From a practical standpoint, this raises two main questions:

1. What constitutes a "loss of expression" that is more specific to an underlying CDC73 mutation?
2. Does the "loss of parafibromin expression" without underlying detected CDC73 alteration carry diagnostic or prognostic significance? This point will be covered when discussing the role of parafibromin immunohistochemistry (IHC) in the diagnosis and prognosis of PCs, see below.

As for the first question, it is widely accepted that complete loss of nuclear parafibromin immunoreactivity is a surrogate marker of underlying CDC73 alterations and can be used to distinguish PCs and HPT-JT-associated adenomas (**Fig. 1**).[6,20,24,27,31] Nevertheless, some authors

Fig. 1. (*A–C*) Examples of nuclear parafibromin loss in parathyroid tumors. Retained nuclear staining in nonneoplastic cells can be seen in (*A*). Note the high cytoplasmic background staining especially (*A*) and (*B*). There are scattered cells with positive nuclear staining in (*C*) admixed with the tumor cells. This represents an area of vascular invasion in parathyroid carcinoma.

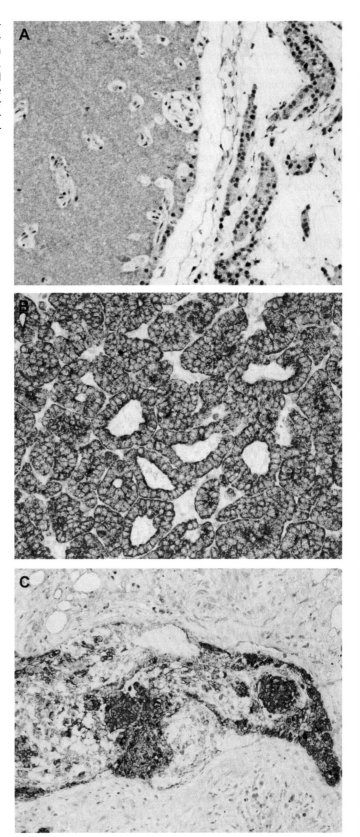

accepted focal nuclear immunoreactivity reaching approximately 5% to 10% of tumor cells,[16,32] and some of the cases with established *CDC73* alterations showed partial nuclear immunoreactivity rather than complete loss.[33] Furthermore, as parafibromin has nucleolar localization signals in addition to its nuclear localization ones,[12,34] some reports showed, in a limited number of cases, that complete loss of nucleolar expression can be a surrogate to underlying *CDC73* alterations in cases where there is no complete loss of nuclear immunoreactivity.[33]

CLINICAL FEATURES

1. The most common presentation of HPT-JT syndrome and parathyroid tumors, in general, is hyperparathyroidism.[2,4,35,36] In contrast to other familial hyperparathyroidism syndromes, HPT-JT is a single gland disease in most cases, in the form of an adenoma or parathyroid carcinoma. The age of onset is usually less than 40 year old, but cases in older patients are present in the literature.[2,6,36] They are classically associated with markedly elevated parathyroid hormone (PTH) levels and severe hypercalcemia with its associated sequelae. The associated jaw tumors histologically resemble OFs, they are most commonly asymptomatic and occur in the mandible more often than in the maxilla.[9,10,37] They can share some features with brown tumors of hyperparathyroidism, but the latter is purely lytic lesion and lacks the features of the slow and expansive growth of OFs such as sclerotic rim on imaging.[10] Other reported presentations include kidney tumors such as Wilms tumor and mixed epithelial-stromal tumors as well as uterine pathologies.
2. Sporadic PCs most commonly present with symptoms of severe hypercalcemia manifesting predominantly in bone and kidney abnormalities.[1,35,38,39] As mentioned earlier, most sporadic PCs harbor alteration in *CDC73* similar to HPT-JT syndrome and share similar clinical features, without the other syndromic associations.[3,6,20,21] Indeed, some reports describe that approximately 30% of clinically "sporadic" PCs have germline mutations in *CDC73* and might represent unrecognized HPT-JT syndrome.[6]
3. PDPTs share most of the clinical features of parathyroid carcinomas and HPT-JT-associated PAs. The severity of symptoms, although not consistent, is more commonly lower than those of PCs with slightly smaller size and weight. Even their long-term outcome

is more akin to PCs than their parafibromin intact counterparts as will be discussed below.

MORPHOLOGIC FEATURES

Akin to other tumors of the endocrine organs, histologic features of parathyroid tumors run on a spectrum between adenomas on one end and carcinoma on the other without clear unequivocal demarcation. This paradigm also applies for parafibromin-deficient/*CDC73* altered parathyroid tumors, but it has been reported that these tumors show distinct morphology of more abundant eosinophilic cytoplasm with perinuclear clearing surrounding a large nucleus as well as prominent dilated branching "hemangiopericytoma-like" vasculature and a thick capsule as well as variably sized cystic spaces (**Figs. 2 and 3**).[6]

1. In addition to the distinctive morphologic features mentioned above, the diagnosis of PAs in the setting of HPT-JT should still be made after careful examination for features of invasive behavior (see PC discussion below) and other atypical features such as necrosis and increased mitotic counts. Fibrosis can be seen, but broad fibrous bands should prompt a more thorough examination for other atypical features. Border irregularities, hemorrhage with hemosiderin deposition, or cholesterol clefts are frequently encountered, especially in larger adenomas.[4]
2. In the current WHO classification, the diagnosis of PCs requires unequivocal evidence of invasive behavior (Lymphovascular invasion, perineural invasion, direct invasion of surrounding structures, and/or pathologically documented metastatic disease) (**Fig. 4**).[4] This criterion applies to both sporadic and HPT-JT-associated PCs. It is important to assess for lymphatic or vascular invasion outside the tumor substance to avoid overcalling and to be mindful of the fact that focal extension of the tumor into broad fibrotic bands or surrounding connective tissue is not diagnostic of malignancy and this is critical, especially in previously manipulated lesions (eg, fine needle aspiration).
3. The current WHO classification paradigm acknowledges that features such as monotonous sheet-like or trabecular growth, marked cytologic atypia, band-like fibrosis, increased mitotic activity (>5/~10 mm^2), and adherence to adjacent structures, are more commonly seen in PCs but are not pathognomonic.[5,6]

Fig. 2. This is an example of a parafibromin-deficient parathyroid tumor (see **Fig.** 1B is corresponding parafibromin IHC). Note the characteristic features of abundant eosinophilic cytoplasm with perinuclear clearing, large nuclei, and conspicuous nucleoli.

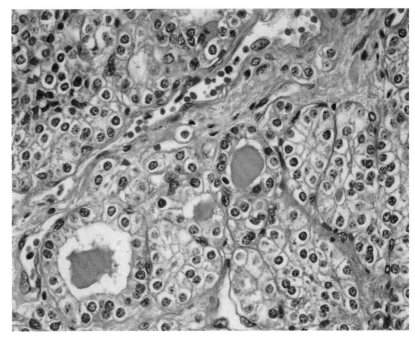

Fig. 3. This is a case of hyperparathyroidism-jaw tumor syndrome associated parathyroid tumor. Note the cystic spaces, large nuclei with prominent nucleoli, and the abundant eosinophilic cytoplasm.

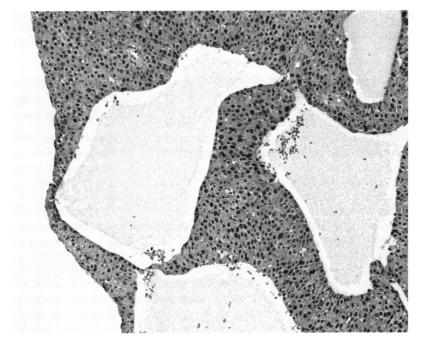

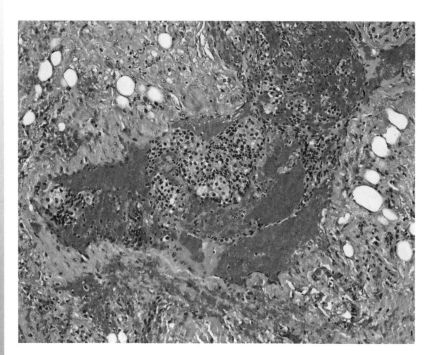

Fig. 4. This is an example of vascular invasion, diagnostic of parathyroid carcinoma in a parafibromin-deficient parathyroid tumor (see **Fig.** 1C for corresponding IHC).

Given that the diagnosis of PCs requires unequivocal evidence of invasive or metastatic behavior, tumors with worrisome features that lack these unequivocal findings are classified as APTs. PDPTs are a subset of APTs, as discussed below, with more aggressive clinical behavior.

PROGNOSTIC SIGNIFICANCE

The outcome for patients with PC is mostly favorable with a reported 10-year survival of 70% to 80% and disease-free survival of approximately 55%.[1,20,40] Multiple studies with a limited number of cases showed a worse clinical outcome for parafibromin-deficient PCs;[7,23,24] this was also validated by a more recent meta-analysis by Zhu and colleagues.[20] They showed that complete loss of parafibromin is a significant predictor of a worse outcome, but they failed to show the same significant effect with *CDC73* alterations. The possible reasons for the inconsistency between parafibromin expression and *CDC73* status were discussed above.

The category of APT (formerly atypical PA) is a testimony to the shortcomings of morphologic features to fully delineate malignant behavior in parathyroid tumors. APT is not a distinct entity, but rather a heterogeneous group that defies conclusive classification.[41] Most of the APTs behave indolently, but some will locally recur or even metastasize.[6,7,20,41] This is especially true for

parafibromin-deficient/*CDC73* altered tumors. Multiple reports have shown that parafibromin-deficient APTs behave more aggressively than their parafibromin intact counterparts with a higher rate of recurrence and metastasis.[7] Furthermore, there are rare parafibromin-deficient cases in the literature designated as adenomas with no worrisome features at all that showed subsequent recurrence and/or metastasis.[6]

ROLE OF PARAFIBROMIN IMMUNOHISTOCHEMISTRY IN CLINICAL PRACTICE

Based on the discussion above, the current literature discusses a role for parafibromin IHC and *CDC73* mutation testing in three scenarios:

1. A parathyroid tumor with histologic features that meet the WHO criteria for carcinoma. Parafibromin IHC is indicated as a prognostic indicator as well as screening for potential syndromic association with HPT-JT syndrome. As mentioned above, some reports describe that approximately 30% of seemingly sporadic PCs harbor a germline alteration in *CDC73*. HPT-JT syndrome association has a role in determining the need for longer follow-up surveillance as well as familial screening.[36,42]
2. A parathyroid tumor with worrisome histologic features that fall short of the WHO criteria for carcinoma, aka APTs. These tumors are not

Fig. 5. A proposed algorithmic approach for the use of parafibromin IHC in the evaluation of parathyroid tumors. [a]Reports of *CDC73* altered PCs with intact parafibromin staining are reported in the literature. If other clinical features of HPT-JT are present or the morphologic features of PDPTs are present, genetic testing can still be considered on a case-by-case basis even with retained parafibromin expression. [b]Adherence to adjacent structures, monotonous sheet-like growth, cytologic atypia, broad fibrous bands, necrosis, and mitotic activity (>5 per 50 high-power field). [c]Abundant eosinophilic cytoplasm with perinuclear staining and large nuclei, cystic spaces, and dilated branching hemangiopericytoma-like vasculature. HPT-JT, hyperparathyroidism-jaw tumor syndrome; PA, parathyroid adenoma; PC, parathyroid carcinoma; PDPT, parafibromin-deficient parathyroid tumor.

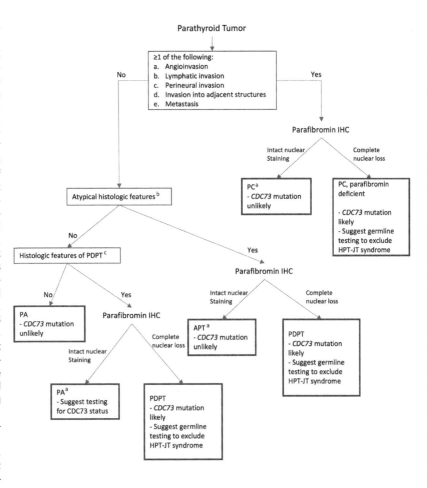

all created equal and loss of nuclear parafibromin expression has been established in the literature to infer a potentially malignant behavior more akin to parathyroid carcinoma.

3. A PA with the distinct morphologic features, recently described of parafibromin-deficient parathyroid tumor. Literature on their behavior is evolving with only rare cases described in the literature with recurrence and even metastasis. Parafibromin testing in this scenario can also be viewed as a screening test for HPT-JT.

The current WHO recommendation for interpreting parafibromin IHC is to look for complete nuclear loss of expression, whereas more data are needed to verify the significance of focal nuclear loss or nucleolar loss.[5]

Fig. 5 summarizes a proposed approach to the use of parafibromin immunohistochemistry in the evaluation of parathyroid tumors. There are a few caveats. First, it has been reported that parafibromin immunohistochemistry can be difficult to deploy and interpret.[17,27] In addition, as discussed above, cases with *CDC73* mutation and retained parafibromin expression are reported in the literature. Therefore, the threshold to suggest *CDC73* genetic testing in cases with typical morphologic features of PDPTs is low even when parafibromin expression is retained. Second, although some reports accept focal retained nuclear staining or only nucleolar loss in PDPTs, a more strict definition with complete loss of parafibromin expression is preferred. Nonetheless, any pattern of loss should be conveyed in the pathology report with potential consideration for genetic testing on a case-by-case basis.

SUMMARY

CDC73 alterations play a vital role in the pathogenesis of parathyroid tumors associated with HPT-JT syndrome as well as in the sporadic setting as they are present in most PCs. The loss of nuclear expression of parafibromin is a good surrogate marker for CDC73 alterations and can be used in clinical practice to screen morphologically distinct PTs and PCs for potential germline mutations as well as identify APTs with a propensity for more clinically aggressive behavior even when definitive morphologic features are lacking, such as in APTs.

CLINICS CARE POINTS

- Performing parafibromin immunohistochemistry can be helpful in screening for an underlying syndrome in parathyroid adenomas with cystic spaces, dilated branching blood vessels, and enlarged nuclei with perinuclear halos.

- We recommend performing parafibromin immunohistochemistry on all atypical parathyroid tumors as the data suggests that parafibromin-deficient atypical parathyroid tumors behave similarly to parathyroid carcinomas.

DISCLOSURE AND CONFLICTS OF INTEREST

The authors have no disclosures or conflicts of interest to disclose.

REFERENCES

1. Asare EA, Sturgeon C, Winchester DJ, et al. Parathyroid carcinoma: an update on treatment outcomes and prognostic factors from the national cancer data base (NCDB). Ann Surg Oncol 2015;22(12):3990–5.
2. Machado Wilhelm. Parathyroid cancer: a review. Cancers 2019;11(11):1676.
3. Cardoso L, Stevenson M, Thakker RV. Molecular genetics of syndromic and non-syndromic forms of parathyroid carcinoma. Hum Mutat 2017;38(12):1621–48.
4.. Organisation mondiale de la santé, Centre international de recherche sur le cancer. In: WHO classification of Tumours of endocrine organs. 4th edition. Lyon, France: International Agency for Research on Cancer; 2017.
5. Erickson LA, Mete O, Juhlin CC, et al. Overview of the 2022 WHO Classification of Parathyroid Tumors. Endocr Pathol 2022;33(1):64–89.
6. Gill AJ, Lim G, Cheung VKY, et al. Parafibromin-deficient (HPT-JT Type, CDC73 Mutated) Parathyroid Tumors Demonstrate Distinctive Morphologic Features. Am J Surg Pathol 2019;43(1):35–46.
7. Kruijff S, Sidhu SB, Sywak MS, et al. Negative Parafibromin Staining Predicts Malignant Behavior in Atypical Parathyroid Adenomas. Ann Surg Oncol 2014;21(2):426–33.
8. Gill AJ, Clarkson A, Gimm O, et al. Loss of Nuclear Expression of Parafibromin Distinguishes Parathyroid Carcinomas and Hyperparathyroidism-Jaw Tumor (HPT-JT) Syndrome-related Adenomas From Sporadic Parathyroid Adenomas and Hyperplasias. Am J Surg Pathol 2006;1140–9. https://doi.org/10.1097/01.pas.0000209827.39477.4f.
9. Turchini J, Gill AJ. Hereditary Parathyroid Disease: Sometimes Pathologists Do Not Know What They Are Missing. Endocr Pathol 2020;31(3):218–30.
10. du Preez H, Adams A, Richards P, et al. Hyperparathyroidism jaw tumour syndrome: a pictoral review. Insights Imaging 2016;7(6):793–800.
11. Carpten JD, Robbins CM, Villablanca A, et al. HRPT2, encoding parafibromin, is mutated in hyperparathyroidism–jaw tumor syndrome. Nat Genet 2002;32(4):676–80.
12. Panicker LM, Zhang JH, Dagur PK, et al. Defective nucleolar localization and dominant interfering properties of a parafibromin L95P missense mutant causing the hyperparathyroidism–jaw tumor syndrome. Endocr Relat Cancer 2010;17(2):513–24.
13. Masi G, Iacobone M, Sinigaglia A, et al. Characterization of a New CDC73 Missense Mutation that Impairs Parafibromin Expression and Nucleolar Localization. PLoS ONE 2014;9(5):e97994.
14. Howell VM. HRPT2 mutations are associated with malignancy in sporadic parathyroid tumours. J Med Genet 2003;40(9):657–63.
15. Shattuck TM, Välimäki S, Obara T, et al. Somatic and Germ-Line Mutations of the HRPT2 Gene in Sporadic Parathyroid Carcinoma. N Engl J Med 2003;349(18):1722–9.
16. Cetani F, Banti C, Pardi E, et al. CDC73 mutational status and loss of parafibromin in the outcome of parathyroid cancer. Endocr Connect 2013;2(4):186–95.
17. Gill AJ. Understanding the Genetic Basis of Parathyroid Carcinoma. Endocr Pathol 2014;25(1):30–4.
18. Cinque L, Pugliese F, Salcuni AS, et al. Molecular pathogenesis of parathyroid tumours. Best Pract Res Clin Endocrinol Metab 2018;32(6):891–908.
19. Juhlin C, Larsson C, Yakoleva T, et al. Loss of parafibromin expression in a subset of parathyroid adenomas. Endocr Relat Cancer 2006;13(2):509–23.
20. Zhu R, Wang Z, Hu Y. Prognostic role of parafibromin staining and CDC73 mutation in patients with parathyroid carcinoma: A systematic review and meta-analysis based on individual patient data. Clin Endocrinol (Oxf) 2020;92(4):295–302.
21. Pyo JS, Cho WJ. Diagnostic and prognostic implications of parafibromin immunohistochemistry in parathyroid carcinomaT. Biosci Rep 2019;39(4). BSR20181778.

22. Hu Y, Liao Q, Cao S, et al. Diagnostic performance of parafibromin immunohistochemical staining for sporadic parathyroid carcinoma: a meta-analysis. Endocrine 2016;54(3):612–9.

23. Hu Y, Bi Y, Cui M, et al. The Influence of Surgical Extent and Parafibromin Staining on The Outcome of Parathyroid Carcinoma: 20-Year Experience From a Single Institute. Endocr Pract 2019;25(7):634–41.

24. Witteveen JE, Hamdy NAT, Dekkers OM, et al. Downregulation of CASR expression and global loss of parafibromin staining are strong negative determinants of prognosis in parathyroid carcinoma. Mod Pathol 2011;24(5):688–97.

25. Tan MH, Morrison C, Wang P, et al. Loss of Parafibromin Immunoreactivity Is a Distinguishing Feature of Parathyroid Carcinoma. Clin Cancer Res 2004;10(19):6629–37.

26. Wang O, Wang C, Nie M, et al. Novel HRPT2/CDC73 Gene Mutations and Loss of Expression of Parafibromin in Chinese Patients with Clinically Sporadic Parathyroid Carcinomas. PLoS ONE 2012;7(9):e45567.

27. Guarnieri V, Battista C, Muscarella LA, et al. CDC73 mutations and parafibromin immunohistochemistry in parathyroid tumors: clinical correlations in a single-centre patient cohort. Cell Oncol 2012;35(6):411–22.

28. Papathomas TG, Nosé V. New and Emerging Biomarkers in Endocrine Pathology. Adv Anat Pathol 2019;26(3):198–209.

29. Guarnieri V, Muscarella LA, Verdelli C, et al. Alterations of DNA methylation in parathyroid tumors. Mol Cell Endocrinol 2018;469:60–9.

30. Hahn MA, Howell VM, Gill AJ, et al. CDC73/HRPT2 CpG island hypermethylation and mutation of 5′-untranslated sequence are uncommon mechanisms of silencing parafibromin in parathyroid tumors. Endocr Relat Cancer 2010;17(1):273–82.

31. Juhlin CC, Nilsson IL, Lagerstedt-Robinson K, et al. Parafibromin immunostainings of parathyroid tumors in clinical routine: a near-decade experience from a tertiary center. Mod Pathol 2019;32(8):1082–94.

32. Silva-Figueroa AM, Bassett R, Christakis I, et al. Using a Novel Diagnostic Nomogram to Differentiate Malignant from Benign Parathyroid Neoplasms. Endocr Pathol 2019;30(4):285–96.

33. Juhlin CC, Haglund F, Obara T, et al. Absence of nucleolar parafibromin immunoreactivity in subsets of parathyroid malignant tumours. Virchows Arch 2011;459(1):47–53.

34. Hahn MA, Marsh DJ. Nucleolar localization of parafibromin is mediated by three nucleolar localization signals. FEBS Lett 2007;581(26):5070–4.

35. Ryhänen EM, Leijon H, Metso S, et al. A nationwide study on parathyroid carcinoma. Acta Oncol 2017;56(7):991–1003.

36. Torresan F, Iacobone M. Clinical Features, Treatment, and Surveillance of Hyperparathyroidism-Jaw Tumor Syndrome: An Up-to-Date and Review of the Literature. Int J Endocrinol 2019;2019:1–8.

37. Carpenter TO, Kelly HR, Sherwood JS, et al. Case 32-2021: A 14-Year-Old Girl with Swelling of the Jaw and Hypercalcemia. N Engl J Med 2021;385(17):1604–13.

38. Guilmette J, Sadow PM. Parathyroid Pathology. Surg Pathol Clin 2019;12(4):1007–19.

39. Akirov A, Asa SL, Larouche V, et al. The Clinicopathological Spectrum of Parathyroid Carcinoma. Front Endocrinol 2019;10:731.

40. Harari A, Waring A, Fernandez-Ranvier G, et al. Parathyroid Carcinoma: A 43-Year Outcome and Survival Analysis. J Clin Endocrinol Metab 2011;96(12):3679–86.

41. Cetani F, Marcocci C, Torregrossa L, et al. Atypical parathyroid adenomas: challenging lesions in the differential diagnosis of endocrine tumors. Endocr Relat Cancer 2019;26(7):R441–64.

42. Sarquis MS, Silveira LG, Pimenta FJ, et al. Familial hyperparathyroidism: surgical outcome after 30 years of follow-up in three families with germline HRPT2 mutations. Surgery 2008;143(5):630–40.

On the Chopping Block
Overview of *DICER1* Mutations in Endocrine and Neuroendocrine Neoplasms

Carl Christofer Juhlin, MD, PhD*

KEYWORDS

- DICER1 • Mutation • Endocrine tumor • Neuroendocrine neoplasia • Review

Key points

- *DICER1* is a tumor suppressor gene encoding a micro-RNA (miRNA) master regulator, and mutations disrupting this function may have consequences on global miRNA maturation and hence propagate tumor development in various endocrine organs.

- When present in germline, *DICER1* mutations cause the DICER1 syndrome, a multitumor syndrome including a wide array of organs, including thyroid follicular nodular disease and thyroid carcinoma.

- *DICER1* mutations may also arise in somatic tissues, and subsets of well-differentiated thyroid carcinoma and poorly differentiated thyroid carcinoma in pediatric patients seem particularly enriched for this genetic aberrancy.

- In this review, the prevalence of *DICER1* mutations in endocrine and neuroendocrine tumors and the eventual effect on tumor progression and clinical outcome is discussed.

ABSTRACT

Mutational inactivation of the *DICER1* gene causes aberrant micro-RNA maturation, which in turn may have consequences for the posttranscriptional regulation of gene expression, thereby contributing to tumor formation in various organs. Germline *DICER1* mutations cause DICER1 syndrome, a pleiotropic condition with an increased risk of various neoplastic conditions in the pleura, ovaries, thyroid, pituitary, pineal gland, and mesenchymal tissues. Somatic *DICER1* mutations are also frequently observed in a wide variety of solid tumors, thereby highlighting the importance of this gene in tumor development. In this review, the importance of *DICER1* inactivation in endocrine tumors is discussed.

OVERVIEW

MICRO-RNAs AND THE DICER1 GENE

Micro-RNAs (miRNAs) are small molecules with the ability to regulate gene expression on the posttranscriptional level via binding of complimentary sequences in the messenger RNA (mRNA) single-strand.[1] The binding may cause mRNA degradation or impaired translation at the ribosomal level, with a similar end-result—less translated protein products.[2] Since their initial discovery, miRNAs have been associated with a multitude of biological processes, including key regulatory functions in embryology, organ differentiation, DNA repair, and tumor development.[1] Their influence on biology is well reflected through sequence conservation across species, including both animals and plants alike, thus implying a crucial and preserved mechanism of gene regulation through evolution.[3] Approximately 2500 human miRNAs have hitherto been identified, and they are thought to regulate one-third of the collective pool of genes—thus further reflecting the importance of these molecules in biology.[4]

Given the various key roles of miRNA in determining cellular fate, the regulation of miRNA processing and maturation is tightly regulated. In the human cell, miRNAs are encoded by nuclear

Department of Oncology-Pathology, Karolinska Institutet, Stockholm, Sweden
* Corresponding author. Department of Pathology and Cancer Diagnostics, Karolinska University Hospital, Radiumhemmet P1:02, Stockholm, 17177.
E-mail address: christofer.juhlin@ki.se

Surgical Pathology 16 (2023) 107–118
https://doi.org/10.1016/j.path.2022.09.010
1875-9181/23/

Regulation of micro-RNA maturation

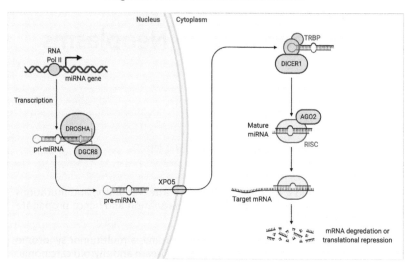

Fig. 1. Overview of the cellular regulation of miRNA maturation. The left part of the illustration depicts the nuclear compartment, in which a miRNA gene encoded by nuclear DNA is transcribed via RNA polymerase II (RNA Pol II). This creates a hairpin-containing primary transcript (pri-miRNA) molecule, which is further processed into a shorter pre-miRNA by the miRNA regulators DROSHA and DGCR8. The pre-miRNA can escape the nuclear compartment via the shuttling protein XPO5, and subsequently associate to DICER1 and TRBP in the cytosol (right part of the illustration). This allows the formation of mature miRNA, which can be used to target a specific mRNA molecule using the RNA-induced silencing complex (RISC) and AGO2. (Created using BioRender.com.)

DNA and are transcribed via RNA polymerase type II (**Fig. 1**). The product, called a pri-miRNA molecule, is then cleaved and further processed by the proteins DROSHA and DGCR8 into a pre-miRNA.[5] This pre-miRNA is then allowed to escape the nuclear compartment via the XPO5 shuttling protein.[6] Once in the cytosol, the DICER1 protein (encoded by the *DICER1* gene) will act in concert with the TAR DNA-binding protein (TRBP) to further cleave the pre-miRNA into a ~22 nucleotide-long, mature miRNA molecule, and the target RNA sequence is then targeted and degraded via the RNA-induced silencing complex (RISC) complex.[5,7] The role of DICER1 in this maturation process is imperative because this protein exhibits a riboendonuclease (RNAse) function with the ability to cleave double-stranded RNA molecules into shorter fragments.[7,8]

DICER1 is a 27 exon-long gene positioned at chromosome 14q32.13 that encodes the DICER1 protein, a ubiquitously expressed, 1922 amino acid protein with various functional domains (**Fig. 2**). Given the miRNA-processing abilities, DICER1 exhibits helicase and double-stranded (ds)RNA-binding domains required for recognition of certain dsRNAs,[9] as well as an RNAse function allocated to 2 functionally important regions entitled RNAse IIIa and IIIb, respectively.[10,11] The RNAse ability of DICER1 allows for the catalytic conversion of pre-miRNA to mature miRNA, and specific metal-ion–binding residues at specific amino acid positions within these RNAse III

domains are especially important for this task (most notably codons 1705, 1709, 1809, 1810, and 1813; see **Fig. 2**).[10] Given the biological importance of these codons for DICER1 function, it may come as little surprise that these amino acid positions constitute so called hotspots for somatic *DICER1* missense mutations in various neoplasms.[12–17] The mutations are thought to impair the catalytic activity of the RNAse IIIb domain, thereby making the DICER1 protein unable to process miRNAs to their mature state. Any eventual target mRNA would thereby escape degradation/ribosomal blockade, and the effects on the proteome could therefore be immense. In theory, subsets of oncoproteins may also escape downregulation, thereby possibly stimulating tumor development. However, germline mutations (causing DICER1 syndrome) often are deleterious and may therefore occur all along the *DICER1* gene, although often upstream of the functionally important RNAse III domains.[14,18–20] It has been shown that the *DICER1* gene fulfills the criteria of the Knudson 2-hit hypothesis, in which both alleles need to be impaired in order to stimulate tumor formation.[21] For example, syndromic patients with DICER1 recurrently display a truncating germline mutation and a second, somatic mutation (very often allocated to the RNAse IIIb hotspot regions) in the arising tumors.[21] Alternatively, the trans allele may also be deleted entirely in some tumors, as noted in pineoblastoma.[22] In sporadic tumors arising in non-DICER1 patients, biallelic

DICER protein structure and common mutational sites

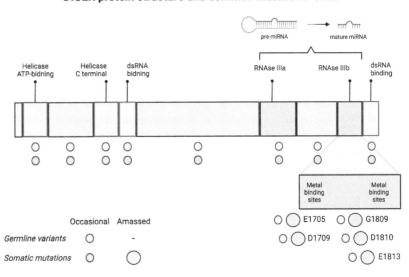

Fig. 2. DICER1 is a 1922 amino acid protein with several important functional regions, including 2 helicase-binding domains, several domains used for double-stranded RNA binding as well as 2 catalytically active regions (RNAse IIIa and RNAse IIIb) used to cleave the pre-miRNA into mature miRNA. Within the RNAse IIIb region, several metal binding sites are especially sensitive to missense mutations, including codons 1705, 1709, 1809, 1810, and 1813. The crude, spatial distributions of somatic *DICER1* mutations in human tumors and in patients with DICER1 syndromic are shown with pink and green circles, respectively. (Created using BioRender.com.)

mutational inactivation of *DICER1* has also been reported, thereby reinforcing the view of *DICER1* as a *bona fide* tumor suppressor gene.[23,24]

THE DICER1 SYNDROME

The DICER1 syndrome is a tumor predisposition condition, often afflicting patients aged younger than 40 years, and is characterized by an increased risk for several immature as well as differentiated variants of neoplasia.[25] In children aged older than 10 years, common tumors include pleuropulmonary blastoma (PPB), pulmonary cysts, various forms of thyroid carcinoma as well as cystic nephroma.[26] More seldomly, medulloepithelioma of the ciliary body, anaplastic sarcoma of the kidney, embryonal rhabdomyosarcoma of the cervix, pituitary blastoma, pineoblastoma, central nervous system tumors, and presacral malignant teratoid tumors are noted.[27] In DICER1 kindred aged older than 10 years, the spectrum may also include thyroid follicular nodular disease (TFND), thyroblastoma (previously known as thyroid malignant teratoma), nasal chondromesenchymal hamartoma, and ovarian Sertoli-Leydig cell tumors[27] (**Fig. 3**). Apart from neoplastic conditions, an overrepresentation of development-related clinical features, such as macrocephaly and ocular and dental abnormalities, has been reported.[28–30]

SOMATIC DICER1 MUTATIONS IN HUMAN CANCER

When consulting the Catalog of Somatic Mutations In Cancer (COSMIC) for the purpose of this review (https://cancer.sanger.ac.uk/cosmic, database last accessed 26th of April 2022), 1885 out of 63,367 tumors sequenced (~3%) display *DICER1* mutations. Not entirely unexpected, the prevalence of *DICER1* mutations in tumor DNA is highest among tumor types that are also core features of the DICER1 syndrome, including tumors of the pleura (~21% of all interrogated cases, all being PPB apart from a single mesothelioma) and pituitary tumors (~9% of all cases, pituitary blastoma and a single pituitary neuroendocrine tumor [NET]). Moreover, ~9% of all sequenced meningiomas exhibited *DICER1* mutations, with similar frequency for tumors of the endometrium, skin, and nervous system. In terms of endocrine and neuroendocrine tumors, *DICER1* mutations are most frequently reported in various forms of thyroid carcinoma, pituitary blastoma, and pineoblastoma. Although rare in scope, the mutations may have correlations to specific disease phenotypes, patient outcomes, and also consequences for genetic counseling. In the following sections, lesions derived from endocrine organs and their relationship to *DICER1* aberrations are detailed. A schematic overview of

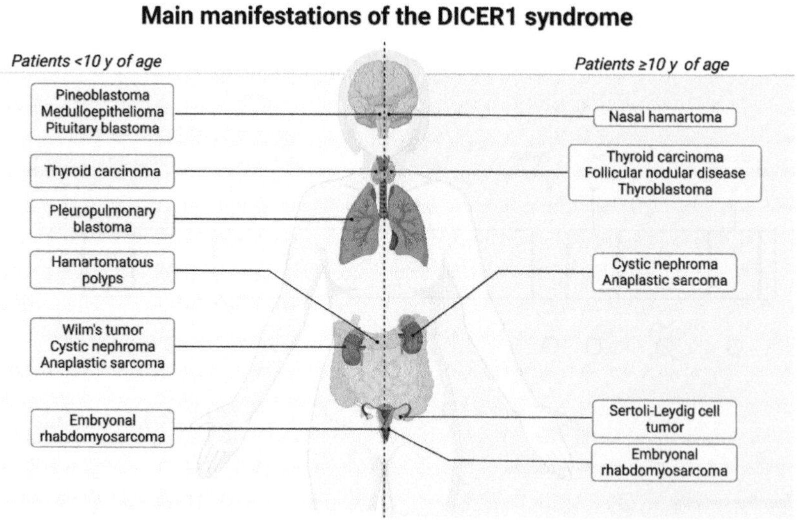

Main manifestations of the DICER1 syndrome

Fig. 3. Overview of DICER1 syndrome-related lesions. Main manifestation in patients aged younger than 10 years are depicted to the left, whereas patients aged 10 years or older are represented to the right. (Created using Bio-Render.com.)

DICER1 mutations in endocrine and neuroendocrine neoplasia is presented in **Table 1** and further illustrated in **Fig. 4**.

DICER1 MUTATIONS IN THYROID FOLLICULAR NODULAR DISEASE

The terminology "thyroid follicular nodular disease" is novel to the upcoming 2022 World Health Organization (WHO) classification of endocrine and neuroendocrine tumors and is thought to encompass the entities previously referred to as "multinodular goiter," "adenomatoid nodule," and "follicular hyperplasia."[31] The reasoning for this restructuring is based on the fact that "goiter" is a clinical term referring to an enlarged thyroid gland, as well as the notion that subsets of cases may exhibit a mixture of benign, nonclonal, and clonal expansions. The latter fact is based on modern genetic analyses, making it almost impossible to separate all entities in this continuous spectrum of nonclonal, hyperplastic, and clonal proliferations—and the former separation seems to lack clinical relevance.[31] Therefore, this review will solely use the terminology TFND for these lesions. Today, TFND is an established component of the DICER1 syndrome.[18,32] In one of the most comprehensive analyses to date, Khan and colleagues investigated 145 patients with a *DICER1* germline mutation and 135 non-DICER1 controls and found that the cumulative incidence of TFND or thyroidectomy was significantly higher in DICER1 syndrome individuals compared with the controls.[33] Patients with DICER1 syndrome had a 16-fold increased risk of thyroid cancer, and most TFND nodules and thyroid carcinoma samples interrogated were positive for somatic pathogenic *DICER1* mutations.[33] Although the finding of

"second hit" alterations in thyroid cancer may have been expected, the occurrence of somatic DNA level *DICER1* variants in TFND was more surprising. In all, the findings strongly suggest that the development of TFND in patients with *DICER1* may to a large part be clonal and driven by aberrant miRNA regulation.[33] A recent Danish study concluded that 6 out of 46 patients (13%) with TFND aged older than 25 years displayed pathogenic (nonsense or frameshift) germline *DICER1* variants.[34] Interestingly, only 2 of these patients (33%) had other DICER1 syndrome-related tumors (1 patient exhibited cysts of the kidney and lung, and a second patient was diagnosed with an ovarian Sertoli-Leydig cell tumor. The authors conclude that patients with TFND aged younger than 21 years and patients aged younger than 25 years with a family history of TFND should be referred to genetic counselling and *DICER1* sequencing in constitutional tissues. Moreover, all patients with TNFD also exhibiting other components of the DICER1 syndrome should similarly be referred.[34] A histologic example of TFND in a DICER1 syndrome patient is illustrated in **Fig. 5**.

DICER1-MUTATED FOLLICULAR-Cell–Derived THYROID CARCINOMA

Today, somatic and germline *DICER1* mutations are established in specific subgroups of thyroid cancer. Approximately 2.5% of all thyroid carcinoma subtypes carry *DICER1* mutations according to the COSMIC database, including both differentiated forms (papillary thyroid carcinoma [PTC] and follicular thyroid carcinoma [FTC]) but also subsets of poorly differentiated and anaplastic thyroid carcinoma (ATC).[35–38] In a comprehensive report of 829 malignant thyroid tumors assessed via next-

Table 1
Overview of *DICER1* aberrant endocrine and neuroendocrine tumors

Lesion Type	Somatic *DICER1* Mutational Frequency (%)	Seen in Patients with Germline *DICER1* Mutations
Thyroid lesions		
TFND	Often reported (>50%)	Yes
Pediatric PTC	Reported (>10%)	Yes
Adult PTC	Very rarely reported (<1%)	Yes
Pediatric FTC	Reported (>10%)	Yes
Adult FTC	Rarely reported (5%–10%)	Yes
Oncocytic carcinoma	Rarely reported (<5%)	N.d.
Pediatric PDTC	Often reported (>50%)	Yes
Adult PDTC	Rarely reported (<5%)	N.d.
ATC	Rarely reported (<5%)	N.d.
Blastoma	Often reported (>50%)	Yes
Parathyroid lesions		
Carcinoma	Very rarely reported (<1%)	No
Pituitary lesions		
Blastoma	Often reported (>50%)	Yes
Pineal lesions		
Blastoma	Not reported	Yes
Adrenal lesions		
ACA	Not reported	No
ACC	Not reported	No
Other		
MCC	Not reported	No
GEP-NENs	Not reported	No

Abbreviations: ACA, adrenal cortical adenoma; ACC, adrenal cortical carcinoma; ATC, anaplastic thyroid carcinoma; FTC, follicular thyroid carcinoma; GEP-NEN, gastroenteropancreatic neuroendocrine neoplasia; MCC, Merkel cell carcinoma; N.d, Not determined; PDTC, poorly differentiated thyroid carcinoma; PTC, papillary thyroid carcinoma; TFND, thyroid follicular nodular disease.

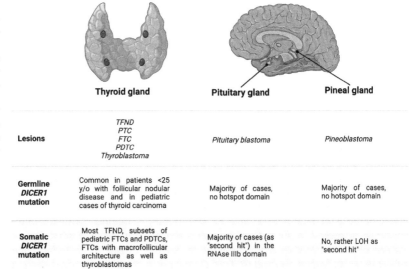

Fig. 4. *DICER1*-mutated lesions in endocrine glands. PTC; papillary thyroid carcinoma, FTC; follicular thyroid carcinoma, PDTC; poorly differentiated thyroid carcinoma, y/o; year-old, TFND; thyroid follicular nodular disease (replacing the previous terminology "multinodular goiter"). (Created using BioRender.com.)

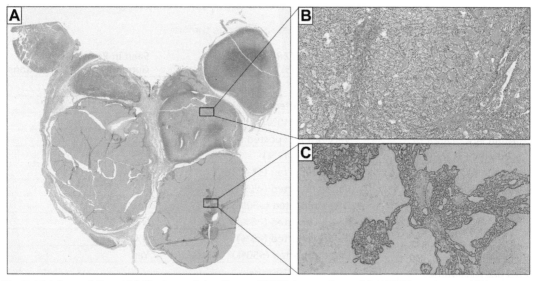

Fig. 5. Histology of thyroid follicular nodular disease (TFND) in a patient with DICER1 syndrome. All images are hematoxylin-eosin stains. (*A*) Low power overview highlighting the heterogenous nature of TFND in a DICER1 syndrome setting, with colloid nodules intermingled with hyperplastic lesions (of which some may be clonal with somatic *DICER1* second-hit mutations). (*B*) High-power magnification of a hyperplastic area depicting microfollicular growth but no nuclear atypia and lack of invasive growth. (*C*) Areas with prominent papillae are evident but papillary thyroid carcinoma nuclear features are absent.

generation sequencing, *DICER1* mutations were found in 14 cases (1.7%).[38] The frequency was highest in FTC (6.7%) and oncocytic thyroid carcinoma (previously known as Hürthle cell carcinoma; 4%), followed by poorly differentiated thyroid carcinoma (PDTC) and differentiated high-grade thyroid carcinoma (2.5%), ATC (1.4%), and PTC (0.8%). However, when only assessing pediatric thyroid carcinoma, the pooled prevalence of *DICER1* mutations is 12.5%, making it one of the most common genetic alterations in this demographic group.[39]

In one of the first studies, de Kock and colleagues detected somatic *DICER1* mutations in 3 PTCs arising in patients with DICER1 syndrome carrying pathogenic germline variants.[35] The somatic mutations all affected the critical metal-binding residues of the RNase IIIb domain, thereby constituting "second hits" in *DICER1* tumorigenesis. This proposed mechanism has been validated by independent investigators in which patients with DICER1 syndrome with thyroid cancer have been found to exhibit biallelic *DICER1* inactivation.[40] Interestingly, sporadic PTC and FTC cases have also been reported with assumed biallelic inactivation on the somatic level, further solidifying the notion that *DICER1* could be considered a driver of subgroups of thyroid neoplasia.[23,41] Also arguing in favor for a tumor driver status is the fact that somatic *DICER1* mutations are observed in subsets of pediatric PTCs absent of other credible driver alterations (such as *BRAF* V600E mutations and *RET::PTC* fusions).

In one particular study, *DICER1* mutations were found in 3 of 18 (16.7%) pediatric PTC cases lacking conventional genetic events and should thus be considered a fairly common genetic alteration in driver-negative PTC among patients aged younger than 18 years.[42] Similarly, *DICER1* mutations have been reported in unusual cases of pediatric FTC but given the rarity of FTC among patients aged younger than 18 years, the true prevalence of *DICER1* mutations in this patient group is not known.[43,44] In a recent NGS-based study of 41 pediatric patients with follicular-patterned tumors (follicular thyroid adenomas [FTAs], FTCs, oncocytic adenomas, encapsulated follicular variant PTCs, and noninvasive follicular thyroid neoplasms with papillary-like nuclear features (NIFTPs), *DICER1* emerged as the top altered gene with 22% of cases (mostly FTAs and FTCs) exhibiting hotspot missense variants in the RNAse IIIb region.[45] Moreover, the *DICER1* mutations were mutually exclusive with oncogenic *RAS* mutations, further emphasizing the potential driver role of the former aberrancy in thyroid neoplasia. The germline status of the cohort was not assessed but all patients with a *DICER1* variant in the tumor tissue lacked other manifestations related to the DICER1 syndrome.[45] The fact that subsets of FTAs may exhibit somatic *DICER1* mutations suggests that *DICER1* gene aberrancies may constitute an early event in thyroid tumorigenesis.[23,45–47] Indeed, from a functional perspective, *DICER1* has been shown to exhibit tumor suppressor functions in both PTC and FTC cell lines, thereby providing a mechanistic link between mutational inactivation and increased proliferation.[44,48]

Apart from pediatric PTCs and FTCs either arising through somatic *DICER1* mutations in patients with pathogenic germline *DICER1* variants or via somatic mutations on both alleles, somatic *DICER1* mutations seem to be particularly amassed in pediatric PDTCs and follicular thyroid tumors with a macrofollicular architecture. PDTCs are rare tumors in the pediatric population, displaying invasive features, solid/trabecular/insular growth patterns as well as an increased mitotic index and/or tumor necrosis. Recently, an NGS analysis of such lesions identified *DICER1* mutations in the RNAse IIIb region in 5 out of 6 cases (83%), and one case was found to harbor an additional germline variant, whereas another case displayed loss of heterozygosity (LOH) for the *DICER1* locus.[49] Intriguingly, 3 patients died of disease shortly after diagnosis, thereby possibly reflecting a severe clinical course. Although based on few cases overall, the data suggest that pediatric and adolescent patients with PDTC should undergo germline *DICER1* sequencing.

Follicular thyroid tumors with a macrofollicular architecture are neoplastic lesions often arising in young female patients.[23,41] The tumors exhibit a well-demarcated, often thick capsule, and are composed of tumor cells with dilated follicles, scattered papillae, and areas suggestive of tumor infarction[23] (**Fig. 6**). The tumors are often very similar to the colloid nodules characterizing TFND, and fine-needle aspiration biopsies of such lesions often render a Bethesda II category diagnosis preoperatively.[41] If capsular invasion is present, a diagnosis of FTC is favored according to standard WHO guidelines.[31] Angioinvasion has not yet been reported, and the prognosis is excellent.[23,41] In recent years, follicular thyroid tumors with a macrofollicular architecture have been found to exhibit biallelic *DICER1* mutations, of which subsets were also verified in the germline setting, thus possibly motivating constitutional sequencing of these rare patients.[23,41,50]

DICER1-MUTATED BLASTOMA OF THE THYROID, PITUITARY, AND PINEAL GLANDS

Blastoma is an immature neoplasm arising in progenitor cells of various lineages, and patients with

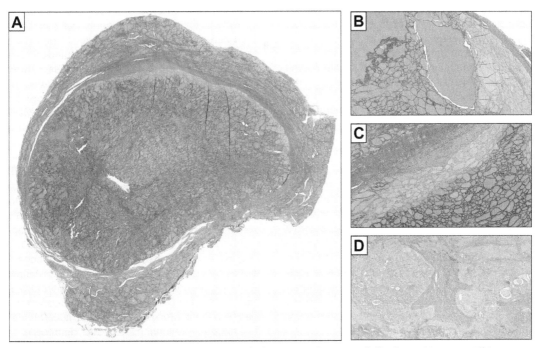

Fig. 6. Morphologic hallmarks of a follicular thyroid adenoma with a macrofollicular architecture. All images are hematoxylin-eosin stains. (*A*) Well-demarcated and encapsulated lesion is observed on low power. Note the macrofollicular structures and the focal papillary growth. (*B, C*) Areas of degeneration (infarction-like) are present, mostly accentuated directly underneath the tumoral capsule. (*D*) High-power overview of a degenerative area simulating geographic necrosis. This tumor lacked invasive behavior. Sequencing of tumor DNA identified 2 different somatic mutations in the RNAse IIIb region. The patient was negative for germline involvement.

DICER1 syndrome have an increased risk of developing such tumors in several endocrine organs, including the thyroid, pituitary, and pineal glands. Thyroblastoma (previously referred to as "malignant thyroid teratoma") occur mainly in adolescent and adult patients, and are poor-prognosis, triphasic tumors with a primitive, often neurectodermal-derived component displaying classic hallmarks of malignant tumors (frequent mitotic figures, elevated Ki-67 indices and tumor necrosis), scattered spindled cells with frequent rhabdomyoblastic differentiation as well as teratoid epithelial tubules suggestive of primitive thyroid follicles that may exhibit various growth patterns.[31,51,52] From an immunohistochemical perspective, the heterogenous nature of this tumor is highlighted by the various staining patterns, including SALL4 and TTF1 positivity in the primitive component, whereas the rhabdomyoblastic component is highlighted by myogenin and desmin and the thyroid epithelial component stains for TTF1 and PAX8.[51] Although only a handful of cases have been sequenced to date, there seems to be a massive overrepresentation of somatic DICER1 hotspot mutations in these lesions, whereas the frequency of germline involvement is not established.[52–54]

Pituitary blastoma was first described in a 13-month-old female patient with Cushing syndrome and ACTH elevation,[55] and subsequent genetic analyses of an unrelated case series revealed a very-high frequency of germline DICER1 mutations along with a "second-hit" somatic event (most often mutations in the RNAse IIIb region, and some with LOH of the DICER1 locus).[56] Pituitary blastomas are composed of 3 separate components, including primitive blastoid cells, cuboidal or columnar Rathke's pouch epithelium with rosette or glandular structures, as well as neuroendocrine cells, mostly with a corticotroph cell differentiation.[57] ACTH secretion from the latter cells is thought to give rise to the often observed hypercortisolism in these patients.[57,58]

Pineoblastoma is a primitive, malignant neuroectodermal tumor of the pineal gland primarily affecting children aged 0 to 4 years.[59] Germline DICER1 mutations along with second-hit LOH of the DICER1 locus have been reported in most cases.[22,60] In this way, pineoblastoma is different from other DICER1-related endocrine neoplasia in that no RNAse IIIb region mutations are found but rather loss of the unmutated allele.

DICER1 MUTATIONS IN OTHER ENDOCRINE TUMORS

Apart from the lesions discussed above, DICER1 mutations in other endocrine and neuroendocrine tumors are exceedingly rare. Most parathyroid tumors are usually driven by MEN1 alterations (adenomas) or CDC73 gene mutations (carcinomas),[61] and only single cases of parathyroid carcinoma have been reported to exhibit deleterious DICER1 mutations.[62] Adrenal cortical adenomas (ACAs) are driven by mutations in ion channel genes (aldosteronoma) or the protein kinase A pathway (cortisol-producing tumors), whereas the genetic background of adrenal cortical carcinoma (ACC) is more heterogenous and includes P53 and Wnt pathway gene mutations.[63] No DICER1 mutations have been reported in adrenal cortical tumors but previous efforts have mostly targeted the RNAse IIIb region.[64] Similarly, pheochromocytoma and abdominal paraganglioma are driven by mutations in genes encoding proteins regulating the citric acid cycle, pseudohypoxic and protein kinase-related pathways, and have not been reported to exhibit DICER1 mutations.[65,66]

NON-MUTATIONAL DICER1 ABERRATIONS IN ENDOCRINE AND NEUROENDOCRINE TUMORS

Apart from DICER1 mutations, there are other molecular mechanisms at play in endocrine neoplasia interfering with DICER1 function (Fig. 7). FTAs recurrently exhibit DICER1 mRNA downregulation, similarly to their malignant counterparts, FTC.[44] It has been shown that the transcription factor GA-binding protein alpha chain (GABPA) binds directly to the DICER1 promoter and enhances DICER1 mRNA output.[44] Interestingly, GABPA levels are also reduced in follicular thyroid tumors, providing a plausible explanation to the observed DICER1 mRNA downregulation in these lesions.[44] In ACCs, the mRNA levels of DICER1 and the binding partner TRBP have been found upregulated when compared with ACA, and the inhibition of TRBP expression resulted in the induction of apoptosis in an ACC cell line.[67] Interestingly, although the reason for higher expression of the tumor suppressor DICER1 in malignant adrenal cortical tumors compared with benign ones in not known, lower DICER1 expression was intimately associated to worse outcome within the ACC group.[64] Finally, in Merkel cell carcinomas (MCCs), recent study indicates that the DICER1 mRNA may be stabilized via HSC70 and Merkel cell polyoma virus (MCPyV) T antigen, preventing it from degradation.[68] Although the possible effects on tumor propagation need to be further explored, the findings are fascinating given the important roles of miRNA in MCC.[69] Whether or not DICER1 could exert oncogenic functions in addition to the bona fide tumor suppressor roles is not well-known but the

Fig. 7. Molecular, non-mutational aberrancies involving DICER1 in endocrine tumors. Top row: The GABPA-dependent downregulation of *DICER1* mRNA in follicular thyroid tumors (right) compared with normal thyroid tissue (left). In the latter group, the transcription factor GABPA is downregulated (for unknown reasons), causing a reduction in *DICER1* gene transcription, which will lead to proliferation. Middle row: The DICER1 and TRBP proteins are responsible for processing pre-miRNA into mature miRNA sequences, and both proteins have been

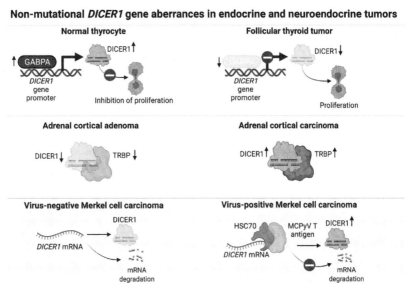

Non-mutational *DICER1* gene aberrances in endocrine and neuroendocrine tumors

found to be downregulated in adrenal cortical adenoma (left) compared with adrenal cortical carcinoma (right). Interestingly, within the carcinoma group, the cases with lowest DICER1 expression exhibit poorer outcome. Bottom row: Merkel cell carcinomas (MCCs) with Merkel cell polyoma virus T antigen expression (right) demonstrate stabilization of *DICER1* mRNA levels via assistance of the HSC70 protein, whereas MCCs lacking the virus T antigen (left) are thought to degrade *DICER1* mRNA to a larger extent. However, the effect on miRNA global output and MCC tumor formation needs to be further elucidated. (Created using BioRender.com.)

stabilization of *DICER1* mRNA in virus-positive MCC is intriguing.

THE EMERGING ROLE OF MICRO-RNA ABERRATIONS UNRELATED TO DICER1 IN THYROID CANCER

Although *DICER1* enjoys an established role in thyroid tumorigenesis, there is data emerging that other miRNA-regulating genes involved in miRNA maturation and processing also may play a role in the development of benign and malignant lesions of the thyroid. For example, p.E518K mutations of the *DGCR8* gene underly the autosomal dominant tumor susceptibility syndrome familial multinodular goiter with schwannomatosis, in which the afflicted develop early-onset TFND and multiple schwannomas, and the same mutation was also found in 2 unrelated PTCs.[70] After this discovery, recurrent E518K *DGCR8* mutations were found in 2 out of 11 FTCs, and *DGRC8* mRNA expression is reduced in most FTCs studied.[71] The 2 *DGCR8*-mutated FTCs also exhibited a distinct global miRNA profile, suggesting that the mutations are impactful. Apart from *DGCR8*, single cases with mutations in the miRNA processing gene *DROSHA* have also been reported in thyroid cancer,[72] and a recent fusion involving the miRNA shuttling protein gene *XPO5* has been implied in

ATC, although the functional consequences remain to be established.[73]

DISCUSSION

Dysregulation of miRNA has been recurrently reported in various endocrine neoplasia for decades, with consequences on tumor phenotype and clinical outcome. However, with the identification of the DICER1 syndrome and inactivating *DICER1* gene mutations, a plausible genetic mechanism arose that possibly could help the scientific community interpret many of the aberrant miRNA patterns observed across endocrine tumors.

Given the association between the *DICER1* syndrome and specific tumor types presenting in very young ages, it comes as little surprise to find that somatic *DICER1* mutations also explain subsets of these tumors arising in sporadic settings. Moreover, the finding of biallelic inactivation (either via two mutations or mutations and LOH) strongly supports a tumor suppressive function of *DICER1* in most affected endocrine tumors. Moreover, an interesting genotype–phenotype correlation seems evident as well, in which germline pathogenic variants seem to be truncating or frameshift alterations distributed across the *DICER1* coding sequences, whereas somatic mutations are highly congregated missense alterations in hotspot codons of the catalytically important RNAse IIIb region. Given the increased proportion of genetic testing performed on tumor DNA as part of the pathology routine practice in recent years, it is expected that the number of tumors with known *DICER1* genotypes will increase, and the need for subsequent germline testing will probably intensify as a consequence. Indeed, given the strong coupling between *DICER1* mutations, TFND in adolescents and thyroid cancer in the pediatric population, it is expected that these patient categories routinely will undergo germline DNA sequencing in the future in order to detect syndromic patients at an early stage.

CLINICS CARE POINTS

- DICER1 syndrome is an emerging, early-onset multitumor entity with various manifestations in endocrine tissues, including the thyroid, pituitary, and pineal glands.

- The syndrome is caused by germline mutations in the *DICER1* tumor suppressor gene, a master regulator of miRNA processing, and is often accompanied by somatic mutations or gene deletions of the remaining allele. The subsequent DICER1 protein deficit is expected to disturb the global output of miRNA and hence interfere with posttranscriptional gene regulation, thereby driving tumor development.

- In the nonsyndromic setting, somatic *DICER1* mutations are especially pronounced among pediatric thyroid carcinomas, including PTCs, FTCs and poor-prognosis PDTCs. A specific coupling to follicular thyroid tumors with a macrofollicular architecture and immature and aggressive thyroblastomas is also noted.

- Young individuals with thyroid follicular nodular disease should undergo *DICER1* gene sequencing of germline tissues because a large subset of patients will exhibit constitutional mutations. The same is also true for patients with pediatric thyroid cancer, although the proportion of cases with germline involvement is smaller.

DISCLOSURE

The author has no disclosures to report.

REFERENCES

1. Ameres SL, Zamore PD. Diversifying microRNA sequence and function. Nat Rev Mol Cell Biol 2013;14(8):475–88.
2. Lin R, Avery L. RNA interference. Policing rogue genes. Nature 1999;402(6758):128–9.
3. Ibáñez-Ventoso C, Vora M, Driscoll M. Sequence relationships among C. elegans, D. melanogaster and human microRNAs highlight the extensive conservation of microRNAs in biology. PLoS One 2008;3(7):e2818.
4. Hammond SM. An overview of microRNAs. Adv Drug Deliv Rev 2015;87:3–14.
5. Dexheimer PJ, Cochella L. MicroRNAs: From Mechanism to Organism. Front Cell Dev Biol 2020;8:409.
6. Wu K, He J, Pu W, et al. The Role of Exportin-5 in MicroRNA Biogenesis and Cancer. Genomics Proteomics Bioinformatics 2018;16(2):120–6.
7. Bernstein E, Caudy AA, Hammond SM, et al. Role for a bidentate ribonuclease in the initiation step of RNA interference. Nature 2001;409(6818):363–6.
8. Knight SW, Bass BL. A role for the RNase III enzyme DCR-1 in RNA interference and germ line development in Caenorhabditis elegans. Science 2001;293(5538):2269–71.
9. Welker NC, Maity TS, Ye X, et al. Dicer's helicase domain discriminates dsRNA termini to promote an altered reaction mode. Mol Cell 2011;41(5):589–99.
10. Takeshita D, Zenno S, Lee WC, et al. Homodimeric structure and double-stranded RNA cleavage activity of the C-terminal RNase III domain of human dicer. J Mol Biol 2007;374(1):106–20.
11. Ohishi K, Nakano T. A forward genetic screen to study mammalian RNA interference: essential role of RNase IIIa domain of Dicer1 in 3' strand cleavage of dsRNA in vivo. FEBS J 2012;279(5):832–43.
12. Brenneman M, Field A, Yang J, et al. Temporal order of RNase IIIb and loss-of-function mutations during development determines phenotype in pleuropulmonary blastoma/DICER1 syndrome: a unique variant of the two-hit tumor suppression model. F1000Res 2015;4:214.
13. Lee M, Kim T-I, Jang SJ, et al. Pleuropulmonary Blastoma with Hotspot Mutations in RNase IIIb Domain of DICER 1: Clinicopathologic Study of 10 Cases in a Single-Institute Experience. Pathobiology 2021;88(3):251–60.
14. Hill DA, Ivanovich J, Priest JR, et al. DICER1 mutations in familial pleuropulmonary blastoma. Science 2009;325(5943):965.
15. Heravi-Moussavi A, Anglesio MS, Cheng S-WG, et al. Recurrent somatic DICER1 mutations in nonepithelial ovarian cancers. N Engl J Med 2012;366(3):234–42.
16. Wu MK, Sabbaghian N, Xu B, et al. Biallelic DICER1 mutations occur in Wilms tumours. J Pathol 2013;230(2):154–64.

17. de Kock L, Wu MK, Foulkes WD. Ten years of DICER1 mutations: Provenance, distribution, and associated phenotypes. Hum Mutat 2019;40(11): 1939–53.

18. Rio Frio T, Bahubeshi A, Kanellopoulou C, et al. DICER1 mutations in familial multinodular goiter with and without ovarian Sertoli-Leydig cell tumors. JAMA 2011;305(1):68–77.

19. Bahubeshi A, Bal N, Rio Frio T, et al. Germline DICER1 mutations and familial cystic nephroma. J Med Genet 2010;47(12):863–6.

20. Doros L, Yang J, Dehner L, et al. DICER1 mutations in embryonal rhabdomyosarcomas from children with and without familial PPB-tumor predisposition syndrome. Pediatr Blood Cancer 2012;59(3): 558–60.

21. Robertson JC, Jorcyk CL, Oxford JT. DICER1 Syndrome: DICER1 Mutations in Rare Cancers. Cancers (Basel) 2018;10(5):E143.

22. Sabbaghian N, Hamel N, Srivastava A, et al. Germline DICER1 mutation and associated loss of heterozygosity in a pineoblastoma. J Med Genet 2012; 49(7):417–9.

23. Juhlin CC, Stenman A, Zedenius J. Macrofollicular variant follicular thyroid tumors are DICER1 mutated and exhibit distinct histological features. Histopathology 2021;79(4):661–6.

24. Seki M, Yoshida K, Shiraishi Y, et al. Biallelic DICER1 mutations in sporadic pleuropulmonary blastoma. Cancer Res 2014;74(10):2742–9.

25. Slade I, Bacchelli C, Davies H, et al. DICER1 syndrome: clarifying the diagnosis, clinical features and management implications of a pleiotropic tumour predisposition syndrome. J Med Genet 2011;48(4):273–8.

26. Schultz KA, Yang J, Doros L, et al. DICER1-pleuropulmonary blastoma familial tumor predisposition syndrome: a unique constellation of neoplastic conditions. Pathol Case Rev 2014;19(2):90–100.

27. Foulkes WD, Bahubeshi A, Hamel N, et al. Extending the phenotypes associated with DICER1 mutations. Hum Mutat 2011;32(12):1381–4.

28. Choi S, Lee JS, Bassim CW, et al. Dental abnormalities in individuals with pathogenic germline variation in DICER1. Am J Med Genet A 2019;179(9): 1820–5.

29. Huryn LA, Turriff A, Harney LA, et al. DICER1 Syndrome: Characterization of the Ocular Phenotype in a Family-Based Cohort Study. Ophthalmology 2019;126(2):296–304.

30. Khan NE, Bauer AJ, Doros L, et al. Macrocephaly associated with the DICER1 syndrome. Genet Med 2017;19(2):244–8.

31. Baloch ZW, Asa SL, Barletta JA, et al. Overview of the 2022 WHO Classification of Thyroid Neoplasms. Endocr Pathol 2022. https://doi.org/10.1007/s12022-022-09707-3.

32. Rath SR, Bartley A, Charles A, et al. Multinodular Goiter in children: an important pointer to a germline DICER1 mutation. J Clin Endocrinol Metab 2014; 99(6):1947–8.

33. Khan NE, Bauer AJ, Schultz KAP, et al. Quantification of Thyroid Cancer and Multinodular Goiter Risk in the DICER1 Syndrome: A Family-Based Cohort Study. J Clin Endocrinol Metab 2017;102(5): 1614–22.

34. Altaraihi M, Hansen T, van O, et al. Prevalence of Pathogenic Germline DICER1 Variants in Young Individuals Thyroidectomised Due to Goitre - A National Danish Cohort. Front Endocrinol (Lausanne) 2021; 12:727970.

35. de Kock L, Sabbaghian N, Soglio DB-D, et al. Exploring the association Between DICER1 mutations and differentiated thyroid carcinoma. J Clin Endocrinol Metab 2014;99(6):E1072–7.

36. Landa I, Ibrahimpasic T, Boucai L, et al. Genomic and transcriptomic hallmarks of poorly differentiated and anaplastic thyroid cancers. J Clin Invest 2016; 126(3):1052–66.

37. Cancer Genome Atlas Research Network Integrated genomic characterization of papillary thyroid carcinoma. Cell 2014;159(3):676–90.

38. Ghossein CA, Dogan S, Farhat N, et al. Expanding the spectrum of thyroid carcinoma with somatic DICER1 mutation: a survey of 829 thyroid carcinomas using MSK-IMPACT next-generation sequencing platform. Virchows Arch 2022;480(2): 293–302.

39. Satapathy S, Bal C. Genomic landscape of sporadic pediatric differentiated thyroid cancers: a systematic review and meta-analysis. J Pediatr Endocrinol Metab 2022. https://doi.org/10.1515/jpem-2021-0741.

40. Rutter MM, Jha P, Schultz KAP, et al. DICER1 Mutations and Differentiated Thyroid Carcinoma: Evidence of a Direct Association. J Clin Endocrinol Metab 2016;101(1):1–5.

41. Bongiovanni M, Sykiotis GP, La Rosa S, et al. Macrofollicular Variant of Follicular Thyroid Carcinoma: A Rare Underappreciated Pitfall in the Diagnosis of Thyroid Carcinoma. Thyroid 2020;30(1):72–80.

42. Wasserman JD, Sabbaghian N, Fahiminiya S, et al. DICER1 Mutations Are Frequent in Adolescent-Onset Papillary Thyroid Carcinoma. J Clin Endocrinol Metab 2018;103(5):2009–15.

43. Nicolson NG, Murtha TD, Dong W, et al. Comprehensive Genetic Analysis of Follicular Thyroid Carcinoma Predicts Prognosis Independent of Histology. J Clin Endocrinol Metab 2018;103(7):2640–50.

44. Paulsson JO, Wang N, Gao J, et al. GABPA-dependent down-regulation of DICER1 in follicular thyroid tumours. Endocr Relat Cancer 2020. https://doi.org/10.1530/ERC-19-0446.

45. Bae J-S, Jung S-H, Hirokawa M, et al. High Prevalence of DICER1 Mutations and Low Frequency of

Gene Fusions in Pediatric Follicular-Patterned Tumors of the Thyroid. Endocr Pathol 2021;32(3):336–46.

46. Poma AM, Condello V, Denaro M, et al. DICER1 somatic mutations strongly impair miRNA processing even in benign thyroid lesions. Oncotarget 2019; 10(19):1785–97.

47. Costa V, Esposito R, Ziviello C, et al. New somatic mutations and WNK1-B4GALNT3 gene fusion in papillary thyroid carcinoma. Oncotarget 2015; 6(13):11242–51.

48. Yuan X, Mu N, Wang N, et al. GABPA inhibits invasion/metastasis in papillary thyroid carcinoma by regulating DICER1 expression. Oncogene 2019; 38(7):965–79.

49. Chernock RD, Rivera B, Borrelli N, et al. Poorly differentiated thyroid carcinoma of childhood and adolescence: a distinct entity characterized by DICER1 mutations. Mod Pathol 2020. https://doi.org/10. 1038/s41379-020-0458-7.

50. Hellgren LS, Hysek M, Jatta K, et al. Macrofollicular Variant of Follicular Thyroid Carcinoma (MV-FTC) with a Somatic DICER1 Gene Mutation: Case Report and Review of the Literature. Head Neck Pathol 2020. https://doi.org/10.1007/s12105-020-01208-1.

51. Sauer M, Barletta JA. Proceedings of the North American Society of Head and Neck Pathology, Los Angeles, CA, March 20, 2022: DICER1-Related Thyroid Tumors. Head Neck Pathol 2022; 16(1):190–9.

52. Agaimy A, Witkowski L, Stoehr R, et al. Malignant teratoid tumor of the thyroid gland: an aggressive primitive multiphenotypic malignancy showing organotypical elements and frequent DICER1 alterations-is the term "thyroblastoma" more appropriate? Virchows Arch 2020;477(6):787–98.

53. Rabinowits G, Barletta J, Sholl LM, et al. Successful Management of a Patient with Malignant Thyroid Teratoma. Thyroid 2017;27(1):125–8.

54. Rooper LM, Bynum JP, Miller KP, et al. Recurrent DICER1 Hotspot Mutations in Malignant Thyroid Gland Teratomas: Molecular Characterization and Proposal for a Separate Classification. Am J Surg Pathol 2020;44(6):826–33.

55. Scheithauer BW, Kovacs K, Horvath E, et al. Pituitary blastoma. Acta Neuropathol 2008;116(6):657–66.

56. de Kock L, Sabbaghian N, Plourde F, et al. Pituitary blastoma: a pathognomonic feature of germ-line DICER1 mutations. Acta Neuropathol 2014;128(1):111–22.

57. Asa SL, Mete O, Perry A, et al. Overview of the 2022 WHO Classification of Pituitary Tumors. Endocr Pathol 2022;33(1):6–26.

58. Solarski M, Rotondo F, Foulkes WD, et al. DICER1 gene mutations in endocrine tumors. Endocr Relat Cancer 2018;25(3):R197–208.

59. Greppin K, Cioffi G, Waite KA, et al. Epidemiology of pineoblastoma in the United States, 2000-2017. Neurooncol Pract 2022;9(2):149–57.

60. de Kock L, Sabbaghian N, Druker H, et al. Germ-line and somatic DICER1 mutations in pineoblastoma. Acta Neuropathol 2014;128(4):583–95.

61. Juhlin CC, Erickson LA. Genomics and Epigenomics in Parathyroid Neoplasia: from Bench to Surgical Pathology Practice. Endocr Pathol 2021;32(1):17–34.

62. Kang H, Pettinga D, Schubert AD, et al. Genomic Profiling of Parathyroid Carcinoma Reveals Genomic Alterations Suggesting Benefit from Therapy. Oncologist 2019;24(6):791–7.

63. Juhlin CC, Bertherat J, Giordano TJ, et al. What Did We Learn from the Molecular Biology of Adrenal Cortical Neoplasia? From Histopathology Translational Genomics Endocr Pathol 2021; 32(1):102–33.

64. de Sousa GRV, Ribeiro TC, Faria AM, et al. Low DICER1 expression is associated with poor clinical outcome in adrenocortical carcinoma. Oncotarget 2015;6(26):22724–33.

65. Juhlin CC. Challenges in Paragangliomas and Pheochromocytomas: from Histology to Molecular Immunohistochemistry. Endocr Pathol 2021;32(2): 228–44.

66. Buffet A, Burnichon N, Favier J, et al. An overview of 20 years of genetic studies in pheochromocytoma and paraganglioma. Best Pract Res Clin Endocrinol Metab 2020;34(2):101416.

67. Caramuta S, Lee L, Ozata DM, et al. Clinical and functional impact of TARBP2 over-expression in adrenocortical carcinoma. Endocr Relat Cancer 2013;20(4):551–64.

68. Gao J, Shi H, Juhlin CC, et al. Merkel cell polyomavirus T-antigens regulate DICER1 mRNA stability and translation through HSC70. IScience 2021; 24(11):103264.

69. Kumar S, Xie H, Shi H, et al. Merkel cell polyomavirus oncoproteins induce microRNAs that suppress multiple autophagy genes. Int J Cancer 2020; 146(6):1652–66.

70. Rivera B, Nadaf J, Fahiminiya S, et al. DGCR8 microprocessor defect characterizes familial multinodular goiter with schwannomatosis. J Clin Invest 2020; 130(3):1479–90.

71. Paulsson JO, Rafati N, DiLorenzo S, et al. Whole-genome sequencing of follicular thyroid carcinomas reveal recurrent mutations in microRNA processing subunit DGCR8. J Clin Endocrinol Metab 2021;dgab471. https://doi.org/10.1210/clinem/dgab471.

72. Paulsson JO, Backman S, Wang N, et al. Whole-genome sequencing of synchronous thyroid carcinomas identifies aberrant DNA repair in thyroid cancer dedifferentiation. J Pathol 2020;250(2):183–94.

73. Stenman A, Yang M, Paulsson JO, et al. Pan-Genomic Sequencing Reveals Actionable CDKN2A/2B Deletions and Kataegis in Anaplastic Thyroid Carcinoma. Cancers (Basel) 2021;13(24): 6340.

Back to Biochemistry
Evaluation for and Prognostic Significance of SDH Mutations in Paragangliomas and Pheochromocytomas

Sounak Gupta, MBBS, PhD, Lori A. Erickson, MD*

KEYWORDS
- Paraganglioma • Pheochromocytoma • Succinate dehydrogenase • *SDHA* • *SDHB* • *SDHC*
- *SDHD* • *SDHAF2*

ABSTRACT

There is increasing recognition of the high prevalence of hereditary predisposition syndromes in patients diagnosed with paraganglioma/pheochromocytoma. It is widely acknowledged that germline pathogenic alterations of the succinate dehydrogenase complex genes (*SDHA, SDHB, SDHC, SDHD, SDHAF2*) contribute to the pathogenesis of most of these tumors. Herein, we have provided an update on the biology and diagnosis of succinate dehydrogenase-deficient paraganglioma/pheochromocytoma, including the molecular biology of the succinate dehydrogenase complex, mechanisms and consequences of inactivation of this complex, the prevalence of pathogenic alterations, and patterns of inheritance.

PREVALENCE OF HEREDITARY PREDISPOSITION SYNDROMES IN PATIENTS WITH PHEOCHROMOCYTOMA/ PARAGANGLIOMA

Up to 30% to 40% of patients diagnosed with paraganglioma/pheochromocytoma (PGL/Pheo) have an underlying hereditary predisposition syndrome.[1,2] Common germline associations include multiple endocrine neoplasia type 2 (*RET*), von Hippel Lindau syndrome type 2 (*VHL*), neurofibromatosis type 1 (*NF1*), paraganglioma-pheochromocytoma syndrome (succinate dehydrogenase complex genes: *SDHA, SDHB, SDHC, SDHD, SDHAF2*), Pacak Zhuang syndrome (*HIF2A*), and nonsyndromal cases (*TMEM127* and *MAX*).[3] Of these, germline alterations of genes encoding for constituent members of the succinate dehydrogenase complex account for most of these tumors.[1,2] Specifically, it is estimated that germline alterations of succinate dehydrogenase genes account for 15% of all cases of PGL/ Pheo, and as much as half of all cases occurring in the setting of a hereditary predisposition syndrome.[4]

Pathogenic alterations of the succinate dehydrogenase genes are thought to account for an even higher number of PGL/Pheo occurring in pediatric patients.[3] In a German cohort of 88 patients and a French cohort of 81 patients, germline variants were detected in 77% to 83% of patients, and alterations of succinate dehydrogenase genes accounted for 29% to 51% of these cases.[5,6] In addition, a study conducted by the National Institutes of Health (Bethesda, Maryland, United States) showed that the contribution of succinate dehydrogenase genes was elevated in pediatric patients with PGL/Pheo that present with metastatic disease.[7] Specifically, among 32 patients with metastatic PGL/Pheo who were diagnosed with a primary tumor before the age of 20 years, germline alterations of succinate dehydrogenase genes accounted for approximately 81% of cases.[7]

In this context, depending on the availability of resources, some form of screening for relevant germline alterations (including for succinate

Sources of Support: None.
Department of Laboratory Medicine and Pathology, Mayo Clinic, Rochester, MN, USA
* Corresponding author. Department of Laboratory Medicine and Pathology, Mayo Clinic, 200 First Street, Southwest, Rochester, MN 55905.
E-mail address: Erickson.Lori@mayo.edu

Surgical Pathology 16 (2023) 119–129
https://doi.org/10.1016/j.path.2022.09.011

dehydrogenase complex genes) is recommended for all patients diagnosed with PGL/Pheo.[1]

THE SUCCINATE DEHYDROGENASE COMPLEX

Entry of electrons into the electron transport chain primarily involves electrons donated by NADH to complex I, whereas complex II represents an additional point of entry.[8] Complex II is a multiprotein complex that includes anchoring proteins (SDHC and SDHD), catalytic units (SDHA and SDHB), and succinate dehydrogenase complex assembly factor 2 (SDHAF2), which is required for flavination of SDHA.[8,9] The first step in electron transport through complex II involves oxidation of succinate to fumarate by SDHA. This is followed by transfer of electrons by SDHB to the anchoring proteins SDHC/SDHD, which are located on the inner mitochondrial membrane. Transfer of electrons reduces ubiquinone (bound to SDHC/SDHD) to ubiquinol.[8] These electrons are then transferred to cytochrome C through complex III.[8] Loss of function alterations involving any subunit of the succinate dehydrogenase complex leads to an unstable protein complex. Subunits such as SDHB once released into the cytosol from this mitochondrial complex undergo rapid degradation.[4,10]

In addition, loss of the succinate dehydrogenase complex leads to an accumulation of succinate, which has significant downstream metabolic consequences.[8,9] Succinate accumulation within the cytosol can inhibit the prolyl hydroxylase (PHD) enzyme. PHD plays an important role in hypoxia-induced signaling. Under steady state conditions, PHD hydroxylates hypoxia inducible factor 1 subunit alpha (HIF-1A), which then undergoes polyubiquitination by the von Hippel Lindau ubiquitin ligase complex, thereby facilitating proteasome-mediated degradation.[8,9] Therefore, inhibition of PHD function by succinate accumulation leads to stabilization of HIF-1A and constitutively increased oncogenic signaling.[8,9,11]

In addition, accumulation of succinate can lead to inhibition of ten-eleven translocation dioxygenases and consequent epigenetic reprogramming by the development of a DNA hypermethylator phenotype.[12]

MECHANISMS OF SUCCINATE DEHYDROGENASE COMPLEX INACTIVATION

Loss of function alterations of the genes encoding for components of the succinate dehydrogenase complex typically involve biallelic inactivation. Biallelic somatic inactivation of succinate dehydrogenase genes have been reported only in rare instances such that identification of a succinate dehydrogenase-deficient tumor is considered an indication for confirmatory germline testing.[13] Therefore, surgical pathologists play an important role in the management of patients with PGL/Pheo, being involved not just in providing an accurate diagnosis but also in identifying patients for subsequent genetic counseling.

It is also important to note that, germline DNA sequencing may occasionally yield a false negative result for patients diagnosed with a succinate dehydrogenase-deficient tumor. For instance, patients presenting with Carney triad: PGL/Pheo, gastrointestinal stromal tumor (GIST), and pulmonary chondroma, often lack mutations in the coding regions of the succinate dehydrogenase genes. Instead, gene silencing typically occurs through hypermethylation of the SDHC gene promoter as a postzygotic event.[14–16] Other rare causes of a false negative test result include deep intronic variants (as noncoding DNA is usually not interrogated by most commercial test platforms), as well as in patients with mosaicism as the alteration may be present at low variant allele frequencies that may be below the reporting range of a given assay.[17]

MECHANISMS OF INHERITANCE OF SUCCINATE DEHYDROGENASE-DEFICIENT CANCER

In addition to PGL/Pheo, the spectrum of succinate dehydrogenase-deficient tumors includes GIST, renal cell carcinoma, pulmonary chondroma, and pituitary neuroendocrine tumors/pituitary adenoma.[13,18–22] Hereditary paraganglioma pheochromocytoma syndromes (PGL1-5) are inherited in an autosomal dominant manner (Table 1).[23]

AUTOSOMAL DOMINANT (PGL3–5)

Of the hereditary paraganglioma pheochromocytoma syndromes, PGL5, PGL4, and PGL3 occur secondary to alterations of the SDHA, SDHB, and SDHC genes, respectively.[23] Consistent with an autosomal dominant pattern of inheritance, carriers with a (heterozygous) pathogenic alteration of an SDHA/SDHB/SDHC gene have a 50% risk of passing on the risk allele to an affected child, and conversely a 50% risk of having an unaffected child.[24]

Alterations of SDHA were initially described in the context of autosomal recessive juvenile encephalopathy.[25] More recently SDHA has been implicated in GIST/pituitary adenomas, although it is infrequently identified as a cause of PGL/Pheo.[23,26,27] SDHB mutations, however, are frequently associated with thoraco-abdominal

Table 1
Succinate dehydrogenase-deficient tumor syndromes

Gene Name	Syndromal Association	Patterns of Inheritance and Penetrance	Common Tumor Associations	Immunohistochemistry
SDHA	PGL5	Autosomal dominant. Low penetrance	Gastrointestinal stromal tumor and pituitary adenomas (infrequently associated with PGL/Pheo)	Loss of SDHA and SDHB
SDHB	PGL4	Autosomal dominant	Thoraco-abdominal PGL/Pheo	Loss of SDHB (retained SDHA)
SDHC	PGL3	Autosomal dominant	Head and neck PGL (carotid body tumors). Rarely multifocal	Loss of SDHB (retained SDHA)
SDHC (Promoter Hypermethylation)	Carney Triad	Nonhereditary syndrome	PGL/Pheo, gastrointestinal stromal tumor, and pulmonary chondroma	Loss of SDHB (retained SDHA)
SDHD	PGL1	Autosomal dominant with maternal imprinting. Highly penetrant	Head and neck PGL. Frequently multifocal	Loss of SDHB (retained SDHA)
SDHAF2	PGL2	Autosomal dominant with maternal imprinting. Highly penetrant	Head and neck PGL (less frequent compared with PGL with *SDHD* alterations) Frequently multifocal	Loss of SDHB (retained SDHA)

Abbreviations: PGL(1–5): hereditary paraganglioma pheochromocytoma syndromes; PGL/Pheo: paraganglioma/pheochromocytoma.

PGL/Pheo (as opposed to a head and neck tumor location). Furthermore, PGL/Pheo in close to a third of patients with *SDHB* pathogenic alterations exhibit malignant behavior.[28–31] *SDHC* alterations are associated with carotid body tumors.[23] Unlike head and neck PGL that commonly occur secondary to alterations of *SDHD/SDHAF2*, tumors with *SDHC* alterations are rarely multifocal.[23,32]

AUTOSOMAL DOMINANT WITH MATERNAL IMPRINTING (PGL1–2)

The hereditary paraganglioma pheochromocytoma syndromes PGL2 and PGL1 occur secondary to alterations of the *SDHAF2*, and *SDHD* genes, respectively.[23] Although PGL1–2 are inherited in an autosomal dominant manner, they differ from PGL3–5 as their inheritance is affected by maternal imprinting/silencing.[23,33,34] Therefore, paternal transmission of an affected allele is associated with tumor development, whereas silencing of the *SDHAF2* and *SDHD* gene locus on the maternal allele through epigenetic changes such as DNA methylation or histone modification is typically not associated with disease transmission.[34,35] Furthermore, paternal transmission provides a logical explanation for why PGL1–2 often "skips" a generation.[23]

PGL1 and PGL2 are highly penetrant diseases that usually affect 75% of carriers and are associated with multifocal disease.[23,28,32,36–38] However, *SDHAF2*-associated PGL have been infrequently reported compared with *SDHD* associated head and neck PGL.[23]

NONHEREDITARY (CARNEY TRIAD)

The Carney triad involves syndromal manifestations of PGL/Pheo, GIST, and pulmonary chondroma.[14–16] As opposed to PGL1–5, Carney triad is characterized by a female predilection, lacks mutations in the coding regions of the succinate dehydrogenase genes, and silencing of the *SDHC* gene occurs through hypermethylation of the gene promoter.[14–16] This is a nonhereditary disorder as *SDHC* silencing in these patients characteristically occurs as a postzygotic event.[14] In practical terms, as somatic biallelic inactivation of the succinate dehydrogenase genes is a rare phenomenon, patients are presumed to have Carney triad if they present with a succinate dehydrogenase-deficient tumor and no germline pathogenic alteration of *SDHA/SDHB/SDHC/SDHD/SDHAF2* genes is identified.

PENETRANCE (SDHA)

In contrast to PGL1–2, which are highly penetrant disorders, PGL5 (secondary to pathogenic alterations of *SDHA*) is characterized by extremely low penetrance.[23] In a study of an Australian cohort of 575 patients and a UK cohort of 1240 subjects, 94 different pathogenic variants were identified in the *SDHA*, *SDHB*, and *SDHC* genes.[39] Of these 94 variants, 13 were present in the exome aggregate consortium (ExAC) database.[39] Allelic frequencies in patients (cases) were compared with the frequencies for these 13 variants in the general population (ExAC) to calculate disease penetrance. This revealed a relatively higher penetrance for *SDHB* variants (22%), compared with that for *SDHC* (8.3%), and *SDHA* (1.7%).[39] Consistent with this finding, a separate study demonstrated that the estimated prevalence of missense or loss-of-function *SDHA* variants in the general population was as high as 0.1% to 1.0%, with a much lower penetrance of 0.1% to 4.9%.[40] Therefore, many patients with a germline *SDHA* variant may not manifest with an SDHA-deficient tumor, and thus the role of surveillance in this patient population is unclear.[40]

IMMUNOHISTOCHEMISTRY-BASED SCREENING FOR HEREDITARY PREDISPOSITION SYNDROMES IN PATIENTS WITH PHEOCHROMOCYTOMA/PARAGANGLIOMA

As access to next-generation sequencing for germline alterations of succinate dehydrogenase genes is restricted in resource-limited settings, immunohistochemistry represents an important, easily accessible, and cost-effective screening tool for such tumors. Some common immunohistochemistry-based surrogates for PGL/Pheo in hereditary tumor predisposition syndromes include screening for loss of SDHB/SDHA proteins in succinate dehydrogenase-deficient tumors, loss of fumarate hydratase (FH) coupled with increased S-(2-succino)-cysteine (2SC) in fumarate hydratase-deficient tumors, loss of MAX protein expression in *MAX*-mutated tumors, and constitutive overexpression of carbonic anhydrase 9 in von Hippel Lindau disease associated lesions.[1,4,13,18,41–48] Because biallelic somatic inactivation of succinate dehydrogenase genes have been reported only in rare instances, identification of a succinate dehydrogenase-deficient tumor using immunohistochemistry is considered an indication for confirmatory germline testing.[13]

As mentioned earlier, biallelic loss-of-function alterations involving any subunit of the succinate dehydrogenase protein complex (including *SDHA*, *SDHB*, *SDHC*, *SDHD*, or *SDHAF2*) leads to an unstable protein complex, and thus SDHB once released into the cytosol from this mitochondrial complex undergoes rapid degradation.[4,10] Although SDHB protein expression is retained in nonneoplastic elements, SDHB-deficient tumors such as PGL/Pheo show loss of expression.[1,4,13,18,43,44] This has been demonstrated in **Fig. 1**, which shows a biopsy of a succinate dehydrogenase-deficient paraganglioma. These tumors typically show positivity for neuroendocrine markers (Fig. B: synaptophysin; Fig. C: chromogranin), and the presence of S100-positive sustentacular cells (Fig. E). In addition, it is important to document the absence of staining with keratins (Fig. F), which is seen in neuroendocrine carcinomas, an important differential diagnostic consideration. Screening immunohistochemistry for SDHB in this case reveals loss of expression in lesional cells, coupled with retained expression in vascular endothelial cells, which serve as an internal positive control (Fig. D).

Furthermore, tumors with biallelic pathogenic *SDHA* variants show loss of the SDHA protein in addition to loss of SDHB, in contrast to SDHB/SDHC/SDHD-deficient tumors that show retained expression of SDHA.[26,49,50] SDHA immunohistochemistry is therefore an useful diagnostic tool given the low penetrance of germline pathogenic *SDHA* variants and the high level of sequence similarity with 3 pseudogenes (*SDHAP1*, *SDHAP2*, and *SDHAP3*), which make it challenging to distinguish alterations in the *SDHA* gene from homologous regions in pseudogenes.[23]

THERANOSTIC IMAGING

An area of considerable advancement in the management of PGL/Pheo involves theranostic

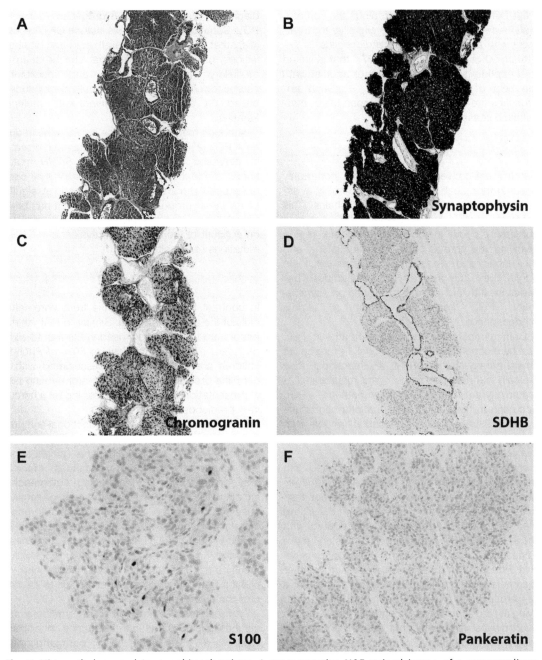

Fig. 1. Histopathology and Immunohistochemistry. A representative H&E-stained image of a paraganglioma diagnosed on a biopsy specimen, and corresponding immunohistochemistry for synaptophysin (*B*), chromogranin (*C*), and SDHB (*D*) is shown (100× magnification). SDHB shows loss of expression within the paraganglioma, with nonneoplastic vascular elements serving as an internal positive control. S100 highlights sustentacular cells (*E*, 400× magnification), whereas pancytokeratin is negative (*F*, 200× magnification).

imaging. Therapeutic nuclear medicine is defined as "administration of radionuclides to achieve a transfer of radiation energy" to target tissues.[51] Here, tumor-specific transporters, receptors or antigens are targeted with radionuclides for diagnostic or therapeutic use. For instance, meta-iodo-benzyl-guanidine (MIBG) labeled with ^{123}I is used for diagnostic imaging of PGL/Pheo with increased norepinephrine transporters on lesional cells, which can then be targeted using ^{131}I MIBG for therapeutic purposes.[51,52] Other agents used in theranostic imaging include the use of

[68]GA-DOTA-Octreotate, which binds the somatostatin receptor and determines eligibility for treatment with agents such as a "radionuclide ([90]Y—Yttrium 90 or [177]Lu—Lutetium 177)" that is linked to a peptide (somatostatin receptor agonist) with the help of a chelator (DOTA).[51,52] Such approaches are often favored for inoperable or metastatic disease.[51,52]

PARAGANGLIOMA

Neural crest-derived sympathetic PGL commonly occur in thoracoabdominal sites and rarely in association with cervical sympathetic chains. This contrasts with parasympathetic PGL, which commonly occur in the head and neck region involving the carotid body, the middle ear, and the vagus and glossopharyngeal nerves.[53] In adults, these tumors are typically diagnosed between the fifth and sixth decades, and parasympathetic PGL frequently exhibit a female predominance.[54–56]

Both sympathetic and parasympathetic PGL can be biochemically nonfunctional. In rare cases where parasympathetic PGL are functional, they typically express dopamine or its metabolite, 3-methoxytyramine.[57,58] Parasympathetic PGL occurring in head and neck locations can cause symptoms based on their location (middle ear: tinnitus, hearing abnormalities; cranial nerve symptoms).[59,60]

Many head and neck PGL are associated with hereditary predisposition, which are frequently due to alterations of succinate dehydrogenase genes.[1,4] At this location, alterations of *SDHD* are identified much more frequently compared with those of *SDHB*, with the latter being more frequently associated with thoracoabdominal PGL/Pheo.[54,61] With regards to risk factors other than hereditary predisposition, a higher incidence of carotid body PGL has been associated with living at high altitudes and in patients with cyanotic heart disease and is thought to be secondary to the effects of hypoxia.[62–64]

Histologically, PGL comprises cells with pale eosinophilic cytoplasm organized in a nested/zellballen architecture with a peripheral rim of sustentacular cells. The lesional cells typically express neuroendocrine markers (synaptophysin, chromogranin, INSM1), and GATA3, whereas the peripheral sustentacular cells show positive staining with S100/SOX10.[65–67] Some reports have documented expression of somatostatin receptors in PGL.[68,69] The role of SDHA/SDHB immunohistochemistry has been discussed in a prior section, and loss of SDHB expression in lesional cells can serve as an important screening tool for the diagnosis of succinate dehydrogenase-deficient PGL. Some diagnostic pitfalls include GATA3 positivity that can be seen in parathyroid and pituitary lesions, calcitonin positivity that can be seen in medullary thyroid carcinoma, and importantly neuroendocrine carcinomas should be excluded based on absence of staining with multiple keratins.[70–73]

Although metastatic disease is rare in head and neck PGL (2%–6%), the risk of metastatic disease is increased in the presence of *SDHB* mutations.[74–76] In contrast, PGL at abdominal sites have been reported to metastasize in a significantly larger proportion of cases, and it has been hypothesized that this higher frequency may be on account of the increased prevalence of *SDHB* mutations at this site.[77]

PHEOCHROMOCYTOMA

In contrast to PGL, Pheo arise from chromaffin cells of the adrenal medulla. Similar to PGL, these tumors are typically diagnosed in the fifth to sixth decades.[78] Importantly, close to 80% of Pheo in children are estimated to be associated with a germline predisposition, and therefore young age at presentation may prompt screening for a hereditary predisposition syndrome.[79,80]

Most Pheo are biochemically functional and present with symptoms of catecholamines excess including hypertension, headache, palpitations, and diaphoresis.[78] In some instances, patients may present with life-threatening emergencies including acute myocardial injury, hypertensive crises, and seizures.[78] On rare occasions, paraneoplastic syndromes secondary to secretion of peptides such as ACTH, CRH, or VIP have been reported.[81–83] Laboratory studies typically involve measurement of 24-hour fractionated urine or plasma-free catecholamine metabolites to identify catecholamine excess.[84]

As mentioned earlier, common germline associations include multiple endocrine neoplasia type 2 (*RET*), *VHL*, *NF1*, paraganglioma-pheochromocytoma syndrome (succinate dehydrogenase complex genes: *SDHA*, *SDHB*, *SDHC*, *SDHD*, *SDHAF2*), and alterations of other genes (including *FH*, *TMEM127*, and *MAX*).[1,3,85] In contrast to genes such as *VHL* that are associated with both hereditary and sporadic Pheo, biallelic somatic inactivation of the succinate dehydrogenase genes have rarely been identified and most succinate dehydrogenase-deficient tumors are associated with a hereditary predisposition.[1,86] Based on the presence of underlying mutations and the biochemical profile, Pheo are categorized into 3 broad groups. Cluster 1 (hypoxia-induced signaling cluster) is characterized by mutations of succinate dehydrogenase genes and *VHL*; cluster 2 (tyrosine kinase induced signaling cluster) includes alterations of *RET*, *NF1*, and the Wnt pathway (*MAML3* fusions and *CSDE1* alterations); and cluster 3 includes adrenergic or mixed adrenergic/noradrenergic Pheo.[84,86–89] Importantly, these clusters may have varied geographic distributions. For instance, there is a high prevalence of cluster 1 Pheo with alterations of succinate dehydrogenase genes/*VHL* in Western populations.[90]

Similar to PGL, Pheo commonly comprise cells with pale eosinophilic cytoplasm organized in a nested/zellballen architecture with a peripheral rim of sustentacular cells and show a similar immunophenotype. In addition to the immunophenotype for PGL, Pheo are positive for tyrosine hydroxylase and dopamine beta hydroxylase, and focal to absent staining of tyrosine hydroxylase expression has been reported in nonfunctional tumors.[91,92] Furthermore, given their location, it may be important to distinguish Pheo from adrenocortical tumors. Pheo are frequently positive for chromogranin, tyrosine hydroxylase, and GATA3.[93] Adrenocortical tumors lack expression of these 3 markers, and typically express melan A and SF1.[93]

Patients with PGL/Pheo are thought to have a permanent risk of developing metastatic disease; however, it is important to distinguish multifocal disease from metastasis.[53] In this context, knowledge of the normal anatomic distribution of the sympathetic and parasympathetic nervous system elements may be helpful.[53] At the molecular level, pathogenic alterations of the *SDHB* gene have been associated with a high risk of metastatic disease.[28–31] At least 4 histology-based scoring systems with multiple variables have been proposed to predict metastatic disease [COmposite Pheochromocytoma/paraganglioma Prognostic Score, Grading system for Adrenal Pheochromocytoma and Paraganglioma (GAPP), modified GAPP, and Pheochromocytoma of the Adrenal gland Scaled Score].[94–97] These scores are interpreted in the context of completeness of tumor resection, underlying molecular alterations, and other relevant clinicopathologic features, and their use is neither recommended nor discouraged.

SUMMARY

It is estimated that germline alterations of succinate dehydrogenase genes account for as much as half of all cases of PGL/Pheo occurring in the setting of a hereditary predisposition syndrome, and likely account for an even higher number of cases occurring in pediatric patients.[3,4] Surgical pathologists play an important role in the management of patients with PGL/Pheo, being involved not just in providing an accurate diagnosis but also in identifying patients for subsequent genetic counseling. As access to next-generation sequencing for germline alterations of succinate dehydrogenase genes is restricted in resource-limited settings, immunohistochemistry represents an important, easily accessible, and cost-effective screening tool for such tumors. Herein, we have summarized our contemporary understanding of the pathogenesis of succinate dehydrogenase-deficient PGL/Pheo, patterns of inheritance, relevant clinicopathologic features, and the use of important diagnostic tools in routine clinical practice.

DISCLOSURE

The authors of this article have no relevant financial relationships with commercial interests to disclose.

ACKNOWLEDGMENTS

The authors have no conflicts of interest or funding to disclose.

REFERENCES

1. Turchini J, Cheung VKY, Tischler AS, et al. Pathology and genetics of phaeochromocytoma and paraganglioma. Histopathology 2018;72:97–105.
2. Gill AJ. Succinate dehydrogenase (SDH) and mitochondrial driven neoplasia. Pathology 2012;44: 285–92.
3. Bholah R, Bunchman TE. Review of Pediatric Pheochromocytoma and Paraganglioma. Front Pediatr 2017;5:155.
4. Gill AJ. Succinate dehydrogenase (SDH)-deficient neoplasia. Histopathology 2018;72:106–16.
5. Redlich A, Pamporaki C, Lessel L, et al. Pseudohypoxic pheochromocytomas and paragangliomas dominate in children. Pediatr Blood Cancer 2021; 68:e28981.
6. de Tersant M, Genere L, Freycon C, et al. Pheochromocytoma and Paraganglioma in Children and Adolescents: Experience of the French Society of Pediatric Oncology (SFCE). J Endocr Soc 2020;4: bvaa039.
7. King KS, Prodanov T, Kantorovich V, et al. Metastatic pheochromocytoma/paraganglioma related to primary tumor development in childhood or adolescence: significant link to SDHB mutations. J Clin Oncol 2011;29:4137–42.

8. Gottlieb E, Tomlinson IP. Mitochondrial tumour suppressors: a genetic and biochemical update. Nat Rev Cancer 2005;5:857–66.

9. King A, Selak MA, Gottlieb E. Succinate dehydrogenase and fumarate hydratase: linking mitochondrial dysfunction and cancer. Oncogene 2006;25:4675–82.

10. van Nederveen FH, Gaal J, Favier J, et al. An immunohistochemical procedure to detect patients with paraganglioma and phaeochromocytoma with germline SDHB, SDHC, or SDHD gene mutations: a retrospective and prospective analysis. Lancet Oncol 2009;10:764–71.

11. Pollard PJ, Briere JJ, Alam NA, et al. Accumulation of Krebs cycle intermediates and over-expression of HIF1alpha in tumours which result from germline FH and SDH mutations. Hum Mol Genet 2005;14:2231–9.

12. Morin A, Goncalves J, Moog S, et al. TET-Mediated Hypermethylation Primes SDH-Deficient Cells for HIF2alpha-Driven Mesenchymal Transition. Cell Rep 2020;30:4551–66.e7.

13. Gill AJ, Toon CW, Clarkson A, et al. Succinate dehydrogenase deficiency is rare in pituitary adenomas. Am J Surg Pathol 2014;38:560–6.

14. Haller F, Moskalev EA, Faucz FR, et al. Aberrant DNA hypermethylation of SDHC: a novel mechanism of tumor development in Carney triad. Endocr Relat Cancer 2014;21:567–77.

15. Killian JK, Miettinen M, Walker RL, et al. Recurrent epimutation of SDHC in gastrointestinal stromal tumors. Sci Transl Med 2014;6:268ra177.

16. Daumova M, Svajdler M, Fabian P, et al. SDHC Methylation Pattern in Patients With Carney Triad. Appl Immunohistochem Mol Morphol 2021;29:599–605.

17. Cardot-Bauters C, Carnaille B, Aubert S, et al. A Full Phenotype of Paraganglioma Linked to a Germline SDHB Mosaic Mutation. J Clin Endocrinol Metab 2019;104:3362–6.

18. Gill AJ, Chou A, Vilain R, et al. Immunohistochemistry for SDHB divides gastrointestinal stromal tumors (GISTs) into 2 distinct types. Am J Surg Pathol 2010;34:636–44.

19. Miettinen M, Wang ZF, Sarlomo-Rikala M, et al. Succinate dehydrogenase-deficient GISTs: a clinicopathologic, immunohistochemical, and molecular genetic study of 66 gastric GISTs with predilection to young age. Am J Surg Pathol 2011;35:1712–21.

20. Fuchs TL, Maclean F, Turchini J, et al. Expanding the clinicopathological spectrum of succinate dehydrogenase-deficient renal cell carcinoma with a focus on variant morphologies: a study of 62 new tumors in 59 patients. Mod Pathol 2021;35(6):836–49.

21. Rodriguez FJ, Aubry MC, Tazelaar HD, et al. Pulmonary chondroma: a tumor associated with Carney triad and different from pulmonary hamartoma. Am J Surg Pathol 2007;31:1844–53.

22. Chatzopoulos K, Fritchie KJ, Aubry MC, et al. Loss of succinate dehydrogenase B immunohistochemical expression distinguishes pulmonary chondromas from hamartomas. Histopathology 2019;75:825–32.

23. Benn DE, Robinson BG, Clifton-Bligh RJ. 15 YEARS OF PARAGANGLIOMA: Clinical manifestations of paraganglioma syndromes types 1-5. Endocr Relat Cancer 2015;22:T91–103.

24. Rasheed M, Tarjan G. Succinate Dehydrogenase Complex: An Updated Review. Arch Pathol Lab Med 2018;142:1564–70.

25. Bourgeron T, Rustin P, Chretien D, et al. Mutation of a nuclear succinate dehydrogenase gene results in mitochondrial respiratory chain deficiency. Nat Genet 1995;11:144–9.

26. Dwight T, Benn DE, Clarkson A, et al. Loss of SDHA expression identifies SDHA mutations in succinate dehydrogenase-deficient gastrointestinal stromal tumors. Am J Surg Pathol 2013;37:226–33.

27. Burnichon N, Briere JJ, Libe R, et al. SDHA is a tumor suppressor gene causing paraganglioma. Hum Mol Genet 2010;19:3011–20.

28. Benn DE, Gimenez-Roqueplo AP, Reilly JR, et al. Clinical presentation and penetrance of pheochromocytoma/paraganglioma syndromes. J Clin Endocrinol Metab 2006;91:827–36.

29. Gimenez-Roqueplo AP, Favier J, Rustin P, et al. Mutations in the SDHB gene are associated with extra-adrenal and/or malignant phaeochromocytomas. Cancer Res 2003;63:5615–21.

30. Brouwers FM, Eisenhofer G, Tao JJ, et al. High frequency of SDHB germline mutations in patients with malignant catecholamine-producing paragangliomas: implications for genetic testing. J Clin Endocrinol Metab 2006;91:4505–9.

31. Timmers HJ, Kozupa A, Eisenhofer G, et al. Clinical presentations, biochemical phenotypes, and genotype-phenotype correlations in patients with succinate dehydrogenase subunit B-associated pheochromocytomas and paragangliomas. J Clin Endocrinol Metab 2007;92:779–86.

32. Schiavi F, Milne RL, Anda E, et al. Are we overestimating the penetrance of mutations in SDHB? Hum Mutat 2010;31:761–2.

33. Baysal BE. Mitochondrial complex II and genomic imprinting in inheritance of paraganglioma tumors. Biochim Biophys Acta 2013;1827:573–7.

34. Neumann HP, Erlic Z. Maternal transmission of symptomatic disease with SDHD mutation: fact or fiction? J Clin Endocrinol Metab 2008;93:1573–5.

35. Abramowitz LK, Bartolomei MS. Genomic imprinting: recognition and marking of imprinted loci. Curr Opin Genet Dev 2012;22:72–8.

36. Kunst HP, Rutten MH, de Monnink JP, et al. SDHAF2 (PGL2-SDH5) and hereditary head and neck paraganglioma. Clin Cancer Res 2011;17:247–54.

37. Neumann HP, Pawlu C, Peczkowska M, et al. Distinct clinical features of paraganglioma syndromes associated with SDHB and SDHD gene mutations. JAMA 2004;292:943–51.

38. Ricketts CJ, Forman JR, Rattenberry E, et al. Tumor risks and genotype-phenotype-proteotype analysis in 358 patients with germline mutations in SDHB and SDHD. Hum Mutat 2010;31:41–51.

39. Benn DE, Zhu Y, Andrews KA, et al. Bayesian approach to determining penetrance of pathogenic SDH variants. J Med Genet 2018;55:729–34.

40. Maniam P, Zhou K, Lonergan M, et al. Pathogenicity and Penetrance of Germline SDHA Variants in Pheochromocytoma and Paraganglioma (PPGL). J Endocr Soc 2018;2:806–16.

41. Favier J, Meatchi T, Robidel E, et al. Carbonic anhydrase 9 immunohistochemistry as a tool to predict or validate germline and somatic VHL mutations in pheochromocytoma and paraganglioma-a retrospective and prospective study. Mod Pathol 2020;33:57–64.

42. Chatzopoulos K, Aubry MC, Gupta S. Immunohistochemical expression of carbonic anhydrase 9, glucose transporter 1, and paired box 8 in von Hippel-Lindau disease-related lesions. Hum Pathol 2022;123:93–101.

43. Gupta S, Zhang J, Rivera M, et al. Urinary Bladder Paragangliomas: Analysis of Succinate Dehydrogenase and Outcome. Endocr Pathol 2016;27:243–52.

44. Gupta S, Swanson AA, Chen YB, et al. Incidence of succinate dehydrogenase and fumarate hydratase-deficient renal cell carcinoma based on immunohistochemical screening with SDHA/SDHB and FH/2SC. Hum Pathol 2019;91:114–22.

45. Trpkov K, Siadat F. Immunohistochemical screening for the diagnosis of succinate dehydrogenase-deficient renal cell carcinoma and fumarate hydratase-deficient renal cell carcinoma. Ann Transl Med 2019;7:S324.

46. Seabrook AJ, Harris JE, Velosa SB, et al. Multiple Endocrine Tumors Associated with Germline MAX Mutations: Multiple Endocrine Neoplasia Type 5? J Clin Endocrinol Metab 2021;106:1163–82.

47. Cheung VKY, Gill AJ, Chou A. Old, New, and Emerging Immunohistochemical Markers in Pheochromocytoma and Paraganglioma. Endocr Pathol 2018;29:169–75.

48. Korpershoek E, Koffy D, Eussen BH, et al. Complex MAX Rearrangement in a Family With Malignant Pheochromocytoma, Renal Oncocytoma, and Erythrocytosis. J Clin Endocrinol Metab 2016;101:453–60.

49. Korpershoek E, Favier J, Gaal J, et al. SDHA immunohistochemistry detects germline SDHA gene mutations in apparently sporadic paragangliomas and pheochromocytomas. J Clin Endocrinol Metab 2011;96:E1472–6.

50. Wagner AJ, Remillard SP, Zhang YX, et al. Loss of expression of SDHA predicts SDHA mutations in gastrointestinal stromal tumors. Mod Pathol 2013;26:289–94.

51. Taieb D, Pacak K. Molecular imaging and theranostic approaches in pheochromocytoma and paraganglioma. Cell Tissue Res 2018;372:393–401.

52. Satapathy S, Mittal BR, Bhansali A. Peptide receptor radionuclide therapy in the management of advanced pheochromocytoma and paraganglioma: A systematic review and meta-analysis. Clin Endocrinol (Oxf) 2019;91:718–27.

53. Asa SL, Ezzat S, Mete O. The Diagnosis and Clinical Significance of Paragangliomas in Unusual Locations. J Clin Med 2018;7.

54. Smith JD, Harvey RN, Darr OA, et al. Head and neck paragangliomas: A two-decade institutional experience and algorithm for management. Laryngoscope Investig Otolaryngol 2017;2:380–9.

55. Berends AMA, Buitenwerf E, de Krijger RR, et al. Incidence of pheochromocytoma and sympathetic paraganglioma in the Netherlands: A nationwide study and systematic review. Eur J Intern Med 2018;51:68–73.

56. Erickson D, Kudva YC, Ebersold MJ, et al. Benign paragangliomas: clinical presentation and treatment outcomes in 236 patients. J Clin Endocrinol Metab 2001;86:5210–6.

57. Eisenhofer G, Goldstein DS, Sullivan P, et al. Biochemical and clinical manifestations of dopamine-producing paragangliomas: utility of plasma methoxytyramine. J Clin Endocrinol Metab 2005;90:2068–75.

58. Van Der Horst-Schrivers AN, Osinga TE, Kema IP, et al. Dopamine excess in patients with head and neck paragangliomas. Anticancer Res 2010;30:5153–8.

59. Applebaum EL. Images in clinical medicine. Paraganglioma of the middle ear. N Engl J Med 1995;333:1677.

60. Netterville JL, Jackson CG, Miller FR, et al. Vagal paraganglioma: a review of 46 patients treated during a 20-year period. Arch Otolaryngol Head Neck Surg 1998;124:1133–40.

61. Offergeld C, Brase C, Yaremchuk S, et al. Head and neck paragangliomas: clinical and molecular genetic classification. Clinics (Sao Paulo) 2012;67(Suppl 1):19–28.

62. Astrom K, Cohen JE, Willett-Brozick JE, et al. Altitude is a phenotypic modifier in hereditary paraganglioma type 1: evidence for an oxygen-sensing defect. Hum Genet 2003;113:228–37.

63. Cerecer-Gil NY, Figuera LE, Llamas FJ, et al. Mutation of SDHB is a cause of hypoxia-related high-altitude paraganglioma. Clin Cancer Res 2010;16:4148–54.

64. Mak JK, Kay M. Carotid body tumour associated with cyanotic heart disease. BMJ Case Rep 2016; 2016.

65. Kriegsmann K, Zgorzelski C, Kazdal D, et al. Insulinoma-associated Protein 1 (INSM1) in Thoracic Tumors is Less Sensitive but More Specific Compared With Synaptophysin, Chromogranin A, and CD56. Appl Immunohistochem Mol Morphol 2020;28:237–42.

66. Kimura N, Shiga K, Kaneko K, et al. The Diagnostic Dilemma of GATA3 Immunohistochemistry in Pheochromocytoma and Paraganglioma. Endocr Pathol 2020;31:95–100.

67. Zhou YY, Coffey M, Mansur D, et al. Images in Endocrine Pathology: Progressive Loss of Sustentacular Cells in a Case of Recurrent Jugulotympanic Paraganglioma over a Span of 5 years. Endocr Pathol 2020;31:310–4.

68. Duet M, Sauvaget E, Petelle B, et al. Clinical impact of somatostatin receptor scintigraphy in the management of paragangliomas of the head and neck. J Nucl Med 2003;44:1767–74.

69. Kimura N, Tateno H, Saijo S, et al. Familial cervical paragangliomas with lymph node metastasis expressing somatostatin receptor type 2A. Endocr Pathol 2010;21:139–43.

70. Shi Y, Brandler TC, Yee-Chang M, et al. Application of GATA 3 and TTF-1 in differentiating parathyroid and thyroid nodules on cytology specimens. Diagn Cytopathol 2020;48:128–37.

71. Turchini J, Sioson L, Clarkson A, et al. Utility of GATA-3 Expression in the Analysis of Pituitary Neuroendocrine Tumour (PitNET) Transcription Factors. Endocr Pathol 2020;31:150–5.

72. Dermawan JK, Mukhopadhyay S, Shah AA. Frequency and extent of cytokeratin expression in paraganglioma: an immunohistochemical study of 60 cases from 5 anatomic sites and review of the literature. Hum Pathol 2019;93:16–22.

73. Baloch Z, Mete O, Asa SL. Immunohistochemical Biomarkers in Thyroid Pathology. Endocr Pathol 2018;29:91–112.

74. Williams MD. Paragangliomas of the Head and Neck: An Overview from Diagnosis to Genetics. Head Neck Pathol 2017;11:278–87.

75. Ellis RJ, Patel D, Prodanov T, et al. The presence of SDHB mutations should modify surgical indications for carotid body paragangliomas. Ann Surg 2014; 260:158–62.

76. McCrary HC, Babajanian E, Calquin M, et al. Characterization of Malignant Head and Neck Paragangliomas at a Single Institution Across Multiple Decades. JAMA Otolaryngol Head Neck Surg 2019;145:641–6.

77. Turkova H, Prodanov T, Maly M, et al. Characteristics and Outcomes of Metastatic Sdhb and Sporadic Pheochromocytoma/Paraganglioma: An National Institutes of Health Study. Endocr Pract 2016;22:302–14.

78. Ebbehoj A, Stochholm K, Jacobsen SF, et al. Incidence and Clinical Presentation of Pheochromocytoma and Sympathetic Paraganglioma: A Population-based Study. J Clin Endocrinol Metab 2021;106:e2251–61.

79. Babic B, Patel D, Aufforth R, et al. Pediatric patients with pheochromocytoma and paraganglioma should have routine preoperative genetic testing for common susceptibility genes in addition to imaging to detect extra-adrenal and metastatic tumors. Surgery 2017;161:220–7.

80. Pamporaki C, Hamplova B, Peitzsch M, et al. Characteristics of Pediatric vs Adult Pheochromocytomas and Paragangliomas. J Clin Endocrinol Metab 2017;102:1122–32.

81. Nijhoff MF, Dekkers OM, Vleming LJ, et al. ACTH-producing pheochromocytoma: clinical considerations and concise review of the literature. Eur J Intern Med 2009;20:682–5.

82. Bayraktar F, Kebapcilar L, Kocdor MA, et al. Cushing's syndrome due to ectopic CRH secretion by adrenal pheochromocytoma accompanied by renal infarction. Exp Clin Endocrinol Diabetes 2006;114: 444–7.

83. Loehry CA, Kingham JG, Whorwell PJ. Watery diarrhoea and hypokalaemia associated with a phaeochromocytoma. Postgrad Med J 1975;51:416–9.

84. Eisenhofer G, Klink B, Richter S, et al. Metabologenomics of Phaeochromocytoma and Paraganglioma: An Integrated Approach for Personalised Biochemical and Genetic Testing. Clin Biochem Rev 2017;38:69–100.

85. Gupta S, Zhang J, Milosevic D, et al. Primary Renal Paragangliomas and Renal Neoplasia Associated with Pheochromocytoma/Paraganglioma: Analysis of von Hippel-Lindau (VHL), Succinate Dehydrogenase (SDHX) and Transmembrane Protein 127 (TMEM127). Endocr Pathol 2017;28:253–68.

86. Casey R, Neumann HPH, Maher ER. Genetic stratification of inherited and sporadic phaeochromocytoma and paraganglioma: implications for precision medicine. Hum Mol Genet 2020;29:R128–37.

87. Fishbein L, Leshchiner I, Walter V, et al. Comprehensive Molecular Characterization of Pheochromocytoma and Paraganglioma. Cancer Cell 2017;31: 181–93.

88. Kluckova K, Tennant DA. Metabolic implications of hypoxia and pseudohypoxia in pheochromocytoma and paraganglioma. Cell Tissue Res 2018;372: 367–78.

89. Dahia PL, Ross KN, Wright ME, et al. A HIF1alpha regulatory loop links hypoxia and mitochondrial signals in pheochromocytomas. Plos Genet 2005;1:72–80.

90. Jiang J, Zhang J, Pang Y, et al. Sino-European Differences in the Genetic Landscape and Clinical Presentation of Pheochromocytoma and Paraganglioma. J Clin Endocrinol Metab 2020;105.

91. Kimura N. Dopamine beta-hydroxylase: An Essential and Optimal Immunohistochemical Marker for Pheochromocytoma and Sympathetic Paraganglioma. Endocr Pathol 2021;32:258–61.

92. Timmers HJ, Pacak K, Huynh TT, et al. Biochemically silent abdominal paragangliomas in patients with mutations in the succinate dehydrogenase subunit B gene. J Clin Endocrinol Metab 2008;93:4826–32.

93. Mete O, Asa SL, Giordano TJ, et al. Immunohistochemical Biomarkers of Adrenal Cortical Neoplasms. Endocr Pathol 2018;29:137–49.

94. Pierre C, Agopiantz M, Brunaud L, et al. COPPS, a composite score integrating pathological features, PS100 and SDHB losses, predicts the risk of metastasis and progression-free survival in pheochromocytomas/paragangliomas. Virchows Arch 2019;474:721–34.

95. Kimura N, Takayanagi R, Takizawa N, et al, Phaeochromocytoma Study Group in J. Pathological grading for predicting metastasis in phaeochromocytoma and paraganglioma. Endocr Relat Cancer 2014;21:405–14.

96. Koh JM, Ahn SH, Kim H, et al. Validation of pathological grading systems for predicting metastatic potential in pheochromocytoma and paraganglioma. PLoS One 2017;12:e0187398.

97. Thompson LD. Pheochromocytoma of the Adrenal gland Scaled Score (PASS) to separate benign from malignant neoplasms: a clinicopathologic and immunophenotypic study of 100 cases. Am J Surg Pathol 2002;26:551–66.

All Together Now

Standardization of Nomenclature for Neuroendocrine Neoplasms across Multiple Organs

Pari Jafari, MD*, Aliya N. Husain, MBBS, Namrata Setia, MD

KEYWORDS

- Neuroendocrine neoplasm (NEN) • Neuroendocrine tumor (NET) • Small-cell/large-cell neuroendocrine carcinoma (SC/LC NEC) • Typical/atypical carcinoid
- Small-cell lung carcinoma (SCLC)

Key points

- Neuroendocrine neoplasms (NENs) arise across virtually all organ systems but are most common in the gastroenteropancreatic (GEP) tract and lungs.

- NENs across anatomic sites can be grouped into well- and poorly differentiated tiers (neuroendocrine tumors [NETs] and neuroendocrine carcinomas [NECs], respectively) based on morphology and proliferative activity. Underpinning this paradigm are distinct, and often mutually exclusive, molecular and immunohistochemical (IHC) profiles.

- NECs are by definition high-grade and are typically associated with dismal prognoses. In contrast, NETs exhibit a complex spectrum of behavior, necessitating a two- or three-tiered grading rubric, with proliferative activity serving as a crucial parameter.

- Nomenclature and grading of NENs have historically varied across anatomic sites, though efforts toward conceptual unification are underway, most notably with the adoption of a standardized rubric for GEP-NENs.

ABSTRACT

Neuroendocrine neoplasms (NENs) span virtually all organ systems and exhibit a broad spectrum of behavior, from indolent to highly aggressive. Historically, nomenclature and grading practices have varied widely across, and even within, organ systems. However, certain core features are recapitulated across anatomic sites, including characteristic morphology and the crucial role of proliferative activity in prognostication. A recent emphasis on unifying themes has driven an increasingly standardized approach to NEN classification, as delineated in the World Health Organization's *Classification of Tumours* series. Here, we review recent developments in NEN classification, with a focus on NENs of the pancreas and lungs.

OVERVIEW

In 1907, physicians abreast of the literature might have noted a brief but striking report by the German pathologist Siegfried Oberndorfer in the *Frankfurt Journal of Pathology*, describing a new and intriguing class of small bowel neoplasms.[1] These lesions appeared relatively indolent–though Oberndorfer later came to recognize that a subset harbored significant metastatic potential–and were well-circumscribed, submucosal, and composed of relatively bland cells forming

Department of Pathology, The University of Chicago Medicine, 5841 South Maryland Avenue, MC 6101, Room S-638, Chicago, IL 60637, USA
* Corresponding author.
E-mail address: Pari.Jafari@uchicagomedicine.org

Surgical Pathology 16 (2023) 131–150
https://doi.org/10.1016/j.path.2022.09.012
1875-9181/23/© 2022 Elsevier Inc. All rights reserved.

surgpath.theclinics.com

nests or rosettes. Today, Oberndorfer's "benign carcinomas" or *carcinoid tumors* (*Karzinoid Tumoren*) are known to arise from the *neuroendocrine system,* a unique population of cells exhibiting neurosecretory properties and disseminated across multiple anatomic sites, from the pituitary to the pancreas.[1–6] Corresponding neoplasms have been known by a variety of site- and era-specific names over the years (**Box 1**); at present, the more neutral and inclusive term *neuroendocrine neoplasm* is generally favored.[2–8]

Neuroendocrine neoplasms (NENs) represent an unusual class of tumors: at once capacious, yet bound together by many of the distinctive morphologic features that Oberndorfer described (**Fig. 1**, **Table 1**). Indeed, the study of NENs is characterized by several overarching themes, including:

1. Bifurcation of neoplasms into relatively well-differentiated ("neuroendocrine tumor," NET) and poorly differentiated ("neuroendocrine carcinoma," NEC) tiers, each with a distinct clinicopathologic profile.[7,8] NETs exhibit a complex spectrum of behavior, from indolent to relatively aggressive, necessitating a superimposed two- or three-tiered grading scheme (**Figs. 2–4**).[7–11] NECs are invariably aggressive and are high-grade by definition; they are further classified based on small-cell (SC; **Fig. 5**) versus large-cell (LC; **Fig. 6**) morphology.[7,8]
2. The increasingly crucial role of ancillary testing in classification and grading, including molecular and immunohistochemical (IHC) studies.[7–10,12–14]
3. The importance of proliferative activity, as gauged by mitotic count or Ki67 labeling index (LI), in NEN classification and prognostication.[8,15–18]

Despite these common denominators, approaches to NEN classification and nomenclature have long differed across organ systems. This heterogeneity reflects subspecialty preferences and historical associations, and has given rise to persistent concerns about miscommunication between specialties and the challenge of remaining up-to-date with each organ system's evolving classification criteria.[5,7,9] Those concerns are heightened by the rising incidence of NENs, from 1.09 to 6.98 cases per 100,000 between 1973 and 2012 in the United States, likely attributable in large measure to enhanced detection modalities.[19] In response, an expert committee convened by the World Health Organization (WHO)/International Agency for Research on Cancer (IARC) issued a proposal in 2018 for streamlining NEN classification across organ systems, using a 2017 WHO scheme for pancreatic NENs (panNENs) as a conceptual template.[9] As detailed below, this rubric has since been extended, with site-specific adjustments, to include all gastroenteropancreatic (GEP)-NENs as well as NENs of the upper aerodigestive tract and salivary glands.[7,8,16,17,20–22] A similar approach has been discussed in the context of other organ systems, particularly the lungs.[10,15] This unfolding paradigm shift is captured in the WHO's *Classification of Tumours* series (colloquially known as the WHO "Blue Books"), most notably in *Endocrine and Neuroendocrine Tumors* (2022), the first Blue Book to discuss both endocrine and neuroendocrine neoplasms across endocrine and non-endocrine sites.[7,8] Current WHO classification criteria are summarized in **Table 2**.

Box 1
Selected historic nomenclature associated with NENs

Nomenclature reflecting morphology

   Carcinoid/atypical carcinoid (still in use at certain sites, particularly in the thorax)

   Bronchial adenoma

   Oat cell carcinoma/sarcoma

Nomenclature reflecting tumor cell function/hormonal products

   Amine precursor uptake and decarboxylation (APUD)oma

   Glucagonoma, gastrinoma, insulinoma, vasoactive intestinal peptide (VIP)oma, somatostatinoma

Nomenclature reflecting presumptive cell of origin

   Islet cell tumor

   Kulchitsky cell tumor

   Argentaffin/(Entero)chromaffin(-type)/Argyrophil cell tumor

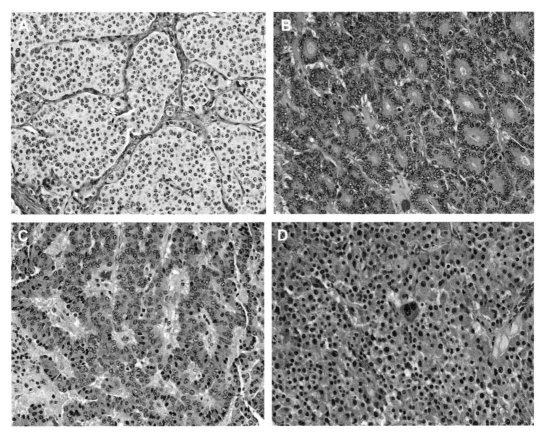

Fig. 1. Neuroendocrine tumors (NETs) classically exhibit organoid growth, as seen here on hematoxylin and eosin (H&E) staining. Common patterns include nests (*A*), rosettes (*B*), and trabeculae (*C*). However, diffuse growth is also observed, as in this atypical carcinoid of the lung (*D*).

In this article, we explore the shifting landscape of NEN classification with an emphasis on the themes described above. Although these principles are perhaps best delineated in NENs of the pancreas and lungs, two organs at the center of NEN clinicopathologic investigation over the years, they are readily applicable to NENs across anatomic sites.[7,8]

Of note, non-epithelial NENs, such as pheochromocytomas/paragangliomas; non-neoplastic entities, such as diffuse idiopathic pulmonary neuroendocrine hyperplasia (DIPNECH); mixed neuroendocrine-non-neuroendocrine neoplasms (MiNENs); and special considerations associated with functional tumors are beyond the scope of this article and will not be discussed here.

NEUROENDOCRINE NEOPLASMS: A TWO-TIERED PARADIGM

Oberndorfer's original article on "carcinoids" described a class of relatively well-differentiated NENs known today as NETs, though the term *carcinoid* is retained at certain anatomic sites, most notably in the thorax.[1,2,4,7,8,15] Under the current schema, NETs are juxtaposed with SC and LC NECs, which are intrinsically high-grade and are associated with poor prognoses. NETs and NECs each exhibit characteristic morphology across anatomic sites (see **Table 1**).[7,8]

WELL-DIFFERENTIATED NEUROENDOCRINE NEOPLASMS: NEUROENDOCRINE TUMORS

The "classic" NET is a well-circumscribed submucosal lesion composed of bland-appearing cells with granular, eosinophilic cytoplasm and round or polygonal contours. The nuclei are typically round with distinctive "salt and pepper" clumping of chromatin and inconspicuous nucleoli.[7,8,23] Atypia and degenerative changes may be present, particularly in higher-grade NETs, but are not in and of themselves worrisome features.[23,24] Crucially, mitoses are relatively infrequent.[7,8,15–17] As described by Soga and Tazawa in their seminal 1971 analysis,

Table 1
Key histologic features of neuroendocrine tumors and neuroendocrine carcinomas (NECs)

		NET	NEC
Morphologic features	Microarchitecture	Organoid (nests, rosettes, trabeculae, and pseudoglands) or solid; mixed phenotypes common	Sheetlike/diffuse
	Necrosis	Absent or punctate	Marked/geographic
	Mitoses	Rare to brisk	Numerous; often atypical
	Cytologic features	Medium-sized, round cells; low N:C ratio; "salt and pepper" chromatin; moderate to abundant eosinophilic cytoplasm; inconspicuous nucleoli	SC NEC: Small cells (<3x size of lymphocyte) with minimal basophilic cytoplasm; granular chromatin and inconspicuous nucleoli; molding and crush artifact often present LC NEC: Large, pleomorphic cells (~3–5x size of lymphocyte) with moderate/abundant amphophilic cytoplasm; prominent nucleoli
IHC profile	*Core neuroendocrine panel*	Cytokeratin 8/18+, CAM5.2+ Chromogranin+ Synaptophysin+ *Less routinely:* CD56+ INSM1+ SSTR2A/5+	CK 8 and 18+/−, CAM5.2+/− [keratins, particularly CAM5.2, may exhibit dot-like staining in SC NECs] Chromogranin ± Synaptophysin+ *Less routinely:* CD56+ INSM1+ SSTR2A/5−/+
	Peptide hormones	Positive staining in functional tumors	Almost uniformly negative (exception: hormone-producing SCLC)
	Ki67	Low (<20% for G1-G2; typically <55% for G3-type tumors)	High (>20%; frequently >55% and often >70%)
	Rb	Rb retention	Rb loss
	p53	Wild-type pattern	p53 mutant pattern (compete loss or diffuse positivity)
	Selected site-specific findings	• Pancreatic origin: ATRX or DAXX loss (panNETs); +ISL1; ± CDX2 • Tubular gastrointestinal tract (particularly mid-gut): +CDX2 • Jejunoileal NET: clusterin− • Lung, thyroid: +TTF-1	
Molecular profile	*Selected site-specific findings*	• 11q13 deletions most common (contains *MEN1* locus) • *MEN1*, *ATRX*, or *DAXX* loss in panNETs • *MEN1* mutations in lung carcinoids; other alterations (eg, *PSIP*, *EIF1AX*, *KMT2*, *ARID1A*) also described	• *RB* and/or *TP53* mutations across anatomic sites • *MYC* amplifications (particularly panNECs) • *ASCL1*, *NEUROD1*, *POU2F3*, *YAP1* alterations in SCLC • NSCLC-type mutations (eg, *KRAS*) in NSCLC-like lung LC NEC

Abbreviations: LC NEC, large-cell neuroendocrine carcinoma; N:C ratio, nuclear:cytoplasmic ratio; NSCLC, non-small-cell lung carcinoma; SC NEC, small-cell neuroendocrine carcinoma; SCLC, small-cell lung carcinoma.

microarchitecture classically assumes one of four patterns, or a combination thereof: type A, nodular/nested; type B, trabecular; type C, pseudoglandular (eg, tubules, acini, and rosettes); and type D, diffuse or otherwise atypical.[25]

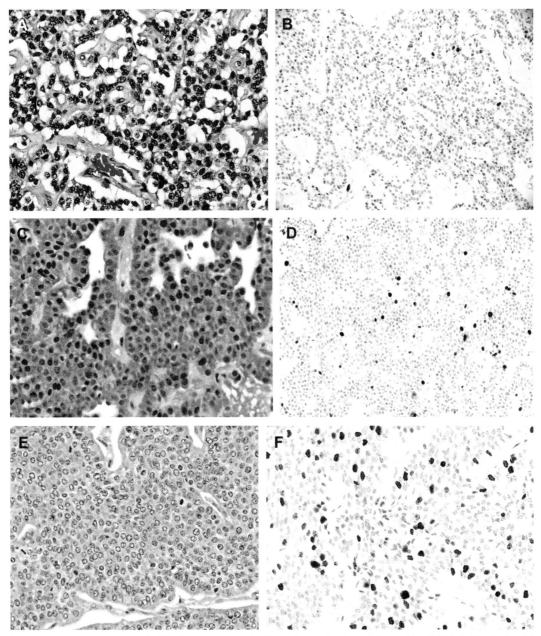

Fig. 2. Gastroentero-pancreatic (GEP)-NETs are graded based on mitotic activity and/or Ki67 labeling index (LI). G1 GEP-NET with a diffuse pattern of growth (H&E, *A*) and <3% Ki67 LI (*B*). Note that Ki67 may also highlight lymphocytes and endothelial cells, serving as a useful positive internal control; however, these non-lesional cells should not be included in the LI assessment. G2 GEP-NET (H&E, *C*) showing trabecular architecture and Ki67 LI of 18% (*D*). G3 GEP-NET exhibiting multiple mitoses (H&E, *E*) and Ki67 LI of 25% (*F*).

Neuroendocrine Tumor Grading: A Three-Tiered Approach

Despite their relatively bland appearance as a whole, NETs exhibit a striking spectrum of behavior, ranging from indolent to aggressive. Prognosis-driven, clinically meaningful stratification of these tumors has proven challenging, as reflected in a series of proposed grading parameters dating from the 1990s.[16,26–28] Though these schemes were originally highly site-specific, the WHO Blue Books have embraced an increasingly unified approach in recent years (see **Table 2**), beginning with the 2019 publication of *Digestive System Tumours,* which extended the existing

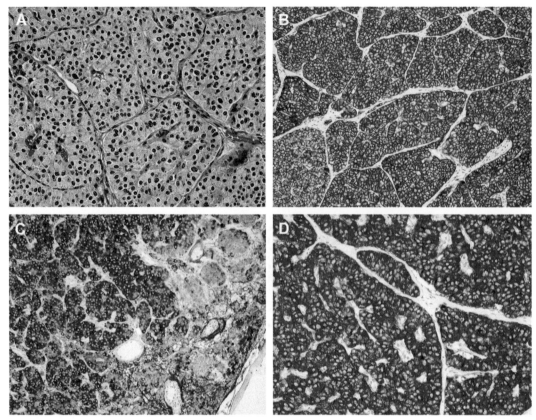

Fig. 3. Typical carcinoid of the lung, demonstrating (H&E, *A*) bland cells with moderate amounts of amphophilic cytoplasm and prominent round nuclei with characteristic "salt and pepper" chromatin. Necrosis is absent, and mitoses are exceedingly rare (<2 mitoses/2 mm²). The cells exhibit diffuse staining for CD56 (*B*; membranous pattern), chromogranin (*C*; cytoplasmic), and synaptophysin (*D*; cytoplasmic).

panNEN rubric to include all GEP-NENs. In this paradigm, NENs are strictly partitioned into NETs and NECs, with NECs considered exclusively high-grade and NETs stratified (G1–G3) based on proliferative activity (see **Fig. 2**).[7,9,16,20,21] This bifurcated approach has since been extended to the upper aerodigestive tract/salivary glands while retaining certain site-specific nuances, such as the inclusion of necrosis as a NET grading parameter and the caveat that G3 NETs have yet to be fully characterized in the head and neck.[7,8,17,22]

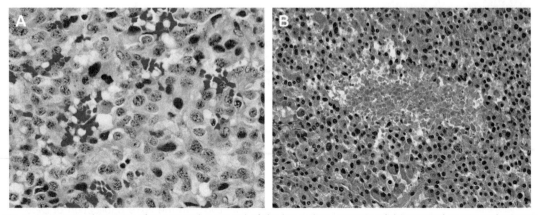

Fig. 4. H&E-stained sections of an atypical carcinoid of the lung, demonstrating (*A*) increased atypia and mitoses as well as (*B*) focal necrosis.

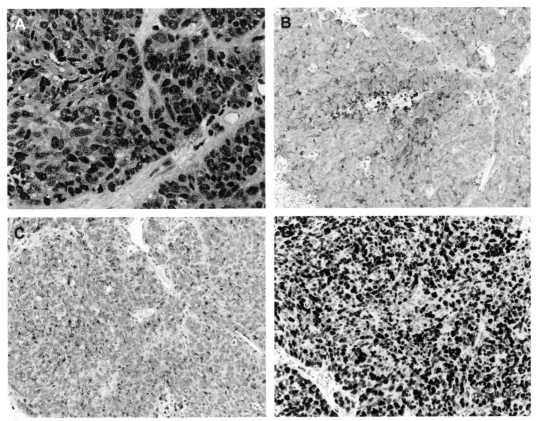

Fig. 5. Small-cell lung carcinoma demonstrating (*A*, H&E) characteristic scant amphophilic cytoplasm, high nuclear:cytoplasmic ratio, and nuclear molding. Staining with (*B*) synaptophysin and (*C*) chromogranin confirms neuroendocrine differentiation. Ki67 LI is 90% (*D*).

The roots of this approach can be traced to the WHO's 2010 panNEN grading rubric, which split tumors into G1/G2 (NET) or G3 (NEC) categories solely based on proliferative activity: G3 tumors were defined by > 20 mitoses/2 mm^2 or Ki67 LI >20%.[26] However, the NEC category was subsequently shown to include both "bona fide NECs"—poorly differentiated neoplasms with either SC or LC morphology–and a vexing subcategory of relatively well-differentiated tumors with

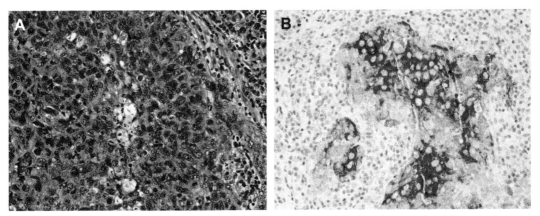

Fig. 6. Large-cell neuroendocrine carcinoma of the lung, showing (*A*) abundant amphophilic cytoplasm and irregularly shaped nuclei with predominantly vesicular or clumped chromatin, arranged here in a sheetlike pattern with focal necrosis. Synaptophysin IHC (*B*) shows patchy positivity.

Table 2
Classification of neuroendocrine neoplasms across selected anatomic sites: World Health Organization criteria (5th edition)[8,15–17]

	Neuroendocrine Tumor	Neuroendocrine Carcinoma
Key histologic features across anatomic sites	Bland cells with round nuclei, salt-and-pepper chromatin, inconspicuous nucleoli; classically arranged in rosettes, nests, or trabeculae; focal necrosis and increased atypia seen with increasing grade	*Small-cell (SC) NEC:* Diameter <3 times that of lymphocyte; scant cytoplasm with high N:C ratio; granular chromatin; inconspicuous nucleoli; sheetlike arrangement with extensive necrosis *Large-cell (LC) NEC:* Diameter ∼3–5 times that of lymphocyte; amphophilic cytoplasm; relatively low N:C ratio; organoid architecture with extensive necrosis

	WHO 5th Edition NET Grading Criteria (G1-G3)		WHO 5th Edition NEC Subclassification Criteria (SC vs LC NEC)	
Gastroentero-pancreatic tract	G1 NET	<2 mitoses/2 mm² *and* Ki67 < 3%	Small-cell NEC	Characteristic small-cell morphology *and* > 20 mitoses/2 mm² *and/or* Ki67 > 20% (typically >70%)
	G2 NET	2–20 mitoses/2 mm² *and/or* Ki67 3–20%		
	G3 NET	>20 mitoses/2 mm² *and/or* Ki67 > 20% (typically <55%)	Large-cell NEC	Characteristic large-cell morphology *and* > 20 mitoses/2 mm² *and/or* Ki67 > 20% (typically > 70%)
Lung and thymus	Typical carcinoid	<2 mitoses/2 mm² *and* no necrosis	Small-cell (lung) carcinoma (SCLC)	Characteristic small-cell morphology *and* >10 mitoses/2 mm²; Ki67 not part of formal criteria but often >30% (typically >75%)
	Atypical carcinoid	2–10 mitoses/2 mm² *and/or* necrosis		
	Emerging category[a]: carcinoids with high proliferative activity	Atypical carcinoid morphology *and* >10 mitoses/2 mm²; Ki67 typically >30%	Large-cell NEC	Characteristic large-cell morphology *and* >10 mitoses/2 mm²; Ki67 not part of formal criteria but often >30% (typically >75%)
Upper aerodigestive tract and salivary glands	G1 NET	<2 mitoses/2 mm² *and* no necrosis; Ki67 typically <20%	Small-cell NEC	Characteristic small-cell morphology *and* >10 mitoses/2 mm² *and/or* Ki67 > 20% (typically >70%)
	G2 NET	2–10 mitoses/2 mm² *and/or* necrosis; Ki67 typically <20%	Large-cell NEC	Characteristic large-cell morphology *and* >10 mitoses/2 mm² *and/or* Ki67 > 20% (typically >50%)
	Emerging category[a]: G3 NET	Relatively well-differentiated histology *and* >10 mitoses/2 mm²; Ki67 > 20%		

Abbreviations: N:C ratio, nuclear:cytoplasmic ratio.

[a] Lung/thymic carcinoids with high proliferative activity (analogous to G3 GEP-NETs) are discussed, but not formally categorized, in the fifth edition of the WHO *Classification of Tumours* series. Similarly, G3 NETs of the upper aerodigestive tract/salivary glands are mentioned as a potential category, but have yet to be fully delineated.

an elevated Ki67 LI (typically 30–40%; generally <55%), prompting a default diagnosis of NEC.[11,29–41] Interestingly, several studies noted comparatively low (<20 mitoses/2 mm^2) mean mitotic counts for this subgroup, despite the elevated Ki67 LI.[11,31,32,36,37] Prognosis fell somewhere between that of G2 NETs and the bona fide (poorly -differentiated) NECs, with reduced amenability to cisplatin-based therapy relative to NECs.[11,29–41] Crucially, ancillary testing revealed a molecular and IHC profile relatively similar to that of G1/G2 NETs.[31,32,34,42] In response to these findings, the WHO's 2017 *Classification of Tumours of Endocrine Organs* refashioned panNETs into three tiers (G1, G2, and G3), with G3 serving to house the former "well-differentiated NEC" subcategory. This change broadened the definition of panNET to include all relatively well-differentiated tumors, regardless of proliferative activity, while narrowing the panNEC category to include only those "true" carcinomas that united poorly differentiated histology with high proliferative activity.[43,44] This rubric was subsequently expanded to encompass all GEP-NENs.[16,20,21]

A similar reappraisal is currently underway across other organ systems, most notably in the lungs, where NETs (known in the thorax as *carcinoids*) have traditionally been bifurcated into typical and atypical carcinoids (TCs and ACs, respectively) based on mitotic count and presence of necrosis (see **Table 2**).[10,15] However, this paradigm has been challenged by the recent identification of "highly proliferative carcinoids," which combine the morphology of ACs with the marked proliferative activity characteristic of NECs (>10 mitoses/2 mm^2; Ki67 LI typically 20–40%). Though available data are limited, outcomes appear to be intermediate between those of lung ACs and NECs, whereas the associated molecular and IHC profile is similar to that of carcinoids.[7,8,10,45–52] These findings suggest that lung carcinoids may be amenable to G1-G3 stratification, analogous to GEP-NETs.[7,10,15] Such a change would mark another key step toward the unification of NEN nomenclature and categorization.

Of note, as the diagnostic criteria for G3 NETs/ highly proliferative carcinoids include a threshold for mitotic activity, but no ceiling, histology plays a pivotal role in diagnosis. By definition, G3 NET histology falls somewhere between that of G1/G2 NETs and (LC) NECs; in practice, this distinction may be quite challenging, as G3 NETs may exhibit high-grade, NEC-like features, such as nuclear atypia and necrosis (punctate or even geographic).[8,24,32,50] It has been suggested that identification of lower-grade (G1-G2) NET components supports a diagnosis of G3 NET, whereas the presence of interspersed non-neuroendocrine elements (eg, adenocarcinoma, squamous cell carcinoma) favors NEC.[24,33] **Table 3** summarizes these and other "rules of thumb" for differentiating between G3 NETs and NECs.

POORLY DIFFERENTIATED NEUROENDOCRINE NEOPLASMS: NEUROENDOCRINE CARCINOMAS

Unlike NETs, all NECs are high-grade by default: as such, there is no role for a superimposed grading scheme. Instead, NECs are subdivided based on SC versus LC morphology.[7,8] Of note, pulmonary SC NECs are traditionally known as small-cell lung carcinomas (SCLCs), as not all express core neuroendocrine markers such as chromogranin and synaptophysin.[10,15] Both SC and LC NECs are characterized by extensive necrosis and marked proliferative activity (see **Figs. 5–6**).[7,8] SC NEC cells measure up to three times the diameter of a lymphocyte and exhibit round, ovoid, or angulated contours; granular chromatin; and scant cytoplasm, resulting in a high nuclear:cytoplasmic ratio. Nuclear molding is common, as is extensive necrosis, and crush artifact and/or encrustation of vessel walls with extruded chromatin may be observed. Growth is classically sheetlike, though organoid microarchitecture has also been described.[7,8,10,53–55] In contrast, large-cell NECs exhibit variable quantities of amphophilic cytoplasm and are approximately three to five times the diameter of a lymphocyte in size. The chromatin may be granular or vesicular; nucleoli are often prominent. The cells typically palisade or form nests, trabeculae, or rosettes, among other patterns.[7,8,10,54]

As noted above, there may be considerable morphologic overlap among high-grade NENs (ie, G3 NETs and SC and LC NECs): indeed, in Tang and colleagues'[32] 2016 evaluation of panNECs and G3 panNETs, diagnostic consensus was reached in just a third of cases.[8,24,50] Both SC and LC NECs also raise the differential of poorly differentiated non-neuroendocrine carcinomas, whereas SC NECs may warrant consideration of other "small round blue cell tumors," such as lymphoma, neuroblastoma, and Ewing sarcoma.[8,10,15,53,55]

CLINICAL IMPLICATIONS OF NEUROENDOCRINE NEOPLASM CLASSIFICATION

Each NEN category–NET versus NEC as well as individual NET tiers–carries substantial clinical

Table 3
Features favoring a diagnosis of G3 neuroendocrine tumor versus neuroendocrine carcinoma

	G3 NET	NEC
Proliferative activity	• Ki67 LI typically 20%-55% • Mitotic count may be discordant (within G2 NET range)	• Ki67 LI >55% strongly favors NEC • Mitotic count typically concordant with Ki67 LI
IHC profile	• Rb1 retained, p53 wild-type expression • Loss of menin ± ATRX/DAXX • Retained SSTR2A	• Rb1 loss and/or p53-mutated pattern (global loss or diffuse positivity) • Menin, ATRX, and DAXX retained • Loss of SSTR2A
Molecular profile	• *MEN1* ± *ATRX* or *DAXX* mutations (panNET) • Mutations in genes associated with chromatin remodeling; *MEN1* mutations most common • *RB* and *TP53* wild-type	• Mutated *RB* and/or *TP53* • Absence of *MEN1* or *ATRX/DAXX* mutations
Other findings	Presence of areas with G1/G2 histology	Presence of areas with non-neuroendocrine differentiation (eg, adenocarcinoma or squamous cell carcinoma)

ramifications. Recently reported median overall survival rates for panNETs, for instance, improve in stepwise fashion from G3 (19–99 months) to G1 (over 100 months), versus approximately 10-16 months for panNECs.[11,29–39,41,56] Each tier also dictates a distinct approach to treatment, as outlined below.

- *NETs:* Resection is generally curative for localized/locoregional NETs (stages I-II).[57–61] Non-resectable/advanced disease is primarily managed with somatostatin analogs (SSAs), which exploit NET overexpression of somatostatin receptors (SSTRs). Examples include octreotide long-acting release (LAR) and lanreotide, which preferentially bind to SSTR2 and SSTR5, exerting an antiproliferative effect while also providing symptomatic relief for functional tumors.[58–65] In patients with a high burden of hepatic metastases, debulking or liver-directed therapies, such as transarterial chemoembolization (TACE), may be appropriate.[59,60,66,67] In the event of disease progression on SSAs, options include peptide receptor radionuclide therapy (PRRT), which consists of an SSA chelated to a radioisotope, such as ^{111}In, ^{90}Y, or ^{177}Lu, enabling enhanced visualization and targeted treatment of lesional tissue.[58–61,68] Although the role of conventional chemotherapy remains under debate, the biologics sunitinib and everolimus have recently shown promise in managing advanced-stage NETs.[59,61,69–72] At this time, optimal therapy for G3 GEP-

NETs and analogous lesions at other sites remains to be more fully defined, as their clinical profile is intermediate between that of G2 NETs and NECs.[10,11,29–41,45–52]

- *NECs:* Treatment of SC NECs across anatomic sites has traditionally followed the template established for SCLC, which is characterized by striking initial sensitivity to platinum-based chemotherapy and radiation.[30,59,73–76] Very early stage SCLCs may undergo resection, though the evidence base is mixed and it should be emphasized that SCLC is typically relatively advanced at presentation, precluding resection.[73,77] Of note, immune checkpoint inhibitors, such as pembrolizumab and nivolumab, are often combined with conventional chemotherapy in extensive-stage SCLC; their role in extrapulmonary SC NECs remains to be explored.[73–75]

Data regarding the management of LC NECs are limited and are largely derived from studies of pulmonary LC NECs. In contrast to SCLCs, pulmonary LC NECs presenting through at least stage II appear relatively amenable to resection and adjuvant chemotherapy.[78–81] More advanced disease is generally treated with platinum-based regimens, following the SCLC model.[30,59,78,79,82] Of note, a subset of pulmonary LC NECs exhibits a molecular profile more similar to that of non-SCLCs (NSCLCs) than to that of SCLCs, suggesting that such cases may be more effectively managed by NSCLC protocols.[10,47,78,79,82–88]

ANCILLARY TESTING IN THE CLASSIFICATION OF NEUROENDOCRINE NEOPLASMS

The molecular and IHC profiles of NETs and NECs are essentially mutually exclusive, reinforcing the dichotomous NEN paradigm. These ancillary studies can be leveraged in diagnostically challenging cases and, in some instances, may offer prognostic insights or clarify therapeutic options.[7–10,12–14,89] Here, we briefly review key facets of ancillary testing (summarized in Table 1), with the pancreas and lungs as prototypes.

MOLECULAR TESTING

Molecular Profile of Neuroendocrine Tumors

Broadly speaking, NETs exhibit relative genomic stability, with significantly lower tumor mutational burden and copy number alterations in comparison to NECs.[10,90–93] Both lung carcinoids and panNETs are classically associated with loss of chromosome 11q (which harbors the *MEN1* locus), though other cytogenetic abnormalities, including gains of 17q, 7q, and 20q and losses of 6q and 11p in panNETs, have also been described.[12,93–96] At the gene-specific level, sporadic panNETs are closely associated with alterations in *MEN1,* which codes for a chromatin remodeling protein (menin): mutations have been reported in up to nearly two-thirds of cases.[96–99] In addition, molecular and IHC studies have demonstrated mutually exclusive mutations in either *DAXX* or *ATRX,* two genes that govern histone interactions, in up to 43% of panNETs; loss of DAXX/ATRX expression leads to alternative lengthening of telomeres (ALT), a senescence escape mechanism.[12,96,97,100–104] Other processes/pathways implicated in panNET tumorigenesis include mTOR signaling (eg, *TSC1/2, PTEN*), histone modification/chromatin remodeling (*SETD2, MLL3*), and DNA damage repair (*MUTYH, CHEK2, BRCA2*).[96,97] Of note, several studies have linked *DAXX* and *ATRX* mutations to more aggressive tumor behavior and poorer prognosis.[12,96,101–106]

In contrast to panNETs, lung carcinoids largely lack consistent, "hallmark" mutations, though nearly half harbor alterations in genes governing chromatin remodeling pathways.[91,107–109] Of these, *MEN1* alterations are most frequent, with rates of up to ~13% across several recent studies; mutations in *PSIP, EIF1AX, KMT2,* and *ARID1A* are also described.[91,93,107–112] Though the evidence is somewhat mixed, *MEN1* mutations appear to occur more commonly in ACs, where they are associated with poorer prognosis.[108,109,111,112]

Molecular profiling and associated IHC-based studies have likewise been instrumental in the delineation of G3 GEP-NETs and their conceptual counterparts in other organ systems. G3 panNETs, for instance, share frequent alterations in *MEN1* (21%) and *ATRX* or *DAXX* (approximately 30%) with G1/G2 panNETs, and generally lack the *RB/TP53* mutations associated with panNECs.[31,32,34,89] Similarly, emerging evidence suggests that highly proliferative carcinoids of the lung lack the *RB/TP53* alterations or broader genomic instability seen in SCLC, supporting their classification as carcinoids (NETs), rather than NECs.[10,45,47,50–52]

Molecular Profile of Neuroendocrine Carcinomas

The genomic landscape of NECs, particularly those with SC morphology, is classically dominated by alterations in *TP53* and *RB*.[31,32,34,47,83–92,108,113,114] Among panNECs, for instance, molecular and IHC surrogate studies have identified *TP53* mutations and *RB* alterations (encompassing both mutations and copy number alterations) in up to 95% and 74% of cases, respectively; in contrast, such alterations are rarely encountered in panNETs.[31,32,34,89] Mutations in a variety of other driver genes, including *APC, KRAS,* and *BRAF,* are also described, and *MYC* and *KDM5A* gains/amplifications have been reported in approximately half of all panNECs.[31,34]

SCLCs are likewise notable for high rates of concurrent *RB1* and *TP53* loss, with reported frequencies ranging from 24% to >90% and 64% to nearly 100%, respectively.[92,108,113,114] As in lung carcinoids, alterations in chromatin-remodeling genes occur in approximately half of all SCLCs, though it is postulated that their tumorigenic impact may be overshadowed by that of *RB1* and *TP53* losses.[91] SCLCs also exhibit *MYC* amplifications and frequent mutations in *NOTCH* and *KMT2D*; the latter is associated with improved prognosis.[91,92,113,114] Interestingly, recent studies have delineated multiple SCLC subgroups based on dominant transcription factor expression profiles, including *ASCL1* (accounting for some 70% of SCLCs), *NEUROD1, POU2F3,* and *YAP1*.[115–118] Emerging evidence suggests that these subtypes exhibit unique clinical profiles, with *YAP1*- and *ASCL1*-dominant cases associated with the most and least favorable outcomes, respectively.[118]

Similarly, molecular profiling of pulmonary LC NECs has delineated two key subtypes, first reported in a key study by Rekhtman and colleagues.[47] The first of these, *SCLC-like*, constitutes approximately 36%-40% of cases and is characterized by dual mutations/losses in *TP53* and *RB1*, often in conjunction with *MYCL* amplification and/or other SCLC-type alterations. In contrast, the *NSCLC-like* subtype, comprising approximately 56% of pulmonary LC NECs, lacks concurrent *TP53/RB1* loss and often exhibits mutations in genes classically associated with NSCLCs (particularly adenocarcinoma), such as *STK11, KRAS,* and *KEAP1*.[47,83,84,86,87] Comparable rates of *TP53/RB* co-alterations have been reported among extrapulmonary LC NECs as well, though available data are quite limited.[87] These distinctions may have important clinical ramifications, with *RB*-wild-type/NSCLC-like tumors potentially benefitting from NSCLC-type management.[10,47,78,79,82–88]

IMMUNOHISTOCHEMICAL STUDIES

IHC plays several valuable roles in the work-up of NENs, as outlined below.

a. *Establishing neuroendocrine differentiation.* Epithelial NENs are characterized by a dual neural and epithelial phenotype. The neural aspect encompasses the production of peptide hormones (eg, insulin and glucagon) or biogenic amines (eg, serotonin), as well as expression of "classic" neuroendocrine markers, such as synaptophysin (more sensitive) and chromogranin A (more specific). These markers, particularly chromogranin, may be lost in NECs; in such cases, a second-line marker, eg, CD56, may be considered, though these are often quite nonspecific.[7,13,14,119] Of note, relatively recent additions to the NEN IHC toolkit include insulinoma-associated protein 1 (INSM1), which is highly specific for NENs across a variety of anatomic sites, and SSTR2A/5, which is significantly more likely to be expressed in GEP-NETs (particularly in low-grade tumors and/or low-stage disease) than in GEP-NECs.[7,13,62,120–122]

In addition to these neural markers, epithelial NENs classically express low-molecular weight keratins (LMWKs), eg, CK8 and CK18, and as such stain with a variety of broad-spectrum/pankeratin markers, including CAM5.2 and AE1/AE3; NECs, particularly SC NECs, may exhibit dot-like staining.[7,8,13,14] CK7 and CK20 are typically negative, though site-specific exceptions do occur.[13] In the rare event of a keratin-negative NET, negativity for tyrosine hydroxylase (highly sensitive for pheochromocytoma and, to a lesser extent, paraganglioma) or S100 (to demonstrate the absence of sustentacular cells) may help to exclude a non-epithelial NEN.[13,14]

Though the vast majority of NENs are nonfunctional (ie, do not produce biologically active peptides), staining for peptide hormones, such as insulin and glucagon, may occasionally be indicated in the appropriate clinical context.[13]

b. *Determining the origin of NEN metastases of uncertain primary.* In approximately one-tenth of metastatic NEN cases, the site of the primary malignancy cannot be determined; IHC studies may offer some clarity, as highlighted below, though the specificity and/or sensitivity of many markers is often greater in NETs than in NECs.[13,119,123–126]

   i. *Thyroid tissue transcription factor-1 (TTF-1):* Highly specific for lung carcinoids (both AC and TC) and thyroid NETs (namely, medullary thyroid carcinoma [MTC]), with positivity for calcitonin or CEA favoring a diagnosis of MTC.[13,14,119,123] In contrast, among NECs, TTF-1 is expressed not only by tumors of pulmonary origin, but also by approximately one-third of extrapulmonary NECs.[13,123]

   ii. *CDX2:* Classically associated with intestinal-type differentiation, and particularly sensitive for tumors originating in the mid-gut.[13,14,123] Notably, some 13%-16% of panNENs stain with CDX2, whereas expression in pulmonary NENs is exceedingly rare.[13,14,123,127,128]

   iii. *Additional stains:* CK7 is expressed in approximately 40% of lung carcinoids and is typically negative in GEP-NENs, whereas *CK20* positivity is seen in approximately 25% of GEP-NETs.[123] Emerging markers include *ISL-1*, highly sensitive for panNETs, though not particularly specific, and *clusterin*, which exhibits strong expression in NETs outside of the jejunum and ileum.[13,14,119,129,130]

c. *Assessing proliferative activity.* Ki67 IHC plays a valuable role in NEN grading, particularly in the GEP tract; see discussion below.[7,8,15–18]

d. *Distinguishing between NET and NEC.* As discussed above, high-grade NETs and SC/LC NECs may overlap morphologically, creating a diagnostic challenge. In tumors of pancreatic origin, loss of *MEN1* and/or *DAXX/ATRX* supports a diagnosis of panNET; across anatomic sites, *Rb1* loss or aberrant *p53* expression favors a diagnosis of NEC.[7,10,13,31,89,97,98] Among GEP-NENs, SSTR2A/5 expression favors a diagnosis of NET over NEC.[7,13,62]

PROLIFERATIVE ACTIVITY: THE CRUX OF NEUROENDOCRINE NEOPLASM GRADING

Across organ systems, proliferative activity has emerged as a powerful common denominator for

---

Box 2
Approaches to evaluation of Ki-67 LI within proliferation "hotspots"

"Eyeballing"(gestalt impression; no counting/assessment of discrete cells):

- Benefits: highly efficient (~1 min/slide); no additional resources required

- Drawbacks: poor interobserver agreement/accuracy

Manual counting at microscope:

- Benefits: highly accurate; no additional resources required

- Drawbacks: time-intensive (~6 min/slide); poor interobserver agreement

Manual counting using printed micrograph:

- Benefits: most accurate method, with highest interobserver agreement

- Drawbacks: time-intensive (~8 min/slide); requires microscope fitted with camera and access to high-quality printer

Digital image analysis (DIA):

- Benefits: increasingly accurate with continued advances in software; relatively efficient (~3–5 min/slide)

- Drawbacks: requires investment in slide scanning technology and image analysis software; persistent concerns regarding under-/over-counting and risk of software failure; current iterations typically require pathologist to screen slides and identify hotspots, raising concerns for inter-observer variability

---

NEN classification: it is the sole parameter for GEP-NET grading and one of just two parameters (in conjunction with necrosis) for thoracic and head and neck NET/carcinoid grading. Likewise, NECs are defined based on proliferative activity and histology.[7,8,15–17]

Proliferative activity can be assessed via either mitotic count or Ki67 LI. Ki67 IHC was initially reserved for biopsies too small for a meaningful mitotic count (ie, less than 2 mm^2 of tissue, or the equivalent of 10 standard high powered fields [HPFs]); however, in a 2010 survey, nearly half of queried pathologists supported incorporation of Ki67 into routine NEN assessment.[131] Today, both Ki67 and mitotic count are included in the WHO grading parameters for GEP-NENs, and Ki67 IHC is recognized as a valuable adjunct (though not a formal parameter) in the work-up and classification of lung NENs.[8,15,16] Among NETs, mitotic count and Ki67 LI exhibit grade-discordance in approximately a quarter to a third of cases; in such instances, the higher grade (usually associated with the Ki67 LI rather than mitotic count) is assigned, as this appears to more accurately reflect tumor behavior.[16,132,133]

Among NENs, as in other tumor types, there may be substantial variability in proliferative activity within a single neoplasm and, indeed, on a single slide. This heterogeneity raises the possibility of sampling error and, by extension, inaccurate grading.[134–137] As such, multiple approaches to the evaluation of mitoses and Ki67 have been proposed; Yang and colleagues[136] reported in 2011

that evaluating metastatic panNETs via proliferative "hotspots" rather than a whole-slide average generated grades that more accurately correlated with prognosis. At present, the WHO endorses the hotspot approach, with grading typically based on the number of mitoses per 2 mm^2 (approximately 10 HPFs) or percent Ki67 positivity across at least 500 hotspot cells.[15,16]

MITOTIC COUNT

Given the prognostic significance of specific NET grades, an accurate, reproducible count is of paramount importance. To this end, the WHO criteria specify that NEN mitoses be counted per 2 mm^2, which equates to approximately 10 HPFs using most standard contemporary microscopes. This approach sidesteps the potential for inter-microscope variability, a concern when count cutoffs are defined on a per-HPF basis.[8,138–140] Mitotic counts near a grade cutoff should prompt evaluation of at least three hotspots, with grade based on an average count.[15] Of note, mitotic figures may be difficult to distinguish from lymphocytes or from pyknotic or hyperchromatic nuclei; as such, the WHO Blue Books offer guidelines for identification of mitoses, such as the presence of basophilic cytoplasm and hairy chromosomal projections.[15,141,142] In addition, emerging evidence suggests that the mitosis-specific IHC marker phosphohistone H3 may be a valuable adjunct in evaluating NEN mitotic counts.[141,142]

KI67 LABELING INDEX

Optimal assessment of Ki67 within a given hotspot remains an area of active discussion. Approaches include "eyeballing" (gestalt impression of Ki67 LI, without counting individual cells) and manual counting, either at the microscope or using a printed photomicrograph. A study by Reid and colleagues[143] in 2015 identified manual counting of photomicrographs as the most accurate, albeit relatively time-intensive (approximately 8 min per slide), method. Recently, digital image analysis (DIA) has emerged as a promising alternative, though further validation and discussion are necessary.[144–147] Benefits and drawbacks of each approach are outlined in **Box 2**.

It should be emphasized that although Ki67 plays a key role in the WHO's grading criteria for GEP-NENs, this is not the case across anatomic sites.[15,17] In the lung, for instance, Ki67 is not included in the WHO's formal grading parameters; this reflects longstanding concerns about overlapping Ki67 ranges between successive diagnostic categories and potential discordance when diagnoses based on Ki67 versus mitotic count are compared.[15,18,148] However, in light of growing evidence that Ki67 LI in lung NENs correlates significantly with prognosis, the use of Ki67 as an alternative to mitotic count is now under discussion.[18,148–151] In addition, there is evidence to support the use of Ki67 as a complement to mitotic count in technically challenging cases, such as carcinoid tumor biopsies that exhibit considerable crush artifact, which may not only obscure mitoses but also raise the morphologic differential of SCLC.[10,18,152]

SUMMARY

In the years since Siegfried Oberndorfer first described the seemingly indolent, histologically unprepossessing *Karzinoid Tumoren* of the small bowel, NENs have emerged as an ever more nuanced clinicopathologic domain, encompassing a disparate array of morphologies and behaviors. In this article, we have explored several key unifying threads, including the presence of two histologic tiers and their distinct clinicopathologic profiles; the role of ancillary testing in corroborating and clarifying current grading schemes; and the primacy of proliferative activity in NET grading. These themes take on heightened significance in light of ongoing efforts to standardize and harmonize NEN classification across organ systems. Just as importantly, they have brought stability and coherence to the century-old NEN narrative, weathering nomenclature changes, shifting classification parameters, and the rise of ancillary testing–and seem likely to do so for decades to come.

CLINICS CARE POINTS

- Neuroendocrine neoplasms (NENs) can be divided into neuroendocrine tumors (NETs) and neuroendocrine carcinomas (NECs), each with a distinct molecular, immunohistochemical, and clinical profile. NETs are relatively indolent, though prognosis worsens in tandem with increasing grade. In contrast, NECs are high-grade by default and typically carry a dismal prognosis.

- Resection is the cornerstone of NET treatment; approaches to disseminated disease include somatostatin analogues, peptide receptor radionuclide therapy, and biologic therapies (eg, sunitinib and everolimus). Hepatic metastases may be managed via debulking and liver-directed therapy, where appropriate.

- Platinum-based chemotherapy and radiotherapy is the bedrock of small-cell lung carcinoma (SCLC) management, with the addition of immune checkpoint inhibitors in extensive-stage disease; resection is generally considered only in very early stage disease. In contrast, early-stage pulmonary large-cell (LC) NECs appear relatively amenable to resection and adjuvant therapy, whereas more advanced disease is typically treated with platinum-based chemotherapy. Of note, there is a paucity of data regarding treatment of extrapulmonary SC and LC NECs, which have typically been managed similarly to their counterparts in the lung.

- Molecular profiling has enabled a more nuanced characterization of NENs, revealing at least two subtypes of lung LC NECs (SCLC-like and NSCLC-like) as well as at least four subtypes of SCLC. These subtypes appear to be clinically distinct, raising the possibility of more tailored management: for instance, NSCLC-like LC NEC may benefit from an NSCLC-type approach.

- An emerging group of NENs is characterized by relatively well-differentiated histology and high proliferative activity (typically between 20% and 55%). Tumor behavior appears to be intermediate between that of G2 NETs and NECs, with less robust response to platinum-based chemotherapy than NECs. Optimal clinical management for these "G3 NETs" remains under investigation.

CONFLICT OF INTEREST

The authors have no funding or conflicts of interest to declare.

REFERENCES

1. Oberndorfer S. Karzinoide tumoren des dunndarms. Frankf Z Pathol 1907;1:426–32.
2. Modlin IM, Shapiro MD, Kidd M. Siegfried Oberndorfer: origins and perspectives of carcinoid tumors. Hum Pathol 2004;35(12):1440–51.
3. Modlin IM, Champaneria MC, Bornschein J, et al. Evolution of the diffuse neuroendocrine system: clear cells and cloudy origins. Neuroendocrinology 2006;84(2):69–82.
4. Klöppel G. Oberndorfer and his successors: from carcinoid to neuroendocrine carcinoma. Endocr Pathol 2007;18(3):141–4.
5. Asa SL, Lloyd RV, Tischler AS. Neuroendocrine neoplasms: historical background and terminologies. In: Asa SL, La Rosa S, Mete O, editors. The spectrum of neuroendocrine neoplasia: a practical approach to diagnosis, classification and therapy. Cham, Switzerland: Springer International Publishing; 2021. p. 1–14.
6. Gosney J. Identification, morphology, and secretory products of the pulmonary endocrine system. In: Pulmonary endocrine pathology: endocrine cells and endocrine tumours of the lung. Oxford (United Kingdom): Butterworth-Heinemann Ltd; 1992. p. 6–24.
7. Rindi G, Mete O, Uccella S, et al. Overview of the 2022 WHO classification of neuroendocrine neoplasms. Endocr Pathol 2022;33(1):115–54.
8. WHO Classification of Tumours Editorial Board. Endocrine and neuroendocrine tumours. 5th edition. Lyon: IARC Press; 2022.
9. Rindi G, Klimstra DS, Abedi-Ardekani B, et al. A common classification framework for neuroendocrine neoplasms: an International Agency for Research on Cancer (IARC) and World Health Organization (WHO) expert consensus proposal. Mod Pathol 2018;31(12):1770–86.
10. Rekhtman N. Lung neuroendocrine neoplasms: recent progress and persistent challenges. Mod Pathol 2022;35(1):36–50.
11. Basturk O, Yang Z, Tang LH, et al. The high-grade (WHO G3) pancreatic neuroendocrine tumor category is morphologically and biologically heterogenous and includes both well differentiated and poorly differentiated neoplasms. Am J Surg Pathol 2015;39(5):683–90.
12. Tirosh A, Kebebew E. Genetic and epigenetic alterations in pancreatic neuroendocrine tumors. J Gastrointest Oncol 2020;11(3):567–77.
13. Bellizzi AM. Immunohistochemistry in the diagnosis and classification of neuroendocrine neoplasms: what can brown do for you? Hum Pathol 2020;96: 8–33.
14. Duan K, Mete O. Algorithmic approach to neuroendocrine tumors in targeted biopsies: practical applications of immunohistochemical markers. Cancer Cytopathol 2016;124(12):871–84.
15. WHO Classification of Tumours Editorial Board. Thoracic tumours. 5th ed. Lyon: IARC Press; 2022.
16. WHO Classification of Tumours Editorial Board. Digestive system tumours. 5th ed. Lyon: IARC Press; 2019.
17. WHO Classification of Tumours Editorial Board. Head and neck tumours. 5th ed. Lyon: IARC Press; 2022.
18. Pelosi G, Rindi G, Travis WD, et al. Ki-67 antigen in lung neuroendocrine tumors: unraveling a role in clinical practice. J Thorac Oncol 2014;9(3):273–84.
19. Dasari A, Shen C, Halperin D, et al. Trends in the incidence, prevalence, and survival outcomes in patients with neuroendocrine tumors in the United States. JAMA Oncol 2017;3(10):1335–42.
20. Nagtegaal ID, Odze RD, Klimstra D, et al. The 2019 WHO classification of tumours of the digestive system. Histopathology 2020;76(2):182–8.
21. Assarzadegan N, Montgomery E. What is new in the 2019 World Health Organization (WHO) Classification of Tumors of the Digestive System: review of selected updates on neuroendocrine neoplasms, appendiceal tumors, and molecular testing. Arch Pathol Lab Med 2020;145(6):664–77.
22. Mete O, Wenig BM. Update from the 5th edition of the World Health Organization Classification of Head and Neck Tumors: overview of the 2022 WHO Classification of Head and Neck Neuroendocrine Neoplasms. Head Neck Pathol 2022;16(1): 123–42.
23. Xue Y, Reid MD, Pehlivanoglu B, et al. Morphologic variants of pancreatic neuroendocrine tumors: clinicopathologic analysis and prognostic stratification. Endocr Pathol 2020;31(3):239–53.
24. Kim H, An S, Lee K, et al. Pancreatic high-grade neuroendocrine neoplasms in the Korean population: a multicenter study. Cancer Res Treat 2020; 52(1):263–76.
25. Soga J, Tazawa K. Pathologic analysis of carcinoids: histologic re-evaluation of 62 cases. Cancer 1971;28(4):990–8.
26. WHO Classification of Tumours Editorial Board. WHO classification of tumours of the digestive system. 4th ed. Lyon: IARC Press; 2010.
27. Capella C, Heitz PU, Höfler H, et al. Revised classification of neuroendocrine tumours of the lung, pancreas and gut. Virchows Archiv A Pathol Anat 1995;425(6).
28. Hochwald S, Sui Z, Conlon K, et al. Prognostic factors in pancreatic endocrine neoplasms: an analysis of 136 cases with a proposal for low-grade

and intermediate-grade groups. J Clin Oncol 2002; 20(11):2633–42.

29. Sorbye H, Welin S, Langer SW, et al. Predictive and prognostic factors for treatment and survival in 305 patients with advanced gastrointestinal neuroendocrine carcinoma (WHO G3): the NORDIC NEC study. Ann Oncol 2013;24(1):152–60.

30. Sorbye H, Strosberg J, Baudin E, et al. Gastroenteropancreatic high-grade neuroendocrine carcinoma. Cancer 2014;120(18):2814–23.

31. Hijioka S, Hosoda W, Matsuo K, et al. RB loss and KRAS mutation are predictors of the response to platinum-based chemotherapy in pancreatic neuroendocrine neoplasm with grade 3: a Japanese multicenter pancreatic NEN-G3 study. Clin Cancer Res 2017;23(16):4625–32.

32. Tang LH, Basturk O, Sue JJ, et al. A practical approach to the classification of WHO grade 3 (G3) well-differentiated neuroendocrine tumor (WD-NET) and poorly differentiated neuroendocrine carcinoma (PD-NEC) of the pancreas. Am J Surg Pathol 2016;40(9):1192–202.

33. Tang LH, Untch BR, Reidy DL, et al. Well-differentiated neuroendocrine tumors with a morphologically apparent high-grade component: a pathway distinct from poorly differentiated neuroendocrine carcinomas. Clin Cancer Res 2016;22(4):1011–7.

34. Venizelos A, Elvebakken H, Perren A, et al. The molecular characteristics of high-grade gastroenteropancreatic neuroendocrine neoplasms. Endocr Relat Cancer 2021;29(1):1–14.

35. Heetfeld M, Chougnet CN, Olsen IH, et al. Characteristics and treatment of patients with G3 gastroenteropancreatic neuroendocrine neoplasms. Endocr Rel Cancer 2015;22(4):657–64.

36. Shi H, Chen L, Zhang Q, et al. Concordance between the Ki-67 index cutoff value of 55% and differentiation in neuroendocrine tumor and neuroendocrine carcinoma in grade 3 pancreatic neuroendocrine neoplasms. Pancreas 2020; 49(10):1378–82.

37. Vélayoudom-Céphise FL, Duvillard P, Foucan L, et al. Are G3 ENETS neuroendocrine neoplasms heterogeneous? Endocr Relat Cancer 2013;20(5):649–57.

38. Jann H, Kayser A, Wiedenmann B, et al. Treatment outcomes of patients with G3 neuroendocrine neoplasms [abstract only]. J Clin Oncol 2020; 38(4_suppl):622.

39. Raj N, Valentino E, Capanu M, et al. Treatment response and outcomes of grade 3 pancreatic neuroendocrine neoplasms based on morphology: well differentiated versus poorly differentiated. Pancreas 2017;46(3):296–301.

40. La Rosa S, Sessa F. High-grade poorly differentiated neuroendocrine carcinomas of the gastroenteropancreatic system: from morphology to proliferation and back. Endocr Pathol 2014;25(2):193–8.

41. Lithgow K, Venkataraman H, Hughes S, et al. Well-differentiated gastroenteropancreatic G3 NET: findings from a large single centre cohort. Sci Rep 2021;11(1):17947.

42. Konukiewitz B, Jesinghaus M, Steiger K, et al. Pancreatic neuroendocrine carcinomas reveal a closer relationship to ductal adenocarcinomas than to neuroendocrine tumors G3. Hum Pathol 2018;77:70–9.

43. WHO Classification of Tumours Editorial Board. WHO classification of tumours of endocrine organs. 4th ed. Lyon: IARC Press; 2017.

44. Rindi G, Klersy C, Albarello L, et al. Competitive testing of the WHO 2010 versus the WHO 2017 grading of pancreatic neuroendocrine neoplasms: data from a large international cohort study. Neuroendocrinology 2018;107(4):375–86.

45. Vivero M, Sholl L. Borderline" neuroendocrine carcinomas of the lung are clinically and genomically distinct from large-cell neuroendocrine carcinoma [abstract only]. Mod Pathol 2016;29:467–88.

46. Megyesi M, Berta M, Khoor A. Endobronchial large-cell neuroendocrine carcinoma. Pathol Oncol Res 2003;9(3):198–200.

47. Rekhtman N, Pietanza MC, Hellmann MD, et al. Next-generation sequencing of pulmonary large-cell neuroendocrine carcinoma reveals small-cell carcinoma-like and non-small-cell carcinoma-like subsets. Clin Cancer Res 2016;22(14):3618–29.

48. Inafuku K, Yokose T, Ito H, et al. Two cases of lung neuroendocrine carcinoma with carcinoid morphology. Diagn Pathol 2019;14(1):104.

49. Hermans BCM, Derks JL, Moonen L, et al. Pulmonary neuroendocrine neoplasms with well differentiated morphology and high proliferative activity: illustrated by a case series and review of the literature. Lung Cancer 2020;150:152–8.

50. Zhang Y, Wang W, Hu Q, et al. Clinic and genetic similarity assessments of atypical carcinoid, neuroendocrine neoplasm with atypical carcinoid morphology and elevated mitotic count and large-cell neuroendocrine carcinoma. BMC Cancer 2022;22(1):321.

51. Sazonova O, Manem V, Orain M, et al. Transcriptomic data helps refining classification of pulmonary carcinoid tumors with increased mitotic counts. Mod Pathol 2020;33(9):1712–21.

52. Quinn AM, Chaturvedi A, Nonaka D. High-grade neuroendocrine carcinoma of the lung with carcinoid morphology: a study of 12 cases. Am J Surg Pathol 2017;41(2):263–70.

53. Nicholson SA, Beasley MB, Brambilla E, et al. Small-cell lung carcinoma (SCLC): a clinicopathologic study of 100 cases with surgical specimens. Am J Surg Pathol 2002;26(9):1184–97.

54. Travis WD. Advances in neuroendocrine lung tumors. Ann Oncol 2010;21:vii65–71.

55. Travis WD. Update on small-cell carcinoma and its differentiation from squamous cell carcinoma and other non-small-cell carcinomas. Mod Pathol 2012;25(1):S18–30.

56. Fahmy JN, Varsanik MA, Hubbs D, et al. Pancreatic neuroendocrine tumors: surgical outcomes and survival analysis. Am J Surg 2021;221(3):529–33.

57. Okereke IC, Taber AM, Griffith RC, et al. Outcomes after surgical resection of pulmonary carcinoid tumors. J Cardiothorac Surg 2016;11:35.

58. Hu Y, Ye Z, Wang F, et al. Role of somatostatin receptor in pancreatic neuroendocrine tumor development, diagnosis, and therapy. Front Endocrinol (Lausanne) 2021;12:679000.

59. Pavel M, Öberg K, Falconi M, et al. Gastroenteropancreatic neuroendocrine neoplasms: ESMO Clinical Practice Guidelines for diagnosis, treatment and follow-up. Ann Oncol 2020;31(7):844–60.

60. Starr JS, Sonbol MB, Hobday TJ, et al. Peptide receptor radionuclide therapy for the treatment of pancreatic neuroendocrine tumors: recent insights. Onco Targets Ther 2020;13:3545–55.

61. Baudin E, Caplin M, Garcia-Carbonero R, et al. Lung and thymic carcinoids: ESMO Clinical Practice Guidelines for diagnosis, treatment and follow-up. Ann Oncol 2021;32(4):439–51.

62. Popa O, Taban SM, Pantea S, et al. The new WHO classification of gastrointestinal neuroendocrine tumors and immunohistochemical expression of somatostatin receptor 2 and 5. Exp Ther Med 2021; 22(4):1–9.

63. Cakir M, Dworakowska D, Grossman A. Somatostatin receptor biology in neuroendocrine and pituitary tumours: part 2—clinical implications. J Cell Mol Med 2010;14(11):2585–91.

64. Rinke A, Müller HH, Schade-Brittinger C, et al. Placebo-controlled, double-blind, prospective, randomized study on the effect of octreotide LAR in the control of tumor growth in patients with metastatic neuroendocrine midgut tumors: a report from the PROMID Study Group. J Clin Oncol 2009;27(28):4656–63.

65. Caplin ME, Pavel M, Ćwikła JB, et al. Lanreotide in metastatic enteropancreatic neuroendocrine tumors. N Engl J Med 2014;371(3):224–33.

66. Gupta S. Intra-arterial liver-directed therapies for neuroendocrine hepatic metastases. Semin Intervent Radiol 2013;30(1):28–38.

67. Baere T de, Deschamps F, Tselikas L, et al. GEP-NETs update: Interventional radiology: role in the treatment of liver metastases from GEP-NETs. Eur J Endocrinol 2015;172(4):R151–66.

68. Camus B, Cottereau AS, Palmieri LJ, et al. Indications of peptide receptor radionuclide therapy (PRRT) in gastroenteropancreatic and pulmonary neuroendocrine tumors: an updated review. J Clin Med 2021;10(6):1267.

69. Wong MH, Chan DL, Lee A, et al. Systematic review and meta-analysis on the role of chemotherapy in advanced and metastatic neuroendocrine tumor (NET). PLoS ONE 2016;11(6):e0158140.

70. Liu IH, Kunz PL. Biologics in gastrointestinal and pancreatic neuroendocrine tumors. J Gastrointest Oncol 2017;8(3):457–65.

71. Yao JC, Shah MH, Ito T, et al. Everolimus for advanced pancreatic neuroendocrine tumors. N Engl J Med 2011;364(10).

72. Faivre S, Niccoli P, Castellano D, et al. Sunitinib in pancreatic neuroendocrine tumors: updated progression-free survival and final overall survival from a phase III randomized study. Ann Oncol 2017;28(2):339–43.

73. AKP Ganti, Loo BW, Bassetti M, et al. Small-cell lung cancer, version 2.2022, NCCN Clinical Practice Guidelines in Oncology. J Natl Compr Canc Netw 2021;19(12):1441–64.

74. Saltos A, Shafique M, Chiappori A. Update on the biology, management, and treatment of small-cell lung cancer (SCLC). Front Oncol 2020;10:1074.

75. Stelwagen J, de Vries EGE, Walenkamp AME. Current treatment strategies and future directions for extrapulmonary neuroendocrine carcinomas: a review. JAMA Oncol 2021;7(5):759–70.

76. Walenkamp AME, Sonke GS, Sleijfer DT. Clinical and therapeutic aspects of extrapulmonary small-cell carcinoma. Cancer Treat Rev 2009;35(3): 228–36.

77. Barnes H, See K, Barnett S, et al. Surgery for limited-stage small-cell lung cancer. Cochrane Database Syst Rev 2017;2017(4):CD011917.

78. Ferrara MG, Stefani A, Simbolo M, et al. Large-cell neuro-endocrine carcinoma of the lung: current treatment options and potential future opportunities. Front Oncol 2021;11:650293.

79. Corbett V, Arnold S, Anthony L, et al. Management of large-cell neuroendocrine carcinoma. Front Oncol 2021;11:653162.

80. Sakurai H, Asamura H. Large-cell neuroendocrine carcinoma of the lung: surgical management. Thorac Surg Clin 2014;24(3):305–11.

81. Raman V, Jawitz OK, Yang CFJ, et al. Outcomes for surgery in large-cell lung neuroendocrine cancer. J Thorac Oncol 2019;14(12):2143–51.

82. Atieh T, Huang CH. Treatment of advanced-stage large-cell neuroendocrine cancer (LCNEC) of the lung: a tale of two diseases. Front Oncol 2021;11.

83. Derks JL, Leblay N, Thunnissen E, et al. Molecular subtypes of pulmonary large-cell neuroendocrine carcinoma predict chemotherapy treatment outcome. Clin Cancer Res 2018;24(1):33–42.

84. George J, Walter V, Peifer M, et al. Integrative genomic profiling of large-cell neuroendocrine

carcinomas reveals distinct subtypes of high-grade neuroendocrine lung tumors. Nat Commun 2018; 9(1):1048.

85. Miyoshi T, Umemura S, Matsumura Y, et al. Genomic profiling of large-cell neuroendocrine carcinoma of the lung. Clin Cancer Res 2017;23(3):757–65.

86. Baine MK, Rekhtman N. Multiple faces of pulmonary large-cell neuroendocrine carcinoma: update with a focus on practical approach to diagnosis. Transl Lung Cancer Res 2020;9(3).

87. Saghaeiannejad Esfahani H, Vela CM, Chauhan A. Prevalence of TP-53/RB-1 co-mutation in large-cell neuroendocrine carcinoma. Front Oncol 2021;11: 653153.

88. Zhuo M, Guan Y, Yang X, et al. The prognostic and therapeutic role of genomic subtyping by sequencing tumor or cell-free DNA in pulmonary large-cell neuroendocrine carcinoma. Clin Cancer Res 2020;26(4):892–901.

89. Yachida S, Vakiani E, White CM, et al. Small-cell and large-cell neuroendocrine carcinomas of the pancreas are genetically similar and distinct from well-differentiated pancreatic neuroendocrine tumors. Am J Surg Pathol 2012;36(2):173–84.

90. van Riet J, van de Werken HJG, Cuppen E, et al. The genomic landscape of 85 advanced neuroendocrine neoplasms reveals subtype-heterogeneity and potential therapeutic targets. Nat Commun 2021;12(1):4612.

91. Simbolo M, Mafficini A, Sikora K, et al. Lung neuroendocrine tumours: deep sequencing of the four World Health Organization histotypes reveals chromatin-remodelling genes as major players and a prognostic role for TERT, RB1, MEN1 and KMT2D. J Pathol 2017;241(4):488–500.

92. Clinical Lung Cancer Genome Project (CLCGP), Network Genomic Medicine (NGM). A genomics-based classification of human lung tumors. Sci Transl Med 2013;5(209):209ra153.

93. Walch AK, Zitzelsberger HF, Aubele MM, et al. Typical and atypical carcinoid tumors of the lung are characterized by 11q deletions as detected by comparative genomic hybridization. Am J Pathol 1998;153(4):1089–98.

94. Capurso G, Festa S, Valente R, et al. Molecular pathology and genetics of pancreatic endocrine tumours. J Mol Endocrinol 2012;49(1):R37–50.

95. Floridia G, Grilli G, Salvatore M, et al. Chromosomal alterations detected by comparative genomic hybridization in nonfunctioning endocrine pancreatic tumors. Cancer Genet Cytogenet 2005;156(1): 23–30.

96. Scarpa A, Chang DK, Nones K, et al. Whole-genome landscape of pancreatic neuroendocrine tumours. Nature 2017;543(7643):65–71.

97. Jiao Y, Shi C, Edil BH, et al. DAXX/ATRX, MEN1, and mTOR pathway genes are frequently altered in pancreatic neuroendocrine tumors. Science 2011;331(6021):1199–203.

98. Corbo V, Dalai I, Scardoni M, et al. MEN1 in pancreatic endocrine tumors: analysis of gene and protein status in 169 sporadic neoplasms reveals alterations in the vast majority of cases. Endocr Relat Cancer 2010;17(3):771–83.

99. Raj NP, Soumerai T, Valentino E, et al. Next-generation sequencing (NGS) in advanced well differentiated pancreatic neuroendocrine tumors (WD pNETs): a study using MSK-IMPACT. J Clin Oncol 2016;34(15_suppl):e15661.

100. Heaphy CM, de Wilde RF, Jiao Y, et al. Altered telomeres in tumors with ATRX and DAXX mutations. Science 2011;333(6041):425.

101. Marinoni I, Kurrer AS, Vassella E, et al. Loss of DAXX and ATRX are associated with chromosome instability and reduced survival of patients with pancreatic neuroendocrine tumors. Gastroenterology 2014;146(2):453–60.e5.

102. Kim JY, Brosnan-Cashman JA, An S, et al. Alternative lengthening of telomeres in primary pancreatic neuroendocrine tumors is associated with aggressive clinical behavior and poor survival. Clin Cancer Res 2017;23(6):1598–606.

103. Singhi AD, Liu TC, Roncaioli JL, et al. Alternative lengthening of telomeres and loss of DAXX/ATRX expression predicts metastatic disease and poor survival in patients with pancreatic neuroendocrine tumors. Clin Cancer Res 2017;23(2):600–9.

104. Park JK, Paik WH, Lee K, et al. DAXX/ATRX and MEN1 genes are strong prognostic markers in pancreatic neuroendocrine tumors. Oncotarget 2017;8(30):49796–806.

105. Chan CS, Laddha SV, Lewis PW, et al. ATRX, DAXX or MEN1 mutant pancreatic neuroendocrine tumors are a distinct alpha-cell signature subgroup. Nat Commun 2018;9(1):4158.

106. Heaphy CM, VandenBussche CJ. Prognostic biomarkers in pancreatic neuroendocrine tumors. Cancer Cytopathol 2021;129(11):841–3.

107. Derks JL, Leblay N, Lantuejoul S, et al. New insights into the molecular characteristics of pulmonary carcinoids and large-cell neuroendocrine carcinomas, and the impact on their clinical management. J Thorac Oncol 2018;13(6):752–66.

108. Simbolo M, Di Noia V, D'Argento E, et al. Exploring the molecular and biological background of lung neuroendocrine tumours. J Thorac Dis 2019; 11(Suppl 9):S1194–8.

109. Fernandez-Cuesta L, Peifer M, Lu X, et al. Frequent mutations in chromatin-remodelling genes in pulmonary carcinoids. Nat Commun 2014;27(5):3518.

110. Debelenko LV, Brambilla E, Agarwal SK, et al. Identification of MEN1 gene mutations in sporadic carcinoid tumors of the lung. Hum Mol Genet 1997;6(13):2285–90.

111. Swarts DRA, Scarpa A, Corbo V, et al. MEN1 gene mutation and reduced expression are associated with poor prognosis in pulmonary carcinoids. J Clin Endocrinol Metab 2014;99(2):E374–8.

112. Rossi G, Bertero L, Marchiò C, et al. Molecular alterations of neuroendocrine tumours of the lung. Histopathology 2018;72(1):142–52.

113. George J, Lim J, Lang S, et al. Comprehensive genomic profiles of small-cell lung cancer. Nature 2015;524(7563):47–53.

114. Peifer M, Fernández-Cuesta L, Sos ML, et al. Integrative genome analyses identify key somatic driver mutations of small-cell lung cancer. Nat Genet 2012;44(10):1104–10.

115. Baine MK, Hsieh MS, Lai WV, et al. Small-cell lung carcinoma subtypes defined by ASCL1, NEUROD1, POU2F3, and YAP1: comprehensive immunohistochemical and histopathologic characterization. J Thorac Oncol 2020;15(12):1823–35.

116. Rudin CM, Poirier JT, Byers LA, et al. Molecular subtypes of small-cell lung cancer: a synthesis of human and mouse model data. Nat Rev Cancer 2019;19(5):289–97.

117. Borromeo MD, Savage TK, Kollipara RK, et al. ASCL1 and NEUROD1 reveal heterogeneity in pulmonary neuroendocrine tumors and regulate distinct genetic programs. Cell Rep 2016;16(5):1259–72.

118. Qi J, Zhang J, Liu N, et al. Prognostic implications of molecular subtypes in primary small-cell lung cancer and their correlation with cancer immunity. Front Oncol 2022;12:779276.

119. Bellizzi AM. An algorithmic immunohistochemical approach to define tumor type and assign site of origin. Adv Anat Pathol 2020;27(3):114–63.

120. Rooper L, Sharma R, LI Q, et al. INSM1 demonstrates superior performance to the individual and combined use of synaptophysin, chromogranin and CD56 for diagnosing neuroendocrine tumors of the thoracic cavity. Am J Surg Pathol 2017; 41(11):1561–9.

121. Rosenbaum JN, Guo Z, Baus RM, et al. INSM1: a novel immunohistochemical and molecular marker for neuroendocrine and neuroepithelial neoplasms. Am J Clin Pathol 2015;144(4):579–91.

122. Juhlin CC, Zedenius J, Höög A. Clinical routine application of the second-generation neuroendocrine markers ISL2, INSM1, and secretagogin in neuroendocrine neoplasia: staining outcomes and potential clues for determining tumor origin. Endocr Pathol 2020;31(4):401–10.

123. Bellizzi A. Assigning site of origin in metastatic neuroendocrine neoplasms: a clinically significant application of diagnostic immunohistochemistry. Adv Anat Pathol 2013;20(5):285–314.

124. Bergsland EK, Nakakura EK. Neuroendocrine tumors of unknown primary: is the primary site really not known? JAMA Surg 2014;149(9):889–90.

125. Catena L, Bichisao E, Milione M, et al. Neuroendocrine tumors of unknown primary site: gold dust or misdiagnosed neoplasms? Tumori 2011;97(5): 564–7.

126. Scoazec JY, Couvelard A, Monges G, et al. Professional practices and diagnostic issues in neuroendocrine tumour pathology: results of a prospective one-year survey among French pathologists (the PRONET study). Neuroendocrinology 2017;105(1): 67–76.

127. Chan ES, Alexander J, Swanson PE, et al. PDX-1, CDX-2, TTF-1, and CK7: a reliable immunohistochemical panel for pancreatic neuroendocrine neoplasms. Am J Surg Pathol 2012;36(5):737–43.

128. Erickson LA, Papouchado B, Dimashkieh H, et al. CDX2 as a marker for neuroendocrine tumors of unknown primary sites. Endocr Pathol 2004;15(3): 247–52.

129. Agaimy A, Erlenbach-Wünsch K, Konukiewitz B, et al. ISL1 expression is not restricted to pancreatic well-differentiated neuroendocrine neoplasms, but is also commonly found in well and poorly differentiated neuroendocrine neoplasms of extrapancreatic origin. Mod Pathol 2013;26(7):995–1003.

130. Czeczok TW, Stashek KM, Maxwell JE, et al. Clusterin in neuroendocrine epithelial neoplasms: absence of expression in a well-differentiated tumor suggests a jejunoileal origin. Appl Immunohistochem Mol Morphol 2018;26(2):94–100.

131. Klimstra DS, Modlin IR, Adsay NV, et al. Pathology reporting of neuroendocrine tumors: application of the Delphic consensus process to the development of a minimum pathology data set. Am J Surg Pathol 2010;34(3):300–13.

132. McCall CM, Shi C, Cornish TC, et al. Grading of well-differentiated pancreatic neuroendocrine tumors is improved by the inclusion of both Ki67 proliferative index and mitotic rate. Am J Surg Pathol 2013;37(11):1671–7.

133. van Velthuysen MLF, Groen EJ, van der Noort V, et al. Grading of neuroendocrine neoplasms: mitoses and Ki-67 are both essential. Neuroendocrinology 2014;100(2–3):221–7.

134. Jannink I, Risberg B, van Diest P, et al. Heterogeneity of mitotic activity in breast cancer. Histopathology 1996;29(5):421–8.

135. Verhoeven D, Bourgeois N, Derde M, et al. Comparison of cell growth in different parts of breast cancers. Histopathology 1990;17(6):505–9.

136. Yang Z, Tang LH, Klimstra DS. Effect of tumor heterogeneity on the assessment of Ki67 labeling index in well-differentiated neuroendocrine tumors metastatic to the liver: implications for prognostic stratification. Am J Surg Pathol 2011;35(6):853–60.

137. Couvelard A, Deschamps L, Ravaud P, et al. Heterogeneity of tumor prognostic markers: a reproducibility study applied to liver metastases of

pancreatic endocrine tumors. Mod Pathol 2009; 22(2):273–81.

138. Cree IA, Tan PH, Travis WD, et al. Counting mitoses: SI(ze) matters. Mod Pathol 2021;34(9):1651–7.

139. Yigit N, Gunal A, Kucukodaci Z, et al. Are we counting mitoses correctly? Ann Diagn Pathol 2013; 17(6):536–9.

140. Facchetti F. A proposal for the adoption of a uniform metrical system for mitosis counting. Int J Surg Pathol 2005;13(2):157–9.

141. Tracht J, Zhang K, Peker D. Grading and prognostication of neuroendocrine tumors of the pancreas: a comparison study of Ki67 and PHH3. J Histochem Cytochem 2017;65(7):399–405.

142. Kim MJ, Kwon MJ, Kang HS, et al. Identification of phosphohistone H3 cutoff values corresponding to original WHO grades but distinguishable in well-differentiated gastrointestinal neuroendocrine tumors. Biomed Res Int 2018;2018:e1013640.

143. Reid MD, Bagci P, Ohike N, et al. Calculation of the Ki67 index in pancreatic neuroendocrine tumors: a comparative analysis of four counting methodologies. Mod Pathol 2015;28(5):686–94.

144. Tang L, Mithat G, Hedvat C, et al. Objective quantification of the Ki67 proliferative index in neuroendocrine tumors of the gastroenteropancreatic system: a comparison of digital image analysis with manual methods. Am J Surg Pathol 2012; 36(12):1761–70.

145. Lea D, Gudlaugsson EG, Skaland I, et al. Digital image analysis of the proliferation markers Ki67 and phosphohistone H3 in gastroenteropancreatic neuroendocrine neoplasms: accuracy of grading compared with routine manual hot spot evaluation of the Ki67 index. Appl Immunohistochem Mol Morphol 2021;29(7):499–505.

146. Hacking SM, Sajjan S, Lee L, et al. Potential pitfalls in diagnostic digital image analysis: experience with Ki-67 and PHH3 in gastrointestinal neuroendocrine tumors. Pathol Res Pract 2020;216(3): 152753.

147. Volynskaya Z, Mete O, Pakbaz S, et al. Ki67 quantitative interpretation: insights using image analysis. J Pathol Inform 2019;10:8.

148. Walts AE, Ines D, Marchevsky AM. Limited role of Ki-67 proliferative index in predicting overall short-term survival in patients with typical and atypical pulmonary carcinoid tumors. Mod Pathol 2012; 25(9):1258–64.

149. Zahel T, Krysa S, Herpel E, et al. Phenotyping of pulmonary carcinoids and a Ki-67-based grading approach. Virchows Arch 2012;460(3):299–308.

150. Grimaldi F, Muser D, Beltrami CA, et al. Partitioning of bronchopulmonary carcinoids in two different prognostic categories by Ki-67 score. Front Endocrinol (Lausanne) 2011;2:20.

151. Skov B, Holm B, Erreboe A, et al. ERCC1 and Ki67 in small-cell lung carcinoma and other neuroendocrine tumors of the lung: distribution and impact on survival. J Thorac Oncol 2010; 5(4):453–9.

152. Aslan D, Gulbahce H, Pambuccian S, et al. Ki-67 immunoreactivity in the differential diagnosis of pulmonary neuroendocrine neoplasms in specimens with extensive crush artifact. Am J Clin Pathol 2005;123(6):874–8.

Light It Up! The Use of DOTATATE in Diagnosis and Treatment of Neuroendocrine Neoplasms

Jason L. Schwarz, MD[a], Jelani K. Williams, MD[a],
Xavier M. Keutgen, MD[b], Chih-Yi Liao, MD[c],*

KEYWORDS

- DOTATATE • Neuroendocrine tumors • Peptide receptor radionuclide therapy (PRRT)
- Radiolabeled somatostatin analogs

Key points

- Somatostatin receptor imaging with ^{68}Ga-DOTATATE PET/CT yields greater sensitivity for neuroendocrine lesion detection compared with other imaging modalities and is recommended for diagnostic workup in several scenarios for patients with known or suspected neuroendocrine tumors.

- Across a range of studies, peptide receptor radionuclide therapy with ^{177}Lu-DOTATATE has demonstrated improvements in survival and quality of life for patients with neuroendocrine tumors.

- Peptide receptor radionuclide therapy only leads to objective response rates of up to 50% at best; thus, research is ongoing to discover methods to improve the efficacy of this treatment.

ABSTRACT

Radiolabeled somatostatin analogs are increasingly used in the diagnosis and treatment of neuroendocrine tumors. Diagnostic imaging with 68Ga-DOTATATE PET/CT has demonstrated the improved sensitivity in detecting primary and metastatic neuroendocrine lesions compared with conventional imaging and prior generation somatostatin receptor imaging. Peptide receptor radionuclide therapy with 177Lu-DOTATATE is now frequently included in the management of neuroendocrine neoplasms, with prospective randomized control studies demonstrating its beneficial impact on survival and quality of life. Nonetheless, peptide rector radionuclide therapy is still considered palliative rather than curative and may be accompanied by adverse effects.

OVERVIEW

Over the last few decades, the incidence of neuroendocrine tumors (NETs) has increased dramatically from just over 1 per 100,000 people in the 1970s to nearly 7 per 100,000 in 2012.[1] This increase can partially be attributed to the invention of radiolabeled somatostatin analogs (RSAs) in the late 1980s that have enhanced diagnostic capabilities for NETs.[2,3] RSAs work by binding somatostatin receptors (SSTRs), of which there are five subtypes (SSTR1-5), located on cell membranes in both healthy tissue and tumors. Although

---

[a] Division of General Surgery and Surgical Oncology, Department of Surgery, University of Chicago, University of Chicago Medicine, 5841 S. Maryland Avenue, MC 6040, Chicago, IL 60637, USA; [b] Division of General Surgery and Surgical Oncology, Department of Surgery, University of Chicago, University of Chicago Medicine, 5841 S. Maryland Avenue, MC 4052, Chicago, IL 60637, USA; [c] Department of Medicine, Section of Hematology/Oncology, University of Chicago, University of Chicago Medicine, 5841 S. Maryland Avenue, MC2115, Chicago, IL 60637, USA
* Corresponding author.
E-mail address: andyliao@medicine.bsd.uchicago.edu

Surgical Pathology 16 (2023) 151–161
https://doi.org/10.1016/j.path.2022.09.013
1875-9181/23/© 2023 Elsevier Inc. All rights reserved.

surgpath.theclinics.com

up to 80% of gastroenteropancreatic (GEP) NETs express SSTRs, SSTR2 is the subtype found most frequently.[4] With greater detection of these tumors, population studies have approximated that 25% of patients present with metastases, whereas up to 60% are diagnosed with metastatic disease during the course of their surveillance.[5,6] Therefore, systemic therapy is an essential component of the treatment of NETs, with peptide receptor radionuclide therapy (PRRT)—which uses RSAs—now considered to be one of the most effective options. This review provides an overview of the role of RSAs in diagnosis and management of NETs.

WHAT IS DOTATATE?

RSAs are compounds composed of three different agents: a somatostatin analog (SSA), a chelating agent, and a radiometal (**Fig. 1**).

The SSA, or "targeting moiety," allows for the specific binding of the compound to cells that express SSTRs. Octreotide is the foundational analog, and its peptide sequence can be altered to create slightly different compounds with varied affinities for the different SSTRs. These analogs are identified by different names and, by convention, are listed last in the overall compound (see **Fig. 1**). For example, octreotide's third amino acid, phenylalanine (Phe), is often converted to a tyrosine (Tyr) to yield $[Tyr^3]$-octreotide, also identified as "TOC." Meanwhile, if octreotide's terminal amino alcohol, threoninol (Thr[ol]), is altered to threonine (Thr), this creates octreotate.[7,8] When these two changes to octreotide are joined to form $[Tyr^3]$-octreotate, the resulting SSA is known as "TATE," which is the agent used in many of the approved imaging and therapeutic compounds. TATE is more specific for SSTR2 and is retained for a longer period within tumors compared with other analogs like TOC.[7]

The chelating agent, of which DOTA (1,4,7-tet-raazacyclododecane-1,4,7,10-tetraacetic acid) is the gold standard, allows for stable binding of the radiometal as well as conjugation of the radiometal to the targeting SSA.[7]

Finally, the radioactive metal determines the functionality of the compound. The choice of radiometal is heavily influenced by the type of emission released on decay as well as the half-life of the agent. Radiometals used in imaging undergo gamma or beta$^+$ (positron) decay, whereas those used in therapy undergo beta$^-$ decay and some possible gamma decay. Radiometals used in imaging emit very penetrating but little ionizing radiation. Contrastingly, those used for PRRT release radiation that is less penetrating but more energetic and ionizing, damaging the DNA within the cells. Common radiometals used today include gallium-68 (^{68}Ga), copper-64 (^{64}Cu), and indium-111 (^{111}In) for imaging; lutetium-177 (^{177}Lu) and yttrium–90 (^{90}Y) are used in PRRT.[7]

DIAGNOSTIC IMAGING WITH RADIOLABELED SOMATOSTATIN ANALOGS

DOTATATE VERSUS OCTREOSCAN

Until recently, [^{111}In-diethylenetriaminepentaace-tic acid-d-phenylalanine (DTPA)^0]-octreotide ([^{111}In]-pentetreotide) single-photon emission computed tomography (SPECT), known commercially as Octreoscan, was the gold standard of somatostatin receptor imaging (SRI).[7] However, compared with newer advancements, drawbacks of Octreoscan include low image quality, high radiation doses, and a lengthy imaging protocol.[9,10] ^{68}Ga-DOTATATE (GaTate) PET/CT scan, which was first used in Europe in 2005 and approved by the US Food and Drug Administration (FDA) in 2017, uses gallium as its radiometal and has become the new benchmark for SRI.[9]

Although the 2.8 day half-life of ^{111}In-DTPA-octreotide requires SPECT imaging be performed 24 hours following compound injection, GaTate, with a 68 minute half-life, minimizes radiation

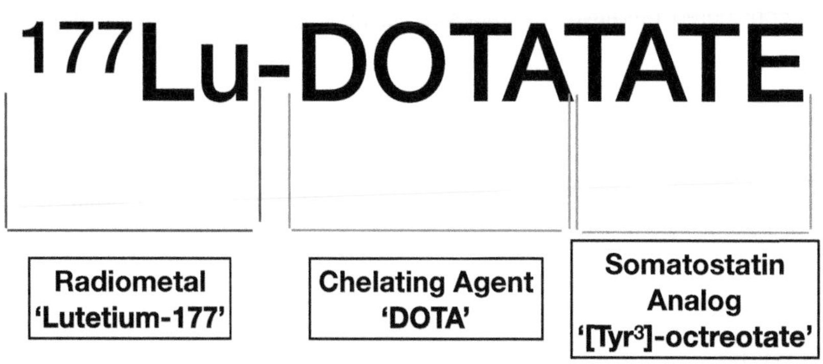

^{177}Lu-DOTATATE

| Radiometal 'Lutetium-177' | Chelating Agent 'DOTA' | Somatostatin Analog '[Tyr³]-octreotate' |

Fig. 1. Components of a radiolabeled somatostatin analog nomenclature.

exposure and can be imaged shortly following injection.[7] More importantly, many studies have demonstrated a greater sensitivity in tumor detection with GaTate. In a retrospective review by Hofman and colleagues,[11] 33 of 40 patients (83%) who underwent GaTate imaging after Octreoscan had additional lesions detected. A larger review by Deppen and colleagues[12] also found that the sensitivity of GaTate PET/CT was higher (97%) compared with those undergoing Octreoscan (83%), whereas specificity was equivalent. Meanwhile, Sadowski and colleagues[13] performed one of the largest prospective reviews comparing the two modalities in which 131 patients underwent both GaTate and Octreoscan imaging, as well as standard anatomic CT or MRI, within a 4 week period. Not only was GaTate superior in detecting the greatest proportion of lesions seen throughout all imaging types (95% of total lesions detected on GaTate vs 31% on Octreoscan vs 45% on CT/MRI), but GaTate also identified 4 of 14 primary tumors not seen on Octreoscan and showed a significantly greater proportion of lesions in patients with NET symptoms but no biochemical evidence of disease (65% vs 26% on Octreoscan, $P = .02$). The higher sensitivity with GaTate is likely secondary to both the improved resolution of PET versus SPECT imaging as well as the stronger affinity for SSTR2 in the octreotate of GaTate versus octreotide.[11] Consequently, both the "Appropriate Use Criteria for Somatostatin Receptor PET Imaging in Neuroendocrine Tumors"[14] and the North American Neuroendocrine Tumor Society (NANETS) guidelines regarding surgical management of pancreatic NETs (PanNETs)[15] have recommended that GaTate PET/CT replace ^{111}In-DTPA-octreotide SPECT in all instances.

EFFECTIVENESS AND INDICATIONS

The goals of SRI at the time of NET diagnosis are four-fold: (1) detect resectable tumor that has gone unrecognized with conventional imaging, (2) adjust surgical management in those with metastases, (3) direct therapy options for inoperable tumors, and (4) select patients for PRRT.[10] With mean sensitivities ranging from 88% to 93% in multiple meta-analyses,[16] GaTate can identify NETs throughout the body, whether it be primary, nodal, or metastatic disease (Fig. 2). In a few single-institutional retrospective reviews, the use of GaTate facilitated discovery of an unknown primary tumor location in 23% (3/13)[17] and 60% (3/5)[9] of patients. In the review by Crown and colleagues[17] with 101 patients, 75% had known metastatic disease with conventional imaging or Octreoscan, but GaTate revealed additional

metastatic tumors—spread throughout lymph nodes, the skeletal system, the peritoneum, and the liver—in 48% of those patients. As surgical resection remains a mainstay of management for localized NETs, it is often essential to accurately map the extent of disease to determine resectability. With preoperative GaTate, Babazadeh and colleagues[9] reported a change in surgical management in 24% of patients, whereas Crown and colleagues[17] reported a surgical adjustment in 50% of patients; changes included primary tumor resection after identifying the location on GaTate, additional hepatic resections for metastases, and pursuance of nonoperative management altogether. In another tertiary center review, Tierney and colleagues[18] reported a management change in 66% of patients undergoing GaTate imaging. More specifically, 73% of these patients experienced an "intermodality" adjustment (eg, switching from surgery to systemic therapy or vice versa) and 27% experienced an "intramodality" adjustment (eg, change in surgical plan or change in surveillance strategy). Overall, across studies, change in management has been demonstrated in approximately one-third of patients following RSA PET scans.[14]

Because diagnostic revelations do not always alter management decisions, a consensus is lacking as to when DOTATATE scans should be performed; but many societal guidelines are adopting broader and more frequent use of such imaging.[14] The European Neuroendocrine Tumor Society (ENETS) radiological guidelines recommend that GaTate should always play a role in tumor staging and preoperative planning, especially given its improved performance in detecting nodal, bone, and peritoneal metastases.[16] The 2018 Appropriate Use Criteria suggest that physicians use DOTATATE imaging for initial staging following histologic diagnosis (Appropriateness Score 9/9), to localize unknown primaries (appropriateness score 9/9), and for preoperative planning (appropriateness score 8/9).[14] With many GEP NETs metastasizing to the liver and being treated with liver cytoreductive surgery, preoperative DOTATATE scans can identify extrahepatic metastases that may preclude surgical intervention or identify further intrahepatic tumors that should be targeted intraoperatively.

Even following surgical resection for localized disease, NET recurrence can be expected in some patients, and therefore, DOTATATE imaging plays a role in recurrence surveillance and post-treatment monitoring.[19] Haug and colleagues, a retrospective study analyzing the use of GaTate following primary tumor resection, reported a sensitivity of 90% and a specificity of 82% in

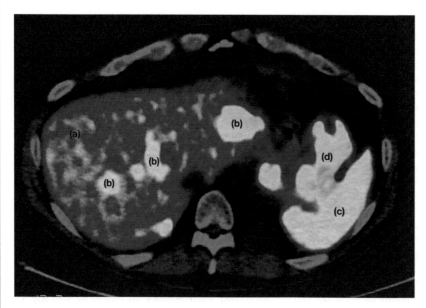

Fig. 2. 68Ga-DOTATATE PET/CT demonstrating (*A*) normal physiologic uptake of the liver, (*B*) neuroendocrine tumor metastatic foci within the liver, (*C*) normal physiologic uptake of the spleen, (*D*) neuroendocrine tumor of the pancreatic tail.

diagnosing recurrent disease.[20] When patients had elevated laboratory values that could hint at recurrence, the specificity of the imaging decreased with more false positives recorded. Expectedly, the specificity improved, albeit at the expense of sensitivity, when reviewers of the scans were blinded to patient clinical data.[20] However, if conventional imaging can readily identify tumors, there is not necessarily a need to perform DOTATATE monitoring on a frequent basis.[14] Importantly, restaging DOTATATE results should be compared with a baseline DOTATATE scan because comparing such results to previous conventional imaging is likely to show increased disease by nature of its greater sensitivity and, thus, may lead to inappropriate management changes.[14] Meanwhile, false-positive reads by DOTATATE reviewers are well-known to occur around the pancreatic uncinate, which can be mistaken for a PanNET, as well as areas of inflammation like fresh postoperative sites.[16,20] Furthermore, SRI may be limited in higher grade NETs (grade 3) because of the decreased SSTR concentration that accompanies greater tumor proliferation. In these tumors with heightened metabolic activity, fluorodeoxyglucose (FDG) PET has shown to be complimentary to GaTate and may be indicated in addition to, or instead of, SRI.[16]

COPPER-64

Although GaTate has become the compound primarily used for SRI, new focus on 64Cu-DOTATATE has arisen with the recent completion of a single-arm phase III study.[21] In this study, the top two radiographic readers of the 64Cu-DOTATATE

PET/CT scans reached 100% sensitivity and 97% specificity, rates on par with those of GaTate. Logistically, however, 64Cu may offer benefits over 68Ga. First, the lower positron energy of 64Cu allows for improved spatial resolution of the images. Second, 64Cu's half-life of 12.7 hours provides a more flexible scanning window for the patients, in which the scans do not necessarily need to be completed immediately following injection of the compound. Last, because of its longer half-life, 64Cu-DOTATATE can be created in a centralized location, making geographic distribution to a multitude of centers a legitimate possibility. In contrast, GaTate requires each individual center to purchase unique generators for storage, creating a financial barrier to widespread use of SRI.[7,21]

FROM IMAGING TO TREATMENT

SRI not only identifies neuroendocrine lesions but also plays a role in selecting NET patients who are likely to benefit from PRRT. Because SSTR concentration in NETs impacts the uptake of RSAs, the higher intensity of a lesion on DOTATATE PET may indicate greater efficacy potential of PRRT due to the increased delivery of radiotherapy to SSTR-rich tumors. Historically, Octreoscan results have been translated into a qualitative Krenning score: 0 for no uptake; 1 for very low uptake; 2 for uptake less than or equal to the liver; 3 for uptake greater than the liver; and 4 for uptake greater than the spleen.[22,23] With the expansion of GaTate, Hope and colleagues[23] compared Octreoscan and GaTate images of the same tumors within a week apart to determine how Krenning scores are impacted based on SRI modality. As expected with the greater sensitivity of GaTate, they found that Krenning scores assigned by radiographic readers were significantly higher in the GaTate images versus the Octreoscan images (2.71 vs 1.23, $P < .001$). This difference was especially pronounced for tumors smaller than 2 cm, signifying that smaller lesions will have higher Krenning scores on GaTate than on Octreoscan. This is pertinent when considering the outcomes of studies evaluating PRRT, including the NETTER-1 phase III randomized control trial.[24] In this trial, the investigators used Octreoscan, not DOTATATE PET, Krenning score results for stratification of assessing PRRT benefits—possibly limiting extrapolation of those results to the many patients currently undergoing GaTate imaging.[23]

To predict PRRT results, other studies measured quantitative imaging metrics, including maximum standardized uptake value (SUVmax), tumor-to-spleen ratio (T/S), and tumor-to-liver ratio (T/L).[22,25] Kratochwil and colleagues[25] retrospectively analyzed 30 patients with metastatic NETs in which 40 lesions responded to PRRT and 20 were nonresponsive. Using pre-PRRT ^{68}Ga-DOTATOC, they found that SUVmax was statistically higher in lesions that were ultimately responsive to PRRT versus those that were nonresponsive (33.55 vs 18.00, $P < .001$). Furthermore, responsive lesions demonstrated larger T/S (1.9 vs 1.2, $P < .05$) and T/L (4.97 vs 3.15, $P < .01$) compared with nonresponsive lesions. Because SUVmax is inherently scanner-dependent, the investigators note that T/S and T/L, as ratios, may be more generalizable as a tool to predict PRRT response and suggest a cutoff of higher than 2.2.[25] Contrastingly, investigators of a different study determined that T/S and T/L were not predictive of PRRT response, but SUVmax correlated with both PRRT efficacy as well as progression-free survival (PFS) for patients with SUVmax greater than 13.0 (45.1 months vs 19.9 months if SUVmax < 13.0).[22,26]

Nevertheless, PRRT would not be a feasible management option without first confirming the presence of SSTR-positive NETs via SRI, for which DOTATATE PET has become the standard.

TREATMENT WITH RADIOLABELED SOMATOSTATIN ANALOGS: PEPTIDE RECEPTOR RADIONUCLIDE THERAPY

HISTORICAL CONTEXT

PRRT was first trialed in the 1990s using [^{111}In-DTPA, Tyr[3]] octreotide. Although symptoms of metastatic tumors reportedly improved, the lack of sufficient tumor response spurred a transition to [^{90}Y-DOTA, Tyr[3]]-octreotide, also known as ^{90}Y-DOTATOC or OctreoTher. An improvement in objective response rate was noted, but this was frequently accompanied by severe renal toxicity that was secondary to the long β-particle path length increasing uptake of the peptides in the proximal convoluted tubules, leading to glomeruli radiation exposure.[8] Finally, the more recent [^{177}Lu-DOTA, Tyr[3]]-octreotate (^{177}Lu-DOTATATE; Lutathera) has demonstrated an improved safety profile and efficacy, making it the only FDA-approved PRRT for advanced GEP NETs.[27]

EFFICACY AND OUTCOMES

Although surgical resection, even in the setting of metastases, remains a key component of NET treatment, medical management is often required for those patients with unresectable, recurrent, or progressive disease. SSAs remain the first-line option for symptomatic control and initial disease management for most NET patients, but PRRT is an effective treatment option for those who progress on first-line SSA therapy.

The NETTER-1 trial[24] led to the FDA approval of PRRT with ^{177}Lu-DOTATATE for patients with advanced gastrointestinal NETs. The trial enrolled 221 patients with progressive, well-differentiated midgut NETs—83% of which had metastasized to the liver—and randomized them to treatment with octreotide long-acting release (LAR) 60 mg or ^{177}Lu-DOTATATE plus octreotide LAR 30 mg. Focusing on PFS as the primary end point, the investigators initially reported a median PFS that was not reached in the PRRT arm at the time of the primary analysis versus 8.4 months in the control group. In adjusted analysis, this translated into a hazard ratio (HR) of 0.18 ($P < .0001$), or 82% lower risk of experiencing disease progression or death while undergoing PRRT compared with octreotide LAR alone.[24,28] This advantage in PFS was not reflected in overall survival (OS) metrics calculated 5 years following initial trial randomization. The recently released results reveal a median OS of 48 months for the PRRT arm versus 36.3 months for the control arm (HR 0.84, $P = .30$). Although no statistically significant improvement in OS was demonstrated, the investigators remark that the 11.7 month difference could still have a clinically meaningful impact for patients.[28] As far as objective tumor response in the 201 patients with subsequent imaging, a statistically higher percentage of patients undergoing PRRT experienced partial or complete tumor response (18% vs 3% SSA only, $P < .001$).[24]

Although the NETTER-1 results were encouraging for small bowel NETs, these may not be generalizable to other sites of NETs for which the data are more restricted to reviews and meta-analyses. In one of the large single-institution, non-comparative reviews from Europe, Brabander and colleagues[29] prospectively analyzed 443 patients who underwent PRRT for NETs of various origins. The reported objective response rate (including partial or complete response) was 39% for the entire cohort, with stable disease found in 43%. Furthermore, the investigators were able to delineate disease control rates (stable and responsive disease) between midgut (84%) and pancreatic tumors (81%). For the entire group, median OS was 63 months and PFS was 29 months. Broken down by tumor origin, patients with NETs of the pancreas reached a median OS of 71 months, whereas those with midgut, bronchial, and unknown primary NETs experienced a median OS of 60, 52, and 53 months, respectively.[29] In another review of PRRT on midgut, pancreatic, and bronchial NETs, investigators discovered progressive disease in only 18% of patients, stable disease in 35%, complete response in 2%, and partially responsive disease in the remaining 45%.[30] A separate single-center review evaluated response rates following two or four cycles of PRRT.[31] The investigators estimated, using logistic regression to model tumor response, that patients with PanNETs who had stable disease after the first two cycles of PRRT were more likely to experience tumor response with the completion of four cycles compared with those with non-pancreatic NETs who had stable disease after two cycles (60% vs 11%).

Across studies, PRRT only leads to objective response rates of up to 50% at best, although patients with PanNETs may have a better chance of response (Fig. 3). Some other factors noted to predict a good response to PRRT in these reviews included high uptake on pretreatment Octreoscan—in other words, high SUVmax or Krenning scores—and limited hepatic tumor burden.[30] Relatedly, tumor size may impact both survival rates and tumor response. In the NETTER-1 subgroup analysis, investigators identified "large" tumors (defined as > 3 cm) and calculated that PFS was improved, regardless of tumor size, in the experimental PRRT arm compared with SSA alone.[32] However, categorizing only the PRRT patients into those with or without a large tumor demonstrated an association between longer PFS and patients lacking a tumor greater than 3 cm (log-rank $P = .02$). Shrinkage of tumor after PRRT was also found to differ depending on baseline tumor size. Possibly, the use of ^{90}Y as the radiometal, instead of ^{177}Lu, could mitigate the effects of tumor size because ^{90}Y particles carry more energy that enables them to penetrate a thicker layer of cells and larger tumors.[7]

Despite apparently beneficial outcomes, the 2017 ENETS guidelines highlight that PRRT should be recognized as a palliative treatment given the low likelihood of an enduring and complete tumor response (Fig. 4).[8] Because of the palliative nature of PRRT, quality of life (QoL) is an important endpoint to consider. As part of the NETTER-1 trial, QoL was measured—on both a functional domain scale and symptom scale—every 12 weeks following therapy until disease progression was recognized.[33] This methodology used time to deterioration (TTD) to determine the point when a functional domain or symptom dropped 10 points below its baseline level, with longer TTD implying improved QoL. TTD was significantly longer in the PRRT arm for overall global health (22.7 months difference in median TTD between the two arms), physical functioning, role functioning, and multiple symptoms such as diarrhea, pain, fatigue, and disease-related worries. Conversely, SSA alone did not show a TTD advantage in any domains.[33] Although the unblinded nature of NETTER-1 limited the measurement of TTD, this trend in QoL improvement with PRRT was supported by a single-institution review analyzing metastatic PanNETs, rather than intestinal NETs. PRRT was again associated with greater improvement in global health status ($P = .08$), social functioning ($P = .049$), fatigue, and appetite loss following the final PRRT cycle.[34]

ELIGIBILITY AND INDICATIONS

Eligibility for PRRT depends on the presence of SSTRs as depicted in SRI modalities. In addition, the primary tumor location influences consensus guideline recommendations. Per the recent joint NANETS/SNMMI (Society of Nuclear Medicine and Molecular Imaging) guidelines, ^{177}Lu-DOTA-TATE should be considered as a top second-line choice for tumors of GEP origin if SSAs alone are insufficient.[35] These NANETS/SNMMI recommendations are strongest for tumors of the midgut (appropriateness score 9/9) following the results of the NETTER-1 trial. PanNETs, having been analyzed mostly in nonrandomized studies that describe overall tumor response rates of 45% to 60%, have also been included by the FDA as an indication for ^{177}Lu-DOTATATE (appropriateness criteria 8/9).[35] Bronchial NETs have demonstrated response to PRRT, but the SSTR concentration is not as robust compared with those of GEP origin. Therefore, consensus guidelines comment that

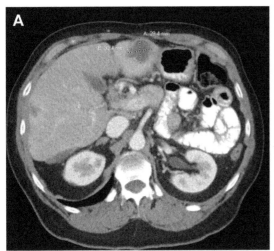
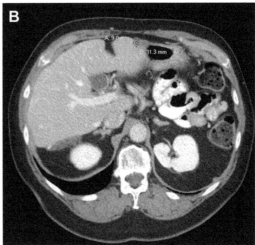

Fig. 3. Surveillance CT scans for a patient with pancreatic neuroendocrine tumor metastatic to the liver demonstrating disease that is responsive to peptide receptor radionuclide therapy (PRRT) during the interval following (*A*) PRRT cycle #1 to (*B*) completion of PRRT cycle #4.

other medical modalities like everolimus may still be preferred after failure of SSAs, with PRRT to follow if disease progression continues (appropriateness criteria 7/9)[35], although optimal choice of PRRT versus other systemic therapies still requires clinical trial validation.

Tumor histologic grade should also be accounted for when considering PRRT. Generally, this treatment has been reserved for grade 1 and 2 tumors, including in the NETTER-1 trial in which all tumors were well-differentiated with a Ki-67 index less than 20%.[24] However, in a retrospective review, Zhang and colleagues[36] analyzed PRRT effects on 69 grade 3 tumors and reported a median PFS of 9.6 months and OS of 19.9 months,

which were generally worse than in many studies analyzing lower grade tumors. When tumors were categorized by a Ki-67 index above or below 55%, the group of patients with Ki-67 greater than 55% had worse median PFS and OS, indicating potentially poorer outcomes with tumors of higher proliferation.[35,36] Nonetheless, other studies have shown preliminary responses in high-grade tumors, especially when patients are given peptide receptor chemoradionuclide therapy—a combo of PPRT and chemotherapy.[8,37]

Beyond tumor characteristics, certain patient-specific variables play a role in selecting patients to undergo PRRT. The ENETS PRRT eligibility guidelines mention characteristics such as

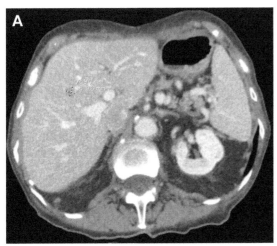
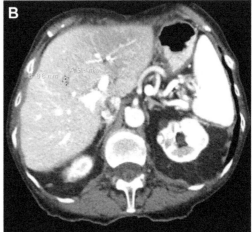

Fig. 4. Surveillance CT scans for a patient with small bowel neuroendocrine tumor metastatic to the liver demonstrating stable/nonresponsive disease to peptide receptor radionuclide therapy (PRRT) during the interval following (*A*) PRRT cycle #2 to (*B*) completion of PRRT cycle #4.

adequate bone marrow reserves, a glomerular filtration rate (GFR) greater than 50, sufficient baseline functioning status, and a survival expectance of at least 3 months.[8] Although these are not strict criteria—NANETS guidelines do not consider GFR less than 50 to be a contraindication—considering these factors when starting patients on PRRT is important to ensure the potential benefits of PRRT outweigh the possible adverse effects.[35]

Importantly, as with many forms of radiation therapy, pregnant and lactating women are not eligible for PRRT and represent an absolute contraindication. In fact, contraception is recommended for the 6 months following completion of PRRT.[8,38]

ADMINISTRATION PROTOCOLS

Dosing and administration protocols for PRRT have been created to ensure patient safety and comfort. Per the NETTER-1 trial and NANETS guidelines on administration, 7.4 GBq (200 mCi) of ^{177}Lu-DOTA-TATE activity is infused peripherally every 8 weeks for a targeted total of 4 doses.[24,38] Despite few reports of renal toxicity with ^{177}Lu compared with ^{90}Y, an amino acid solution of specific arginine and lysine concentrations is run at 320 mL/h concomitantly to the PRRT to prevent reabsorption of the radioactive peptides in the proximal renal tubule. Antiemetics are also provided due to the nausea associated with the amino acids. The 6.6-day half-life of ^{177}Lu allows radiation to persist within patients' systems following treatment. Most of ^{177}Lu-DOTATATE excreted in the urine, medical staff caring for patients should appropriately handle urinary and other bodily samples. For patients who return home immediately, caution should be taken in exposing others to potential radiation, but normal public activities can be resumed safely after 3 days.[38]

TREATMENT SEQUENCING

The optimal sequencing of PRRT in relation to surgical resection remains to be fully explored. The NANETS guidelines on surgical management mention that administering PRRT before hepatic cytoreductive surgery for metastases may provide a couple of advantages.[15] First, reducing the liver tumor burden preoperatively could ease the technical aspects of the operation and enable resection of a larger proportion of tumor. Second, PFS and OS may theoretically increase after systemically treating tumors that otherwise may be left behind following a cytoreduction. Partelli and colleagues[39] evaluated the effects of neoadjuvant

PRRT by matching 23 patients who underwent PanNET resection following PRRT to 23 patients who underwent resection only. Although disease-free survival and PFS were not statistically different between the cohorts, a subgroup analysis of all the patients who underwent a resection with negative margins revealed that those who received PRRT before surgery experienced a longer median PFS (not reached vs 36 months for surgery only, $P < .05$). However, as with any systemic neoadjuvant therapy, it is possible that adverse effects such as bone marrow failure or renal toxicity, as well as the potential for tumor growth while receiving neoadjuvant PRRT, may preclude patients from undergoing the subsequent debulking operation.[15]

Alternatively, studies have also attempted to determine whether up-front surgical resection would alter the outcomes of PRRT. Similar to how preoperative PRRT could improve surgical outcomes by decreasing tumor burden, the same holds true in that surgical resection reduces the amount of remaining tumor needed to be penetrated by PRRT; lower tumor burden has been depicted as a prognostic factor for improved tumor response rate.[30,40] One prospective study by Bertani and colleagues[41] analyzed patients with liver metastases from PanNETs by dividing them into PRRT only versus primary tumor resection followed by PRRT (which included PRRT with ^{177}Lu-DOTATATE or ^{90}Y-DOTATOC). Thirty-one of the 94 patients underwent primary resection followed by PRRT, and the median PFS in this group was 70 months compared with 30 months in the PRRT only group ($P = .002$). Undergoing resection before PRRT was also an independent factor for predicting disease control ($P = .01$). However, a multivariable analysis for OS did not demonstrate primary tumor resection as a prognosticator compared with PRRT alone.[41] A separate retrospective review reported median OS of 140 months versus 58 months for those with Pan-NETs who had primary tumor resection versus no resection before PRRT (HR 2.91, $P < .001$). Patients with small bowel NETs were also found to have improved OS with resection before PRRT (142 months vs 80 months, HR 1.86, $P = .002$).[40]

Overall, these studies suggest that surgery before PRRT, and vice versa, may provide clinical benefit, but the results warrant further investigation and validation in larger studies.

ADVERSE EFFECTS

Nausea and emesis seem to be the most encountered side effects of PRRT as reported in retrospective reviews[30] and the NETTER-1 trial[24] in which 59% and 47% of PRRT patients experienced nausea and emesis, respectively. This is often secondary to the amino acid infusion, which is used to limit the onset of renal toxicity. However, the transition from ^{90}Y to ^{177}Lu has minimized damage to the kidney, now resulting in long-term renal toxicity in less than 2% of patients.[38]

Another documented adverse effect associated with PRRT is hematologic toxicity. This includes transient effects such as neutropenia and lymphopenia, of which 1% and 9% of patients experienced, respectively, in the NETTER-1 trial.[24] Long-lasting complications like acute leukemia and myelodysplastic syndrome are also possibilities.[29] Across a range of reviews, approximately 2% to 3% of patients suffer these serious hematologic complications.[38]

Hepatic dysfunction has also been reported as a potential complication after PRRT, although sporadically. In their single series of 131 patients receiving PRRT, Kwekkeboom and colleagues[30] reported that one patient suffered post-therapy liver failure with development of hepatorenal syndrome and subsequent death. The investigators concluded that this patient's diffuse hepatic metastases severely limited the amount of viable hepatic cells, making the cumulative radiation dose dealt with by those remaining viable cells too extensive. Transaminitis has also been reported, with 3% of patients in a single-institution study experiencing such a side effect.[29] Although these liver-related complications seem uncommon, the 2017 ENETS guidelines for PRRT list severe hepatic impairment as a contraindication to patients receiving PRRT.[8]

Recently, acute small bowel obstructions have been linked to PRRT. Specifically, patients with mesenteric and peritoneal tumor metastases are thought to be at higher risk because of the inflammation caused to these areas by PRRT. The inflammation can subsequently lead to adhesions and tethering of the bowel, creating an obstruction.[42] In a retrospective single-center review of 159 patients, 22 patients were considered at highest risk for developing obstruction due to extensive desmoplastic changes around their mesenteric or peritoneal deposits. The investigators found that five patients (3% of the total) suffered treatment-related bowel obstructions within 3 months of therapy; all of these cases occurred in the "highest risk" patients with significant desmoplastic changes (5/22, 22%).[42] In response to this review, investigators from a separate institution also reported a handful of their PRRT patients who were diagnosed with bowel obstructions.[43] Crucially, these reports depict an acute complication for which closer monitoring in high-risk patients may be warranted to determine need for treatment with steroids or surgical intervention.

FUTURE DIRECTIONS

Modifications to PRRT have been suggested for certain scenarios, with some having already been explored and others being investigated in ongoing trials. First, the delivery of PRRT with a combination of ^{90}Y and ^{177}Lu has been hypothesized to improve outcomes for larger lesions.[8] This combination has demonstrated improved OS compared with just ^{90}Y alone.[44,45] Although ^{90}Y emits beta particles and ^{177}Lu emits both beta and gamma particles, radiometals that emit alpha particles have been used in patients whose tumors seem refractory to standard beta particle PRRT. Results have indicated the heightened killing potential of alpha-emitting particles, and clinical trials of PRRT with alpha particles are underway.[7] Regarding route of administration, infusion of PRRT via the hepatic artery has been described for metastases confined to the liver.[8] Furthermore, ongoing studies are evaluating whether the combination of PRRT with chemotherapy, DNA damage repair targeting agents, or immunotherapy may improve efficacy.[46–49] Last, data directly comparing PRRT to systemic therapies beyond SSAs are lacking. Trials, such as the COMPETE trial,[50] a randomized control trial assessing patient outcomes after receiving PRRT, or everolimus for GEP NETs, are attempting to bridge this gap.

SUMMARY

RSAs, with their affinity for SSTRs that are often found on the surface of NETs, are now commonly used in both the diagnosis and management of these tumors. GaTate PET/CT, compared with other forms of imaging, has demonstrated increased sensitivity and utility for detecting primary tumor location, identifying additional metastatic foci, and predicting responses to therapy. PRRT, most commonly using ^{177}Lu-DOTATATE, can enhance PFS and QoL for patients with NETs. Still, it mainly remains a "palliative" rather than curative option, and investigations to enhance its efficacy are underway.

DISCLOSURE

The authors have no disclosures to declare.

REFERENCES

1. Dasari A, Shen C, Halperin D, et al. Trends in the incidence, prevalence, and survival outcomes in

patients with neuroendocrine tumors in the United States. JAMA Oncol 2017;3(10):1335–42.

2. Günther T, Tulipano G, Dournaud P, et al. International union of basic and clinical pharmacology. CV. somatostatin receptors: Structure, function, ligands, and new nomenclature. Pharmacol Rev 2018;70(4):763–835.

3. Krenning EP, Kwekkeboom DJ, Bakker WH, et al. Somatostatin receptor scintigraphy with [111In-DTPA-d-Phe1]- and [123I-Tyr3]-octreotide: the Rotterdam experience with more than 1000 patients. Eur J Nucl Med 1993;20(8):716–31.

4. Song KB, Kim SC, Kim JH, et al. Prognostic Value of Somatostatin Receptor Subtypes in Pancreatic Neuroendocrine Tumors. Pancreas 2016;45(2):187–92.

5. Riihimäki M, Hemminki A, Sundquist K, et al. The epidemiology of metastases in neuroendocrine tumors. Int J Cancer 2016;139(12):2679–86.

6. Hallet J, Law CHL, Cukier M, et al. Exploring the rising incidence of neuroendocrine tumors: A population-based analysis of epidemiology, metastatic presentation, and outcomes. Cancer 2015;121(4):589–97.

7. Eychenne R, Bouvry C, Bourgeois M, et al. Overview of Radiolabeled Somatostatin Analogs for Cancer Imaging and Therapy. Molecules 2020;25(17).

8. Hicks RJ, Kwekkeboom DJ, Krenning E, et al. ENETS Consensus Guidelines for the Standards of Care in Neuroendocrine Neoplasms: Peptide Receptor Radionuclide Therapy with Radiolabelled Somatostatin Analogues. Neuroendocrinology 2017;105(3):295–309.

9. Babazadeh NT, Schlund DJ, Cornelius T, et al. Should 68Ga-DOTATATE PET/CT be Performed Routinely in Patients with Neuroendocrine Tumors Before Surgical Resection? World J Surg 2020;44(2):604–11.

10. Kwekkeboom DJ, Krenning EP. Somatostatin receptor imaging. Semin Nucl Med 2002;32(2):84–91.

11. Hofman MS, Kong G, Neels OC, et al. High management impact of Ga-68 DOTATATE (GaTate) PET/CT for imaging neuroendocrine and other somatostatin expressing tumours. J Med Imaging Radiat Oncol 2012;56(1):40–7.

12. Deppen SA, Blume JD, Bobbey AJ, et al. 68Ga-DOTATATE Compared with 111 In-DTPA-Octreotide and Conventional Imaging for Pulmonary and Gastroenteropancreatic Neuroendocrine Tumors: A Systematic Review and Meta-Analysis. J Nucl Med 2016;57(6):872–8.

13. Sadowski SM, Neychev V, Millo C, et al. Prospective study of 68Ga-DOTATATE positron emission tomography/computed tomography for detecting gastroentero-pancreatic neuroendocrine tumors and unknown primary sites. J Clin Oncol 2016;34(6):588–97.

14. Hope TA, Bergsland EK, Bozkurt MF, et al. Appropriate use criteria for somatostatin receptor PET imaging in neuroendocrine tumors. J Nucl Med 2018;59(1):66–74.

15. Howe JR, Merchant NB, Conrad C, et al. The North American Neuroendocrine Tumor Society Consensus Paper on the Surgical Management of Pancreatic Neuroendocrine Tumors. Pancreas 2020;49(1):1–33.

16. Sundin A, Arnold R, Baudin E, et al. ENETS Consensus Guidelines for the Standards of Care in Neuroendocrine Tumors: Radiological, Nuclear Medicine and Hybrid Imaging. Neuroendocrinology 2017;105(3):212–44.

17. Crown A, Rocha FG, Raghu P, et al. Impact of initial imaging with gallium-68 dotatate PET/CT on diagnosis and management of patients with neuroendocrine tumors. J Surg Oncol 2020;121(3):480–5.

18. Tierney JF, Kosche C, Schadde E, et al. 68Gallium-DOTATATE positron emission tomography–computed tomography (PET CT) changes management in a majority of patients with neuroendocrine tumors. Surg (United States) 2019;165(1):178–85.

19. Strosberg JR, Halfdanarson TR, Bellizzi AM, et al. The north American neuroendocrine tumor society consensus guidelines for surveillance and medical management of midgut neuroendocrine tumors. Pancreas 2017;46(6):707–14.

20. Haug AR, Cindea-Drimus R, Auernhammer CJ, et al. Neuroendocrine tumor recurrence: Diagnosis with 68Ga-DOTATATE PET/CT. Radiology 2014;270(2):517–25.

21. Delpassand ES, Ranganathan D, Wagh N, et al. 64Cu-DOTATATE PET/CT for imaging patients with known or suspected somatostatin receptor-Positive neuroendocrine tumors: Results of the first U.S. prospective, reader-masked clinical trial. J Nucl Med 2020;61(6):890–6.

22. Liberini V, Huellner MW, Grimaldi S, et al. The challenge of evaluating response to peptide receptor radionuclide therapy in gastroenteropancreatic neuroendocrine tumors: The present and the future. Diagnostics 2020;10(12):1–31.

23. Hope TA, Calais J, Zhang L, et al. 111In-pentetreotide scintigraphy versus 68Ga-DOTATATE PET: Impact on krenning scores and effect of tumor burden. J Nucl Med 2019;60(9):1266–9.

24. Strosberg J, El-Haddad G, Wolin E, et al. Phase 3 Trial of 177 Lu-Dotatate for Midgut Neuroendocrine Tumors. N Engl J Med 2017;376(2):125–35.

25. Kratochwil C, Stefanova M, Mavriopoulou E, et al. SUV of [68Ga]DOTATOC-PET/CT Predicts Response Probability of PRRT in Neuroendocrine Tumors. Mol Imaging Biol 2015;17(3):313–8.

26. Sharma R, Wang WM, Yusuf S, et al. 68Ga-DOTATATE PET/CT parameters predict response to peptide receptor radionuclide therapy in neuroendocrine tumours. Radiother Oncol 2019;141:108–15.

27. Satapathy S, Mittal BR. 177Lu-DOTATATE peptide receptor radionuclide therapy versus Everolimus in advanced pancreatic neuroendocrine tumors: A systematic review and meta-analysis. Nucl Med Commun 2019;40(12):1195–203.

28. Strosberg JR, Caplin ME, Kunz PL, et al. 177Lu-Dotatate plus long-acting octreotide versus high-dose long-acting octreotide in patients with midgut neuroendocrine tumours (NETTER-1): final overall survival and long-term safety results from an open-label, randomised, controlled, phase 3 trial. Lancet Oncol 2021;22(12):1752–63.

29. Brabander T, Van Der Zwan WA, Teunissen JJM, et al. Long-term efficacy, survival, and safety of [177Lu-DOTA0,Tyr3]octreotate in patients with gastroenteropancreatic and bronchial neuroendocrine tumors. Clin Cancer Res 2017;23(16):4617–24.

30. Kwekkeboom DJ, Teunissen JJ, Bakker WH, et al. Radiolabeled somatostatin analog [177Lu-DOTA0, Tyr3] octreotate in patients with endocrine gastroenteropancreatic tumors. J Clin Oncol 2005;23(12):2754–62.

31. Vaghaiwalla T, Ruhle B, Memeh K, et al. Response rates in metastatic neuroendocrine tumors receiving peptide receptor radionuclide therapy and implications for future treatment strategies. Surg (United States) 2021;169(1):162–7.

32. Strosberg J, Kunz PL, Hendifar A, et al. Impact of liver tumour burden, alkaline phosphatase elevation, and target lesion size on treatment outcomes with 177Lu-Dotatate: an analysis of the NETTER-1 study. Eur J Nucl Med Mol Imaging 2020;47(10):2372–82.

33. Strosberg J, Wolin E, Chasen B, et al. Health-related quality of life in patients with progressive midgut neuroendocrine tumors treated with 177 lu-dotatate in the phase III netter-1 trial. J Clin Oncol 2018; 36(25):2578–84.

34. Marinova M, Mücke M, Mahlberg L, et al. Improving quality of life in patients with pancreatic neuroendocrine tumor following peptide receptor radionuclide therapy assessed by EORTC QLQ-C30. Eur J Nucl Med Mol Imaging 2018;45(1):38–46.

35. Hope TA, Bodei L, Chan JA, et al. NANETS/SNMMI consensus statement on patient selection and appropriate use of 177Lu-DOTATATE peptide receptor radionuclide therapy. J Nucl Med 2020;61(2):222–7.

36. Zhang J, Kulkarni HR, Singh A, et al. Peptide receptor radionuclide therapy in grade 3 neuroendocrine neoplasms: Safety and survival analysis in 69 patients. J Nucl Med 2019;60(3):377–85.

37. Kashyap R, Hofman MS, Michael M, et al. Favourable outcomes of 177Lu-octreotate peptide receptor chemoradionuclide therapy in patients with FDG-avid neuroendocrine tumours. Eur J Nucl Med Mol Imaging 2015;42(2):176–85.

38. Hope TA, Abbott A, Colucci K, et al. NANETS/SNMMI procedure standard for somatostatin receptor-based peptide receptor radionuclide therapy with 177Lu-DOTATATE. J Nucl Med 2019; 60(7):937–43.

39. Partelli S, Bertani E, Bartolomei M, et al. Peptide receptor radionuclide therapy as neoadjuvant therapy for resectable or potentially resectable pancreatic neuroendocrine neoplasms. Pancreas 2018;163(4):761–7.

40. Kaemmerer D, Twrznik M, Kulkarni HR, et al. Prior Resection of the Primary Tumor Prolongs Survival After Peptide Receptor Radionuclide Therapy of Advanced Neuroendocrine Neoplasms. Ann Surg 2021;274(1):e45–53.

41. Bertani E, Fazio N, Radice D, et al. Resection of the Primary Tumor Followed by Peptide Receptor Radionuclide Therapy as Upfront Strategy for the Treatment of G1–G2 Pancreatic Neuroendocrine Tumors with Unresectable Liver Metastases. Ann Surg Oncol 2016;23:981–9.

42. Strosberg JR, Al-Toubah T, Pellè E, et al. Risk of bowel obstruction in patients with mesenteric or peritoneal disease receiving peptide receptor radionuclide therapy. J Nucl Med 2021;62(1):69–72.

43. Wee CE, Dundar A, Eiring RA, et al. Bowel obstruction as a complication of peptide receptor radionuclide therapy (PRRT). J Nucl Med 2021;62(9):9–10.

44. Kunikowska J, Królicki L, Hubalewska-Dydejczyk A, et al. Clinical results of radionuclide therapy of neuroendocrine tumours with 90 Y-DOTATATE and tandem 90 Y/177 Lu-DOTATATE: Which is a better therapy option? Eur J Nucl Med Mol Imaging 2011;38(10):1788–97.

45. Dumont RA, Seiler D, Marincek N, et al. Survival after somatostatin based radiopeptide therapy in metastasized gastrinoma. Am J Nucl Med Mol Imaging 2015;5(1):46–55.

46. U.S National Library of Medicine. Personalized CAPTEM Radiopeptide Therapy of Advanced, Non-resectable Neuroendocrine Cancer. Clinical Trials.gov. 2019. https://clinicaltrials.gov/ct2/show/NCT04 194125. Accessed October 28, 2022.

47. Pavlakis N, Turner Ransom D, Wyld D, et al. Australasian Gastrointestinal Trials Group (AGITG) CONTROL NET Study: Phase II study evaluating the activity of 177Lu-Octreotate peptide receptor radionuclide therapy (LuTate PRRT) and capecitabine, temozolomide CAPTEM)—First results for pancreas and upda. J Clin Oncol 2020;38(15 suppl).

48. Lakiza O, Lutze J, Vogle A, et al. Loss of MEN1 function impairs DNA repair capability of pancreatic neuroendocrine tumors. Endocr Relat Cancer 2022;29(4):225–39.

49. Cullinane C, Waldeck K, Kirby L, et al. Enhancing the anti-tumour activity of 177Lu-DOTA-octreotate radionuclide therapy in somatostatin receptor-2 expressing tumour models by targeting PARP. Sci Rep 2020;10(1):1–10.

50. Pavel ME, Rinke A, Baum RP. COMPETE trial: Peptide receptor radionuclide therapy (PRRT) with 177Lu-edotreotide vs. everolimus in progressive GEP-NET. Ann Oncol 2018;29:viii478.

Scarless Surgery
Clinical Indications for Transoral Endocrine Surgery and Implications for Pathologists

Jordan M. Broekhuis, MD[a,b], Benjamin C. James, MD, MS[a,b],
Raymon H. Grogan, MD, MS[c],*

KEYWORDS

- Transoral endocrine surgery • Thyroid cancer • Remote access surgery • Endocrine surgery
- Transoral endoscopic thyroidectomy vestibular approach

Key points

- Transoral endocrine surgery (TES) refers to the endoscopic approach to thyroidectomy and parathyroidectomy via incisions in the oral vestibule.
- The oral vestibular incisions are small, which can limit the size of surgical specimen that can be removed while avoiding fracture and fragmentation.
- Existing observational data suggest TES for parathyroidectomy and thyroidectomy has similar complication profiles compared with open approaches and may result in improved quality of life and satisfaction outcomes for patients.

ABSTRACT

Transoral endocrine surgery (TES) is a scarless approach to thyroidectomy and parathyroidectomy for well-selected patients. Criteria for the TES approach to thyroidectomy include thyroid diameter less than or equal to 10 cm, benign nodule less than or equal to 6 cm, or confirmed or suspected malignant nodule less than or equal to 2 cm. Although fragmentation of surgical specimens has been reported in TES, additional studies are needed to evaluate the implications of TES on pathologic examination.

and bilateral axillo-breast approaches, have been proposed with the goal of eliminating the cervical scar. Although the term "transoral endocrine surgery" is used broadly to describe thyroid and parathyroid operations performed via incisions in the oral vestibule, the technical terms for these operations include transoral endoscopic thyroidectomy vestibular approach and transoral endoscopic parathyroidectomy vestibular approach.

Of the remote-access approaches to thyroid and parathyroid operations, transoral endocrine surgery has emerged as the preferred approach for some patients and surgeons, given the lack of required cutaneous incision and relatively short distance required for creation of a subcutaneous flap compared with other approaches. Use of the transoral approach has increased in Asia and among select high-volume centers in the United States, and data from these centers suggest similar rates of surgical complications.[2] In addition, the elimination of a cutaneous scar may be

OVERVIEW

Transoral endocrine surgery (TES) represents one of the several remote-access approaches to surgery of the thyroid and parathyroid glands.[1] These approaches, which also include the transaxillary

---

[a] Harvard Medical School, Boston, MA, USA; [b] Department of Surgery, Beth Israel Deaconess Medical Center, 330 Brookline Ave, Boston, MA 02215, USA; [c] Michael E. DeBakey Department of Surgery, Baylor College of Medicine, 7200 Cambridge Street, 7th Floor, Room A07-103, Houston, TX 77030, USA
* Corresponding author.
E-mail address: rgrogan@bcm.edu

Surgical Pathology 16 (2023) 163–166
https://doi.org/10.1016/j.path.2022.10.002

preferable to many patients compared with the cervical approach and may be associated with improved quality of life outcomes.[3,4] Society guidelines regarding remote-access endocrine operations contain broad statements recommending that the operation should only be performed by high-volume, experienced surgeons.[5,6] An additional consideration in applying TES is how and when it can be used in cases of known or suspected malignancy. Although data are limited, recommendations have been proposed based on observational data and expert opinion.

Although uptake of transoral endocrine surgery is limited by a substantial learning curve and increased operative time,[7] this approach has grown in popularity in Asia and select US centers, and thus familiarity of this approach and its implications for clinical pathology have become important for pathologists. In this article, the authors review the general approach to TES, its applications in thyroid and parathyroid surgery, and existing data informing the implications of these approaches for pathologists.

OPERATIVE APPROACH

The operative approach to transoral endocrine surgery has been extensively described elsewhere.[8] Here the authors provide an abbreviated summary with emphasis on implications for the surgical and pathologic outcomes described in this article.

Incisions are made on the inner lower lip: a single 5-mm transverse midline incision and 2 stab incisions lateral to the first premolars. Access to the subplatysmal space is gained via the midline port, and this space is dilated before placement of a total of three 5-mm ports. The midline strap muscles are divided and the thyroid isthmus transected. The superior, middle, and lower thyroid vessels are ligated with careful attention to preservation of the recurrent laryngeal nerve. The ligament of Berry is then divided, which frees the thyroid completely from the trachea and surrounding structures. Once the thyroid is resected, the surgeon dilates the central port up to 2 cm in diameter, a bag is placed into the dissection space through this port, and the specimen is removed intact inside the bag.

SOCIETAL GUIDELINES AND EXPERT CONSENSUS ON APPLICATIONS OF TRANSORAL ENDOCRINE SURGERY

Society guidelines addressing remote-access approaches to endocrine surgery contain broad statements about their use and generally do not address specific indications. At the time of a recently published statement by the American Thyroid Association in 2016 on remote-access thyroid surgery, TES was not yet in use in the United States.[6] However, this statement broadly addressed remote access approaches and noted that questions remained regarding operative times, learning curves, and cost. The American Thyroid Association (ATA) recommended that alternative approaches to thyroidectomy (such as TES) could be performed as long as strict selection criteria were met and a high-volume surgeon with experience in the alternative approach was doing the procedure.

In 2020, the American Association of Endocrine Surgeons released guidelines for the surgical management of thyroid disease in adults. These guidelines similarly acknowledged the limited data on improved patient satisfaction and cosmetic results for remote-access endocrine operations and recommended that remote-access thyroidectomy be applied in "carefully selected patients, by surgeons experienced in the approach."[5]

In addition, recommendations for applications of TES based on expert opinion have been suggested in the literature. For applications in thyroidectomy, it has been recommended that TES be applied in patients highly motivated to avoid a cutaneous scar who otherwise meet ATA guidelines for lobectomy or total thyroidectomy.[9] Suggested inclusion criteria include the following: (1) history of hypertrophic scarring or desire to avoid anterior neck scar; (2) maximum thyroid lobe dimension less than or equal to 10 cm or volume less than or equal to 45 mL; (3) benign or indeterminate nodule of size less than or equal to 6 cm; (4) suspicious or malignant nodule of size less than or equal to 2 cm; and (5) substernal goiter above the aortic arch.[10,11] TES has also been applied in cases of symptomatic goiter and Grave disease or Hashimoto thyroiditis within the aforementioned size constraints.[11] Suggested exclusion criteria include the following: (1) poorly differentiated or anaplastic carcinoma; (2) central neck, lateral neck, or extrathyroidal involvement; (3) known recurrent laryngeal nerve injury; (4) prior transcervical neck surgery; (5) oral abscess; and (6) general inability to tolerate surgery or undergo anesthesia.[11]

Application of TES to central neck dissection is limited to cases of small thyroid cancers as discussed earlier, in which evidence of clinical nodal metastasis is identified at the time of surgery. Furthermore, central neck dissection should only be considered by surgeons with sufficient TES experience. TES is not currently considered appropriate for dissection of the lateral neck. In the case of thyroid malignancies, the importance of removing the surgical specimen intact represents a particular challenge in TES, given the small oral vestibular incisions.

Application of TES for parathyroidectomy is less well described, but TES is generally considered an option in cases of primary hyperparathyroidism. Currently secondary and tertiary hyperparathyroidism are considered relative contraindications to the procedure. Although nonlocalized adenomas and multigland hyperplasia have not been suggested to be strict contraindications to TES, a single adenoma that has been localized by preoperative imaging is thought to be the ideal application of TES.[12] In addition, parathyroidectomy of the inferior glands is thought to be less technically challenging compared with the superior glands, as visualization of the lower aspect of the neck is more accessible with the angle of the camera. TES is not recommended in cases of suspected or confirmed parathyroid carcinoma.

EVIDENCE FROM OBSERVATIONAL DATA

Surgical Complications

Since TES was originally described in 2015, it is estimated that at the time of writing there have been more than 5000 cases done worldwide including more than 700 in the United States. A recent review of 689 transoral thyroidectomies found that 99% of cases did not require conversion to an open cervical approach but did require longer operative times compared with the open approach.[13] There were no identified cases of permanent recurrent laryngeal or mental nerve injury and very low rates of hematoma (0.1%) and neck infection (0.1%).

A recent prospective multiinstitutional observational study of 101 consecutive transoral parathyroidectomies found this approach to be safe and efficacious.[2] This study, which included patients with primary hyperparathyroidism who had a single, well-localized adenomas on at least 2 preoperative imaging studies reported a success rate of 98% by immediate normalization of PTH. Furthermore, there were no reported cases of permanent recurrent laryngeal nerve injury or hypoparathyroidism. This study emphasizes the safe application of TES for parathyroidectomy, especially in cases of single, well-localized adenomas.

Implications for Pathologic Evaluation

The most prominent implication of TES for pathologists is the removal of pathologic specimens via the small incisions in the oral vestibule. It is important to note that removing the specimen intact depends on 2 variables, namely the size of the

midline opening that is created and the size of the specimen. The midline opening in the beginning of the operation is usually between 5 and 10 mm; however, it is possible to dilate this opening to 2 cm without negative effects on chin cosmesis. Because the thyroid is relatively soft and pliable, a specimen larger than 2 cm can be extracted intact through a 2 cm opening; however, it is not clear how large that cutoff is or should be. There are also alternative means of removing the specimen. Very limited data exist examining pathologic outcomes in TES. However, one recent study evaluated 50 cases of transoral thyroidectomies for a mean nodule size of 2.6 cm.[14] Of these 50 cases, 34 (68%) reported disruption or fragmentation of the pathologic specimen, although a final diagnosis was achieved in all cases. However, there were 2 cases of papillary carcinomas in which tumor size, microscopic extrathyroidal extension, and margin status could not be determined. An additional small study of 27 cases applied receiver operating characteristic analysis to estimate the safest nodular diameter of 2 cm in order to avoid piecemeal removal.[15] Overall, guidelines suggest that a relative cutoff of 2.0 to 2.5 cm be used for removal of well-differentiated thyroid cancers due to the concern of specimen disruption during extraction. It is likely that even larger cancer specimens can be extracted without any negative impact on histologic diagnosis; however, data are sparse. As the use of TES increases, additional larger studies of the impact of these operations on pathologic specimens are needed to determine to what extent these cases of fragmentation may be eliminated as surgeons gain more experience in this approach.

UPTAKE OF TRANSORAL ENDOCRINE SURGERY APPROACHES

The uptake of TES in the United States has been limited by several factors, including its learning curve and access to appropriate training in the technique. In addition, recent restrictions of elective operations as a result of the COVID-19 pandemic have likely limited the use of TES as well as the ability to train surgeons on its use. An additional proposed reason for the limited uptake of TES is the limited, select group of patients who meet the criteria required for TES. However, a recent cross-sectional study of 1000 consecutive thyroid and parathyroid operations found that 55.8% were eligible for TES based on eligibility criteria as described earlier.[16] As time allows for more surgeons to be trained in this technique pathologists may begin to see more cases of pathologic specimens from TES operations.

SUMMARY

TES is an approach to thyroid and parathyroid surgery that eliminates the cutaneous scar and may provide superior patient satisfaction and quality of life outcomes in well-selected patients. Careful consideration of eligibility for this approach based on the criteria described earlier is important for the application of TES. The pathologic examination of surgical specimens obtained during TES is an additional important consideration, given the size of the oral vestibular incisions and previously described limitations in the setting of specimen fracture or fragmentation. Larger studies evaluating the extend of nodal harvest and successful pathologic evaluation are needed.

CLINICS CARE POINTS

- TES refers to the endoscopic approach to thyroidectomy and parathyroidectomy via incisions in the oral vestibule.

- The oral vestibular incisions are small, which can limit the size of surgical specimen that can be removed while avoiding fracture and fragmentation.

- Existing observational data suggest TES for parathyroidectomy and thyroidectomy has similar complication profiles compared with open approaches and may result in improved quality of life and satisfaction outcomes for patients.

DISCLOSURE

R.H. Grogan received consulting fees from Medtronic. The remaining authors have no personal or financial potential conflicts of interest to disclose.

REFERENCES

1. Udelsman R, Anuwong A, Oprea AD, et al. Transoral Vestibular Endocrine Surgery: A New Technique in the United States. Ann Surg 2016;264(6):e13–6.
2. Grogan RH, Khafif AK, Nidal A, et al. One hundred and one consecutive transoral endoscopic parathyroidectomies via the vestibular approach for PHPTH: a worldwide multi-institutional experience. Surg Endosc 2021. https://doi.org/10.1007/S00464-021-08826-Y.
3. Broekhuis JM, Chen HW, Maeda AH, et al. Public Perceptions of Transoral Endocrine Surgery and their Influence on Choice of Operative Approach. J Surg Res 2021;267:56–62.
4. Choi Y, Lee JH, Kim YH, et al. Impact of postthyroidectomy scar on the quality of life of thyroid cancer patients. Ann Dermatol 2014;26(6):693–9.
5. Patel KN, Yip L, Lubitz CC, et al. The American association of endocrine surgeons guidelines for the definitive surgical management of thyroid disease in adults. Ann Surg 2020;271(3):E21–93.
6. Berber E, Bernet V, Fahey TJ, et al. American Thyroid Association Statement on Remote-Access Thyroid Surgery. Thyroid 2016;26(3):331–7.
7. Razavi CR, Vasiliou E, Tufano RP, et al. Learning Curve for Transoral Endoscopic Thyroid Lobectomy. Otolaryngol - Head Neck Surg (United States) 2018; 159(4):625–9.
8. James BC, Angelos P, Grogan RH. Transoral endocrine surgery: Considerations for adopting a new technique. J Surg Oncol 2020;122(1):36–40.
9. Razavi CR, Tufano RP, Russell JO. Starting a Transoral Thyroid and Parathyroid Surgery Program. Curr Otorhinolaryngol Rep 2019;7(3):204–8.
10. Razavi CR, Fondong A, Tufano RP, et al. Central neck dissection via the transoral approach. Ann Thyroid 2017;2(5):11.
11. Russell JO, Sahli ZT, Shaear M, et al. Transoral thyroid and parathyroid surgery via the vestibular approach-a 2020 update. Gland Surg 2020;9(2): 409–16.
12. Razavi CR, Russell JO. Indications and contraindications to transoral thyroidectomy. Ann Thyroid 2017;2(5):12.
13. Russell JO, Razavi CR, Shaear M, et al. Transoral Vestibular Thyroidectomy: Current State of Affairs and Considerations for the Future. J Clin Endocrinol Metab 2019;104(9):3779.
14. Smith SM, Ahmed M, Carling T, et al. Impact of Transoral Endoscopic Vestibular Approach Thyroidectomy on Pathologic Assessment. Arch Pathol Lab Med 2021. https://doi.org/10.5858/ARPA.2021-0082-OA.
15. Wu YJ, Chi SY, Elsarawy A, et al. What is the Appropriate Nodular Diameter in Thyroid Cancer for Extraction by Transoral Endoscopic Thyroidectomy Vestibular Approach Without Breaking the Specimens? A Surgicopathologic Study. Surg Laparosc Endosc Percutan Tech 2018;28(6):390–3.
16. Grogan RH, Suh I, Chomsky-Higgins K, et al. Patient Eligibility for Transoral Endocrine Surgery Procedures in the United States. JAMA Netw Open 2019; 2(5):e194829.

Applications of Deep Learning in Endocrine Neoplasms

Siddhi Ramesh, BA[a,c], James M. Dolezal, MD[a,c],
Alexander T. Pearson, MD, PhD[a,b,c],*

KEYWORDS
- Machine learning • Deep learning • Endocrine neoplasia • Pathology • Histology

Key points

- Deep learning applications in histopathology have demonstrated the ability to enhance automation to reduce pathologist workloads and to abstract image-related features that are indeterminable from pure human inspection.
- Centralized data repositories must be an emphasis to improve data access and improve the quality and reliability of histopathology-related deep learning studies.
- Standardized reporting and evaluation criteria must be established to improve study interpretability and comparability to ultimately improve clinical adoption of deep learning models.

ABSTRACT

Machine learning methods have been growing in prominence across all areas of medicine. In pathology, recent advances in deep learning (DL) have enabled computational analysis of histological samples, aiding in diagnosis and characterization in multiple disease areas. In cancer, and particularly endocrine cancer, DL approaches have been shown to be useful in tasks ranging from tumor grading to gene expression prediction. This review summarizes the current state of DL research in endocrine cancer histopathology with an emphasis on experimental design, significant findings, and key limitations.

OVERVIEW

In recent years, an exponential increase in data and computational infrastructure across all of medicine has led to significant momentum and interest in developing new methods for data analysis. The use of artificial intelligence (AI) and machine learning (ML) methodologies have continued to grow across many areas within medicine. Specific methodologies such as deep learning (DL) now enable the efficient analysis of complex data to solve issues with large-scale image classification, free text natural language processing, and signal processing.[1]

In medicine, diabetic retinopathy image interpretation,[2] electrocardiogram analysis,[3] and stroke or intracranial hemorrhage[4] are a few examples of areas with FDA-approved AI tools. Within oncology, areas such as cancer radiology, radiation oncology, gynecology-oncology, clinical oncology, and pathology have seen increasing numbers of DL tools undergoing successful FDA approval, with the largest number of DL tools seen in radiology and pathology applications.[5] However, thus far, these FDA-approved tools are

[a] Department of Medicine, Section of Hematology/Oncology, University of Chicago Medical Center, 5841 South Maryland Avenue, MC 2115, Chicago, IL 60637, USA; [b] University of Chicago Comprehensive Cancer Center, Chicago, IL, USA; [c] The University of Chicago Medicine & Biological Sciences, 5841 South Maryland Avenue, Chicago, IL, USA
* Corresponding author.
E-mail address: apearson5@medicine.bsd.uchicago.edu

not viewed as independent substitutes for traditional physician-based diagnostic processes. Instead, they are being used to further augment physician workflows, particularly during diagnosis.[5] Outside of FDA-associated studies, there have been numerous studies of the application of DL in areas outside of diagnostics such as prognosis and treatment response.[6] The cancer subtypes that are experiencing the most growth and focus within DL research include breast, lung, and prostate, which may be attributable to their relatively higher incidence compared with other cancer subtypes.[6]

In this review, we discuss the application of DL methods to histopathologic assessment of endocrine neoplasms, including thyroid, pancreatic, neuroendocrine, parathyroid, pituitary, and adrenal tumors. We will review key studies that characterize the state of pathology-related DL studies within these endocrine neoplasms, discuss strengths and weaknesses of the existing literature, and identify potential areas for future research. Ultimately, this review will assess trends seen across the abstracted literature and highlight areas for methodological improvement for future studies within computational pathology.

WHAT IS MACHINE LEARNING?

Broadly, AI is the domain of study utilizing algorithms to enable a machine to perform tasks with human-like intelligence (**Fig. 1**). ML is a subset of AI encompassing statistical methods that identify of patterns and trends within datasets and enable generation of predictions for novel data. Neural networks (NNs) are ML algorithms that use a series of connected neurons that function in cohesion to identify patterns, loosely resembling the way interconnected neurons function within the brain. NNs are trained on example data through pattern recognition using feedback process known as backpropagation, where the network compares the output it generates to the value that is known to be correct, ultimately using the difference between these values to modify the connections among the units in the network. DL is a methodology utilizing NNs with many layers, enabling the extraction of progressively higher levels of features from input data. There are variations to the structure of DL NNs catered toward the complexity of the underlying data. Although there is a multitude of subclasses of NNs, one example is known as a convolutional neural network (CNN). CNNs include one or more layers of convolutional units,

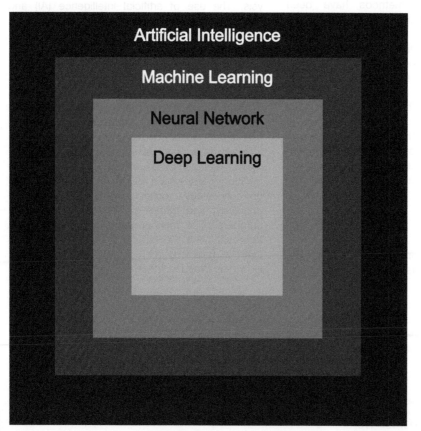

Fig. 1. Relationships between AI terminologies.

which function to receive multiple inputs from a prior layer to create an understanding of proximity, which can often reduce network complexity in cases where data proximity is important (eg, imaging, text, speech). Beyond specific subclasses of NNs, there are additional structural variations such as network depth. For example, shallow NNs (contain less layers) are used to calculate an input and output from one round of processing (eg, clinical scoring algorithms such as CURB-65).[7] In contrast, deep NNs (contain more layers) can represent more complex functions and understand underlying complexity of spatial data that requires more nuance than classical clinical scoring techniques.[7]

The key purpose of ML when compared with traditional statistical approaches is the concept that a model can learn from examples, rather than requiring explicit rules to be defined by a human.[8] During supervised learning, an ML algorithm is trained to predict outcomes through exposure to a large number of labeled data. Most often, these predictions are used for classification tasks in which the target variable is a discrete outcome or in regression tasks where the target variable is a continuous outcome. Algorithms are provided input data, or features, and associated outputs, known as labels (Fig. 2). For applications in pathology, the input data could be a digitized image of a histopathology slide (the pixels of the image

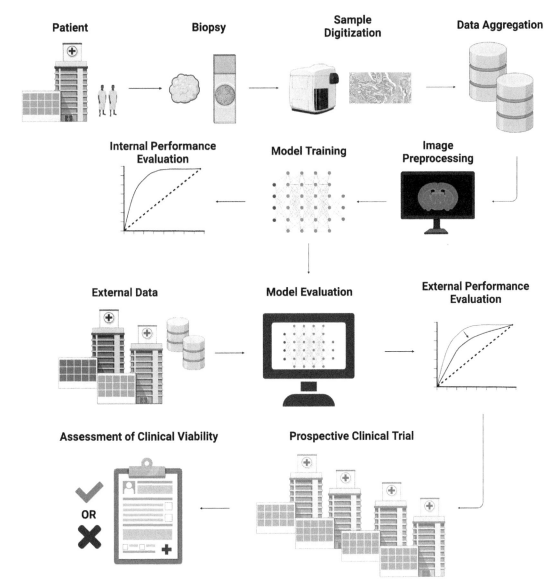

Fig. 2. Digital pathology DL study workflow.

converted into features) labeled with the correct diagnosis. The algorithm then learns to correlate these features to the provided labels through a process known as training. After being exposed to a sufficient number and diversity of examples through training, the model's ability to correctly predict labels on a set of held-out test data is formally assessed. Ideally, the test dataset should be abstracted from a distinct source than the training data so that the model can be evaluated on its ability to generalize to a completely novel setting, ensuring that true underlying and abstractable biological features are driving predictions, rather underlying noise inherent to a particular dataset (see **Fig. 2**).

Conventional ML techniques, such as logistic regression, support vector machine, random forest, and gradient boosting machines, are limited in their ability to process large, complex datasets in unprocessed states.[9] Constructing an effective pattern-recognition system requires significant manual engineering of input data in order to allow the algorithm to effectively extract patterns found throughout the dataset.[9] In comparison, DL methods are able to better learn complex, high-level features within large datasets and are being increasingly investigated for medical applications (eg, histopathology, medical imaging, physician electronic medical record notes).[10]

DEEP LEARNING IN ENDOCRINE PATHOLOGY

One of the many areas DL applications are being increasingly explored is histopathology. In current medical practice, trained pathologists interpret histopathology slides through visual inspection, identifying characteristics that allow for the assessment of a wide range of diseases, from cancer to inflammatory disorders. As medical knowledge of human disease continues to expand, there has been a growing increase in cases requiring pathological interpretation, increasing the need for high-throughput review.[11]

The use of computational analysis to augment tissue sample analysis is known as computational pathology, or CPATH.[11] Early attempts at CPATH utilized feature engineering, or explicitly defined characteristics provided to a computer, such as cell size or shape, in an attempt to help automate pathologist analysis. However, modern CPATH projects often utilize DL techniques that obviate some manual analysis compared with other traditional approaches. Ultimately, DL methodologies can serve as a tool to augment pathologist workflows, enabling more efficiency, while democratizing pathological analysis to areas that may not have dedicated pathologist otherwise.[12]

In this section, we will describe the current state of DL applications in endocrine cancer pathology (**Table 1**), with an emphasis on experimental design, findings, and key limitations. All articles included were abstracted on March 14, 2022.

THYROID NEOPLASIA

Thyroid cancers represent the most common cancer of the endocrine system. The majority of cases within thyroid cancer are of the papillary thyroid carcinoma (PTC) subtype, accounting for 70% to 80% of overall cases,[13] although other subtypes include follicular thyroid carcinoma (FTC), medullary thyroid carcinoma, and anaplastic thyroid carcinoma. There has been some notable progress in CPATH applications in this domain, with applications aimed for tumor identification,[14–16] classification,[17–20] mutation prediction,[20–23] and segmentation[13] from both cytopathologic and histologic samples. Below, we briefly review a sampling of representative studies, summarizing aims, results, and limitations.

A recent study by Lin and colleagues[13] used a CNN for diagnosis and segmentation of PTC with 131 fine needle aspiration and ThinPrep PTC samples digitized as whole slide images (WSIs). All PTC slides were annotated with ground truth annotations by 2 pathologists with 28 slides used for training and 103 slides used for testing. The images were initially processed to remove background noise, and a VCG16-based CNN architecture was developed to identify and segment malignant PTC. The authors demonstrated strong results, showing that their proposed method yielded an accuracy of 99%, precision of 86%, and recall of 98%, outperforming existing architectures.[13] The study is limited largely by the training dataset in which all 131 samples were PTC, making it difficult to assess how such a model might perform when presented benign samples or samples belonging to a different subtype of thyroid malignancy.

Dolezal and colleagues developed a regression model to predict BRAF-RAS gene expression score (BRS) and used the predicted scores to identify noninvasive follicular thyroid neoplasm with papillary-like nuclear features (NIFTP). NIFTP is a diagnostically challenging subtype of follicular thyroid neoplasms known for its high interobserver variability and benign clinical course. It has been associated with RAS mutational profiles, whereas papillary thyroid carcinoma with extensive follicular growth (PTC-EFG) is known to be associated with BRAF^{V600E} mutations.[20] Although not all tumors carry these associated mutations, the authors hypothesized that nonmutant NIFTPs and

Table 1
A survey of neural networks deployed in endocrine neoplasia studies

Manuscript	Disease Area(s)	Task	Method	Number of Slides/ Samples	Type of Data	Validation Strategy
Lin et al,[13] 2021	Thyroid neoplasia	Diagnosis	CNN	131	Cytology	Internal validation
Dolezal et al,[20] 2021	Thyroid neoplasia	Gene expression prediction	CNN	115	Histology	External validation
Böhland et al,[19] 2021	Thyroid neoplasia	Classification (subtype)	CNN	289	Histology	External validation
Kriegsmann et al,[30] 2021	Pancreatic neoplasia	Diagnosis	CNN	201	Histology	Internal validation
Naito et al,[31] 2021	Pancreatic neoplasia	Diagnosis	CNN	532	Histology	Internal validation
Redemann et al,[35] 2020	Neuroendocrine neoplasia	Site of origin prediction	CNN	215	Histology	Internal validation
Govind et al,[36] 2020	Neuroendocrine neoplasia	Grading	CNN	50	Histology	Internal validation
Dum et al,[41] 2022	Adrenal neoplasia	Immune infiltration prediction	CNN	9405	Histology (IHC)	Internal validation

Abbreviations: CNN, convolutional neural network.

follicular-patterned PTCs might still possess differences in BRAF-RAS spectrum gene expression that could be leveraged to train DL models to learn the histologic differences between these classes. They trained a regression model on 386 slides from The Cancer Genome Atlas to predict BRS, and generated BRS predictions on an external dataset of 115 slides of classic PTC, PTC-EFG, NIFTP, and benign follicular adenoma (FA). The authors found that the DL BRS predictions were highly associated with the NIFTP subtype in the external dataset, with RAS-like BRS predictions identifying NIFTP neoplasms with a sensitivity of 97.9% a specificity of 96.6%. The study is limited by the utilization of pathologist-annotated regions of interest and a lack of ground-truth gene expression scores on the external dataset.

Böhland and colleagues[19] explored DL applications in PTC by comparing performance to feature-based classification ML methods to differentiate samples with and without "papillary thyroid carcinoma-like" nuclei. PTC-like nuclei may be seen in NIFTP and follicular variants of papillary thyroid carcinoma (FVPTC); however, FA and FTC are neoplastic subtypes that do not demonstrate PTC-like nuclei. The study used 2 datasets: the Tharun and Thompson dataset (156 samples divided into FTC, FA, NIFTP, FVPTC, and PTC) and the Nikiforov dataset (133 samples divided into benign, FTC, classic PTC, invasive FVPTC, and encapsulated FVPTC). The feature-based classification model included using pretrained model focused on identifying nuclei within the WSIs (trained on a nonthyroid dataset externally), identifying features within the segmented nuclei, and subsequently scoring each slide based on these abstracted features, using an aggregated score threshold to determine a classification of PTC-like versus non-PTC-like. The DL approach also leveraged a model pretrained on ImageNet.[24] Ultimately, the results demonstrate that the feature-based approach achieved an accuracy of 89.7% and 83.5% on the Tharun and Thompson and Nikiforov datasets, respectively, whereas the DL approach yielded results of 83.6% and 89.1%. The study is limited by a limited inclusion of borderline datasets as well as a high-reliance on image preprocessing, in addition to a limited emphasis on results explainability.

PANCREATIC EPITHELIAL NEOPLASIA

Although not strictly endocrine but arising in a mixed exocrine/endocrine organ, pancreatic ductal adenocarcinoma (PDAC) has been a key area of focus in many research disciplines because it is the fourth leading cause of cancer-attributable deaths in the United States and predicted to increase in prevalence during the next decade.[25] Although a multitude of studies have evaluated AI-augmented diagnosis with radiographic image analysis (eg, CT),[26] there are limited examples of applications that use CPATH approaches outside of the studies sampled below.[27–29]

One such example of DL approaches in histopathology within pancreatic neoplasms is a 2021 study by Kriegsmann and colleagues,[30] who developed the first DL-based algorithm to identify key anatomic features and differentiate pancreatic intraepithelial neoplasia (PanIN) from PDAC. The study included 111 patients (201 slides) who were randomly assigned to a training (120 patients), validation (41 patients), and test (40 patients) dataset. Each of the patient-associated slides was manually annotated by a pathologist to show representative regions, or "patches," including endocrine islands, exocrine islands, fatty issue, lymph node metastasis, nontumor fibrosis, normal ducts, tumor-associated stroma, tumor-free pancreatic lymph node, low-grade PanIN, high-grade PanIN, and pancreatic adenocarcinoma. For evaluation of the model, the authors used balanced accuracy (BACC; defined as the arithmetic mean between sensitivity and specificity to correct for class imbalances) and aggregated all benign categories, both PanIN, and malignant categories into 3 individual classes. The study evaluated multiple prediction thresholds to evaluate the model's performance on confident predictions, while mitigating model uncertainty, ultimately finding that a 0.90 prediction cutoff enabled for a BACC output of 92.12% (discarding 53.59% of predictions).[30] Although this study did provide an initial foray into CPATH within the PDAC disease area, it remains experimentally limited. First, the requirement to annotate 11 individual classes during training, while subsequently reaggregating the classes during evaluation raises limitations on results interpretability, particularly when combined with an adjusted evaluation metric such as BACC, which further correct for class imbalances as a single point estimate of accuracy, rather than more traditional uncorrected ML evaluation metrics such as area under the receiver operating curve (AUROC) and precision or recall. Additionally, the use of a 90% threshold in prediction cutoff causes a substantial loss of model robustness as more than half of the sample predictions was discarded. Finally, the most effective method to test model performance and generalizability is to utilize an external validation set that is abstracted from a source distinct from that used in training; however, no external dataset was used in this study.

Naito and colleagues[31] built on these results in their study that used DL predictions to diagnose PDAC versus noncancerous pathology (eg, autoimmune pancreatitis) on endoscopic ultrasound-fine needle biopsy samples. The study used 532 WSIs that were split into 372 slides for training, 40 for validation, and 120 for testing (testing dataset was selected from a subset of 182 WSIs in which all 3 pathologist reviewers agreed on a definitive diagnosis). Additionally, 62 WSIs were discarded after stratification due to pathologist evaluation revealing the diagnosis to be "indeterminate." Before training, the WSIs were annotated by pancreatic pathologists to highlight isolated carcinoma components and invasive ductal carcinoma components. The model demonstrated an AUROC of 0.984, demonstrating significant ability to identify cancer versus noncancer pathologic condition. Although this study shows exceptional performance, there are multiple limitations to the study design. During group stratification, the elimination of all indeterminate diagnoses led to augmented performance that does not mimic real-world clinical scenarios in which many similarly indeterminate diagnoses are present. Additionally, the model was tested on a selected dataset of cases in which a diagnosis was consistent across 3 reviewers, creating a scenario where the model is only tested on more clinically "obvious" cases, while also not utilizing an external dataset for validation. Finally, the manual annotation of regions of interest by human pathologists, necessitated a significant amount manual of input into this workflow, which is an important consideration when considering future real-world application.

NEUROENDOCRINE NEOPLASIA

Neuroendocrine neoplasms (NENs) are rare tumors that can be seen throughout the gastrointestinal (GI) tract, although with lower prevalence and incidence compared with thyroid and pancreatic NENs.[32] Most neuroendocrine tumors (NETs) are well differentiated and can be more localized to a specific organ (eg, pancreas). To date, various biomarkers (mainly in immunohistochemistry [IHC]) have been associated with NENs (eg, Ki-67). To date, there have been several studies that are focused on DL applications within the NEN disease area,[33–35] particularly over the last 3 years; however, as seen in other disease areas, the majority of studies focus on radiomics applications, likely given the ubiquity of radiological datasets relative to other data modalities such as histopathology.[34] A subset of literature with notable findings are highlighted below.

Redemann and colleagues[35] developed a DL model to predict the site of origin for metastatic well-differentiated NETs, given the task is difficult to consistently accomplish even with IHC techniques. The study used 215 well-differentiated NET hematoxylin and eosin-stained slides with a known primary site. Of the overall sample, 130 slides were used for training and 85 slides were used for testing. Compared with IHC (82% accuracy in site-of-origin prediction), the DL model demonstrated an accuracy rate of 72%, ultimately demonstrating that the performance between IHC gold-standard approaches and DL was not statistically significantly different. The study is limited by an overall small sample size and the lack of a discrete external validation set to evaluate model generalizability. Furthermore, there was no emphasis on an analysis of model explainability. Nonetheless, the results do provide an initial proof-of-concept for DL approaches to be used in this disease area.

Another study by Govind and colleagues[36] evaluated the ability for a DL platform to improve the accuracy of GI-NET grading. The study looked to improve GI-NET grading by building on traditional metrics such as the Ki-67 index. The authors used 50 samples derived from various GI sites (8 stomach, 13 small bowel, 5 appendix, 3 colon, 16 rectum, 5 pancreas) with 2 samples discarded due to staining issues.[37] The authors first developed an initial integrated approach termed "Synaptophyin-Ki-67 Index Estimator" where the non-DL model was trained to locate tumor cells, detect hot spots, and calculate the Ki-67 index. The WSIs were cropped into hot-spot-sized tiles and categorized into 4 separate categories of background, nontumor, G1 tumor, and G2 tumor, which served as ground truth for their subsequent DL approach. These tiles were then used to train (42 cases; 15,232 image tiles) and test (6 cases; 9436 image tiles) their DL model. The results demonstrated that when compared with the gold-standard approaches, the study agreed with tumor grade in 45 out of 48 (93.8%) cases and had a Ki-67 index error (difference between GS index and estimated index) of 0.84 ± 1.02%. The study demonstrated an interesting methodology with fully automated "hot-spot detection"; however, it remains constrained in its evaluation. The study is limited overall by its low

sample size and lack of true ground truth metrics for training and evaluation of model performance. Additionally, there was no external dataset used for the evaluation of model performance making it difficult to assess whether this approach can perform effectively in novel settings.

PITUITARY, PARATHYROID, AND ADRENAL NEOPLASIA

When compared with other endocrine neoplasms, pituitary, parathyroid, and adrenal neoplasias are among the least prevalent.[38,39] These neoplasms have been explored with DL applications using radiomics and genomics data[40]; however, there are currently limited examples of studies using histopathology datasets. This may be due to the relative scarcity of data in these domains, particularly given the relative rarity of malignant neoplasms of the pituitary, parathyroid, and adrenal glands.

Dum and colleagues[41] evaluated 90 different tumor entities (including adrenocortical adenoma and pheochromocytoma) to assess the feasibility of a high-throughput analysis of lymphocyte subpopulations by using an AI-supported multiple antibody (cytotoxic T-lymphocyte associated protein 4 [CTLA-4]) approach within multiple tumor subtypes. The study used 2 different CTLA-4 antibodies due to limitations with using a single antibody on formalin-fixed tissue. The study incorporated 9405 images from the 90 tumor types used to train and validate a DL approach for detecting nonspecific staining. The digital images were analyzed using a multistep approach, using a CNN (U-Net) for automated quantification of CTLA-4+ cells and another deep NN (DeepLab3+) for the detection of nonspecific (2) CTLA-4 staining. The results for the density of CTLA-4+ cells in the tumor categories identified clone-dependent unspecific staining pattern in adrenal cortical adenoma (63%) for MSVA-152R and in pheochromocytoma (67%). The authors found that high CTLA-4+ cell density was associated with a low pT category, absent lymph node metastases, and PL-L1 expression in tumor or inflammatory cells. Overall, the study demonstrated the ability for DL-assisted approaches to assist with immunostaining and identified potentially novel biological links between CTLA-4 lymphocytes and prognostic cancer features. The study was limited by sample sizes and potential issues with cross-reactivity that may hinder reproducibility across all tumor subtypes. Moreover, there was no external dataset used for validation of this approach. Finally, prior meta-analyses have indicated that there is no significance in CTLA-4 expression and overall survival in multiple cancer subtypes, contradicting some of this study's findings.[42]

DISCUSSION

Major developments in DL have been enabled by the explosion of data availability and computing power, enabling automated pathology image segmentation analysis to ultimately augment workflows for pathologic assessment of endocrine neoplasms.[43] Despite promising progress, there are still significant shortcomings seen across medical applications of DL, including within the subfield of DL for histopathology in endocrine neoplasms.

First, centralized data repositories must be an area of emphasis across all institutions. Although novel ML and statistical methodologies have shown some promise in mitigating limited datasets during model training through augmentation,[44–46] significant data diversity is necessary to enable accurate assessments of model accuracy. Without multi-institutional datasets, robust algorithms that are exposed to a sufficient diversity of training data will be difficult to generalize, particularly in rare neoplastic subtypes such as pituitary tumors. Furthermore, increased dataset variability will enable for more methodologically rigorous evaluations of models on external, novel datasets to assess generalizability. This concept has been shown to be particularly relevant within the subfield of AI in histopathology, as batch effects can significantly affect results.[47] Although the internal cross-validation-based approaches seen in many of the aforementioned studies can demonstrate some assessment of a model's capabilities, it is insufficient to rely on these results, particularly in areas such a medical diagnosis, which require a tremendous amount of precision and stability before real-world implementation.

Another consideration that can enhance inter-study comparisons is the need for consensus reporting standards and evaluation criteria. Currently, efforts such as the Transparent Reporting of a multivariable prediction model of Individual Prognosis or Diagnosis (TRIPOD) and additional evolving guidelines such as TRIPOD-AI[48] are focused on developing guidelines and standards for reporting prediction models. Currently, studies demonstrate significant variability in how results are reported, making it exceptionally difficult for medical practitioners to assess relative performance across studies. An increased focus on rigorous and standardized metrics will not only enable cross-study comparisons but also serve to increase adoption of DL approaches across medical subspecialties.

DL applications in histopathology have demonstrated the potential to reduce pathologist workloads and increase our understanding of the histologic landscape of endocrine neoplasms. It is important to note that, although AI platforms have demonstrated some promise in the analysis of histopathological samples, they are not in the position to replace pathologist interpretation altogether. Pathologists must integrate clinical context and understanding of disease processes as well as incorporate a patient's individual circumstances to make an informed decision. Ultimately, this multimodal process is not well approximated by existing AI algorithms, which will be best used as tools deployed to work in conjunction with pathologists for the foreseeable future.

Ultimately, to transition from experimental analysis to the clinic, there must be significant progress from federal and institutional levels to ensure that there is clarity on model efficacy as well as clarity surrounding logistical considerations that can drive clinical implementation. Given the growing need for histopathological analysis globally, AI tools have demonstrated promise in enabling more efficient workflows to enhance physician productivity.

DISCLOSURE

This study was supported by the Burroughs Wellcome Fund Early Scientific Training to Prepare for Research Excellence Post-Graduation (BEST-PREP). ATP reports effort support via grans from NIH/NCI U01-CA243075, grants from NIG/NIDCR R56-DE030958, and grants from SU2C (Stand Up to Cancer) Fanconi Anemia Research Fund–Farrah Fawcett Foundation Head and Neck Cancer Research Team Grant during the conduct of the study; ATP reports grants from Abbvie via UChicago–Abbvie Joint Steering Committee Grant, and grants from Kura Oncology. ATP reports personal feeds from Prelude Therapeutics Advisory Board, personal fees from Elevar Advisory Board, and personal fees from Ayala Advisory Board outside of submitted work.

ACKNOWLEDGMENTS

The authors appreciate the opportunity and guidance from Dr. Nicole Cipriani in the composition of this article.

REFERENCES

1. Tran KA, Kondrashova O, Bradley A, et al. Deep learning in cancer diagnosis, prognosis and treatment selection. Genome Med 2021;13:152.

2. Gulshan V, Peng L, Coram M, et al. Development and validation of a deep learning algorithm for detection of diabetic retinopathy in retinal fundus photographs. JAMA 2016;316(22):2402–10.

3. Giudicessi JR, Schram M, Bos JM, et al. Artificial intelligence–enabled assessment of the heart rate corrected qt interval using a mobile electrocardiogram device. Circulation 2021;143(13):1274–86.

4. Ratner M. FDA backs clinician-free AI imaging diagnostic tools. Nat Biotechnol 2018;36(8):673–4.

5. Luchini C, Pea A, Scarpa A. Artificial intelligence in oncology: current applications and future perspectives. Br J Cancer 2022;126(1):4–9.

6. Kleppe A, Skrede OJ, De Raedt S, et al. Designing deep learning studies in cancer diagnostics. Nat Rev Cancer 2021;21(3):199–211.

7. Chary MA, Manini AF, Boyer EW, et al. The Role and Promise of Artificial Intelligence in Medical Toxicology. J Med Toxicol 2020;16(4):458–64.

8. Rajkomar A, Dean J, Kohane I. Machine Learning in Medicine. N Engl J Med 2019;380(14):1347–58.

9. LeCun Y, Bengio Y, Hinton G. Deep learning. Nature 2015;521(7553):436–44.

10. Esteva A, Robicquet A, Ramsundar B, et al. A guide to deep learning in healthcare. Nat Med 2019;25(1):24–9.

11. van der Laak J, Litjens G, Ciompi F. Deep learning in histopathology: the path to the clinic. Nat Med 2021;27(5):775–84.

12. Ahmad Z, Rahim S, Zubair M, et al. Artificial intelligence (AI) in medicine, current applications and future role with special emphasis on its potential and promise in pathology: present and future impact, obstacles including costs and acceptance among pathologists, practical and philosophical considerations. A comprehensive review. Diagn Pathol 2021;16(1):24.

13. Lin YJ, Chao TK, Khalil MA, et al. Deep learning fast screening approach on cytological whole slides for thyroid cancer diagnosis. Cancers (Basel) 2021;13(15):3891.

14. Dov D, Kovalsky SZ, Assaad S, et al. Weakly supervised instance learning for thyroid malignancy prediction from whole slide cytopathology images. Med Image Anal 2021;67:101814.

15. Elliott Range DD, Dov D, Kovalsky SZ, et al. Application of a machine learning algorithm to predict malignancy in thyroid cytopathology. Cancer Cytopathology 2020;128(4):287–95.

16. Sanyal P, Mukherjee T, Barui S, et al. Artificial intelligence in cytopathology: A neural network to identify papillary carcinoma on thyroid fine-needle aspiration cytology smears. J Pathol Inform 2018;9(1):43.

17. Wang Y, Guan Q, Lao I, et al. Using deep convolutional neural networks for multi-classification of thyroid tumor by histopathology: a large-scale pilot study. Ann Transl Med 2019;7(18):468.

18. El-Hossiny AS, Al-Atabany W, Hassan O, et al. Classification of Thyroid Carcinoma in Whole Slide Images Using Cascaded CNN. IEEE Access 2021;9:88429–38.

19. Böhland M, Tharun L, Scherr T, et al. Machine learning methods for automated classification of tumors with papillary thyroid carcinoma-like nuclei: A quantitative analysis. PLoS One 2021;16(9):e0257635.

20. Dolezal JM, Trzcinska A, Liao CY, et al. Deep learning prediction of BRAF-RAS gene expression signature identifies noninvasive follicular thyroid neoplasms with papillary-like nuclear features. Mod Pathol 2021;34(5):862–74.

21. Anand D, Yashashwi K, Kumar N, et al. Weakly supervised learning on unannotated H&E-stained slides predicts BRAF mutation in thyroid cancer with high accuracy. J Pathol 2021;255(3):232–42.

22. Tsou P, Wu CJ. Mapping driver mutations to histopathological subtypes in papillary thyroid carcinoma: applying a deep convolutional neural network. J Clin Med 2019;8(10):1675.

23. Fu Y, Jung AW, Torne RV, et al. Pan-cancer computational histopathology reveals mutations, tumor composition and prognosis. Nat Cancer 2020;1(8):800–10.

24. Deng J, Dong W, Socher R, Li LJ, Li K, Fei-Fei L. ImageNet: A large-scale hierarchical image database. In: 2009 IEEE Conference on Computer Vision and Pattern Recognition. ; 2009:248-255. doi:10.1109/CVPR.2009.5206848.

25. Cancer of the pancreas - cancer stat facts. SEER. Available at: https://seer.cancer.gov/statfacts/html/pancreas.html. Accessed April 5, 2022.

26. Kenner B, Chari ST, Kelsen D, et al. Artificial intelligence and early detection of pancreatic cancer. Pancreas 2021;50(3):251–79.

27. Fu H, Mi W, Pan B, et al. Automatic pancreatic ductal adenocarcinoma detection in whole slide images using deep convolutional neural networks. Front Oncol 2021;11:665929.

28. Wu W, Liu X, Hamilton RB, et al. Graph Convolutional Neural Networks for Histological Classification of Pancreatic Cancer 2022;28. https://doi.org/10.1101/2022.01.26.22269832, 2022.01.26.22269832.

29. Chang YH, Thibault G, Madin O, et al. Deep learning based Nucleus Classification in pancreas histological images. In: 2017 39th Annual International Conference of the IEEE Engineering in Medicine and Biology Society (EMBC). ; 2017:672-675. doi:10.1109/EMBC.2017.8036914.

30. Kriegsmann M, Kriegsmann K, Steinbuss G, et al. Deep learning in pancreatic tissue: identification of anatomical structures, pancreatic intraepithelial neoplasia, and ductal adenocarcinoma. Int J Mol Sci 2021;22(10):5385.

31. Naito Y, Tsuneki M, Fukushima N, et al. A deep learning model to detect pancreatic ductal adenocarcinoma on endoscopic ultrasound-guided fine-needle biopsy. Sci Rep 2021;11(1): 8454.

32. Dasari A, Shen C, Halperin D, et al. Trends in the incidence, prevalence, and survival outcomes in patients with neuroendocrine tumors in the United States. JAMA Oncol 2017;3(10):1335–42.

33. Wallace PW, Conrad C, Brückmann S, et al. Metabolomics, machine learning and immunohistochemistry to predict succinate dehydrogenase mutational status in phaeochromocytomas and paragangliomas. J Pathol 2020;251(4):378–87.

34. Pantelis AG, Panagopoulou PA, Lapatsanis DP. Artificial intelligence and machine learning in the diagnosis and management of gastroenteropancreatic neuroendocrine neoplasms—a scoping review. Diagnostics 2022;12(4):874.

35. Redemann J, Schultz FA, Martinez C, et al. Comparing deep learning and immunohistochemistry in determining the site of origin for well-differentiated neuroendocrine tumors. J Pathol Inform 2020;11:32.

36. Govind D, Jen KY, Matsukuma K, et al. Improving the accuracy of gastrointestinal neuroendocrine tumor grading with deep learning. Sci Rep 2020;10(1):11064.

37. Matsukuma K, Olson KA, Gui D, et al. Synaptophysin-Ki67 double stain: a novel technique that improves interobserver agreement in the grading of well-differentiated gastrointestinal neuroendocrine tumors. Mod Pathol 2017;30(4):620–9.

38. Chen C, Hu Y, Lyu L, et al. Incidence, demographics, and survival of patients with primary pituitary tumors: a SEER database study in 2004–2016. Sci Rep 2021;11(1):15155.

39. Correa P, Chen VW. Endocrine gland cancer. Cancer 1995;75(1 Suppl):338–52.

40. Thomasian NM, Kamel IR, Bai HX. Machine intelligence in non-invasive endocrine cancer diagnostics. Nat Rev Endocrinol 2022;18(2):81–95.

41. Dum D, Henke TLC, Mandelkow T, et al. Semi-automated validation and quantification of CTLA-4 in 90 different tumor entities using multiple antibodies and artificial intelligence. Lab Invest 2022;1–8. https://doi.org/10.1038/s41374-022-00728-4.

42. Hu P, Liu Q, Deng G, et al. The prognostic value of cytotoxic T-lymphocyte antigen 4 in cancers: a systematic review and meta-analysis. Sci Rep 2017; 7(1):42913.

43. Kochanny S, Pearson A. Academics as leaders in the cancer artificial intelligence revolution. Cancer 2020;127. https://doi.org/10.1002/cncr.33284.

44. Sandfort V, Yan K, Pickhardt PJ, et al. Data augmentation using generative adversarial networks (Cycle-GAN) to improve generalizability in CT segmentation tasks. Sci Rep 2019;9(1):16884.

45. Mikołajczyk A, Grochowski M. Data augmentation for improving deep learning in image classification problem. In: 2018 International Interdisciplinary PhD Workshop (IIPhDW). ; 2018:117-122. doi:10.1109/IIPHDW.2018.8388338.

46. Wei J, Suriawinata A, Vaickus L, et al. Generative Image Translation for Data Augmentation in Colorectal Histopathology Images. Proc Mach Learn Res 2019; 116:10–24.

47. Howard FM, Dolezal J, Kochanny S, et al. The impact of site-specific digital histology signatures on deep learning model accuracy and bias. Nat Commun 2021;12(1):4423.

48. Collins GS, Dhiman P, Navarro CLA, et al. Protocol for development of a reporting guideline (TRIPOD-AI) and risk of bias tool (PROBAST-AI) for diagnostic and prognostic prediction model studies based on artificial intelligence. BMJ Open 2021;11(7):e048008.

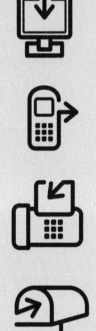

Printed and bound by CPI Group (UK) Ltd, Croydon, CR0 4YY

03/10/2024

01040363-0020